Mechanical Circulatory Support

R. Hetzer · E. Hennig · M. Loebe

Editors

Mechanical Circulatory Support

- In Children
- Towards
  Myocardial Recovery
- Permanent

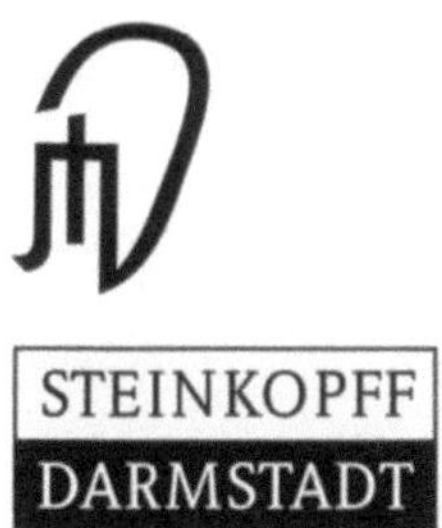

STEINKOPFF
DARMSTADT

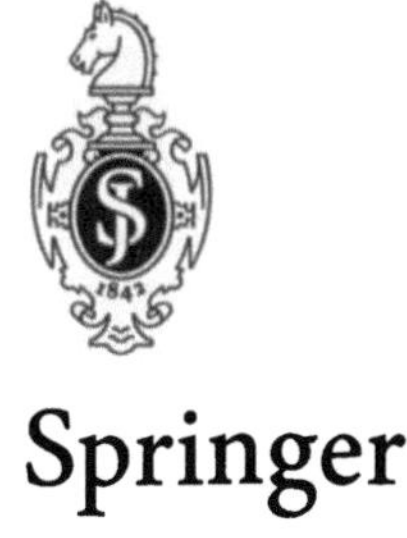

Springer

Editors address:

Prof. Dr. R. HETZER
Dr. E. HENNIG
Dr. M. LOEBE
German Heart Institute Berlin
Augustenburger Platz 1
13353 Berlin, Germany

Die Deutsche Bibliothek – CIP-Einheitsaufnahme

Mechanical circulatory support: In Children, Towards Myocardial Recovery, Permanent / R. Hetzer
... (ed.). – Darmstadt: Steinkopff; Berlin; Heidelberg; New York; London; Paris; Tokyo; Hong
Kong; Barcelona; Budapest: Springer, 1997

NE: Hetzer, Roland [Hrsg.]

© 1997 by Dr. Dietrich Steinkopff Verlag GmbH & Co. KG, Darmstadt
Softcover reprint of the hardcover 1st edition 1997

Medical Editor: Beate Rühlemann – English Editor: James C. Willis – Production: Heinz J. Schäfer
Cover Design: Erich Kirchner, Heidelberg

ISBN-13: 978-3-642-95986-8   e-ISNB-13: 978-3-642-95984-4
DOI: 10.1007/ 978-3-642-95984-4

Introduction

After decades of research and development in animal experimentation and preliminary investigation in the applications in humans, mechanical circulatory support for the failing heart has entered the clinical area. At first, mechanical support systems were used in post-cardiotomy heart failure until adequate recovery of the patient's own myocardium had occurred. When heart transplantation became available as a definite treatment in patients with end-stage heart disease, the primary use of mechanical assist systems became that of bridging to heart transplantation. First experiences with this indication were gained in the late 1980's and since then a growing number of patients has been supported successfully until a suitable donor organ became available. The initial goal, however, in the development of mechanical circulatory support systems was the ultimate replacement of the failing heart with an artificial device. In the mid-80's, Jarvik and DeVries introduced their totally artificial heart into clinical use under extensive international press coverage. The results obtained with this device were disappointing and the general feeling was that mechanical circulatory support would not achieve acceptable results in the near future. The extensive use of artificial devices in the bridge-to-transplant situation, however, produced such a vast amount of insight into the pathophysiology of long-term mechanical support as well as the technical applicability of these devices that, over the last ten years, dramatic improvements in patient selection, device quality and patient management have been achieved.

Today, patients are being supported with these devices for over a year with barely a reduction in quality of life. With the wearable left ventricular assist devices they are discharged home and spend the waiting time with their families. Physical activities such as car driving, bike riding and gardening again become part of their lives. Some patients even return to their professional activities. All these achievements seem to increase the viability of permanent mechanical circulatory support as a definite treatment. If this indeed proves feasible, mechanical circulatory support would then for the first time be a real alternative to heart transplantation and a real answer to the growing shortage of donor organs for these patients. Another exciting aspect is the recovery of the patient's own myocardium under permanent mechanical support. Experiences with this application to date have been collected and are presented in this book. As will be seen, these observations are by and large in accordance with many of the current hypotheses of cardiomyopathic pathophysiology. In addition, they bring back memories of certain "old-fashioned" approaches in treating patients with end-stage heart failure at a time when bed-rest was the only possibility. The potential for myocardial recovery has been demonstrated in both acute myocarditis as well as post-cardiotomy settings. In addition, proposals have been made for the use of support systems in obtaining substantial improvement in heart function in patients with terminal dilated cardiomyopathy.

The development of new assist devices and the total artificial heart, as well as the improvement of the systems already available, do open up new perspectives, especially for permanent support. Be that as it may, the step from animal experiment to use in human patients is somewhat cumbersome and needs careful evaluation. This is why ethical aspects as well as regulatory issues concerning new devices have been included in this volume. Not only through the presentations but during the discussions in particular, many highly interesting insights into the regulatory process and the further development in the field of mechanical circulatory support were disclosed. It goes without saying that with the artificial heart at hand the physician's power to shift the border-line between life and death could have narrowing and perhaps even horrifying effects and, therefore, strict ethical and regulatory considerations are mandatory.

Only very recently have systems became available which are capable of supporting children and newborns for an extended period of time. The world-wide experience with these devices is very limited and they are discussed in this volume by highly-respected experts in the field for the first time. Although pediatric mechanical circulatory support remains still far from being perfect, it is undoubtedly a great step forward in the treatment of small patients otherwise doomed to die from their severe heart disease. With growing experience in the field, indication for assist device implantation in newborns and children will certainly be clarified as technical safety and implantation standards will improve.

Mechanical circulatory support has become an established aspect of cardiac surgery when dealing with patients with severely impaired ventricular function and highly progressed heart disease. Whether it is used to obtain recovery, as a bridge to heart transplantation or as a permanent mechanical replacement of the patient's failing heart, acceptable results have been obtained. Dramatic improvement in system reliability, surgical standards and patient treatment have been accumulated. Rather than giving a summary of what has been done in the past, this book addresses primarily questions of burning interest to investigators and forefront clinical users of mechanical circulatory support systems. The organizers of the symposium were fortunate in attracting the interest of many distinguished experts in the field who have contributed not only the articles included, but in particular, their experience and ideas during the extensive discussions. Therefore, we are confident in having assembled a colorful collage of today's most pressing themes and considerations in the multi faceted field of mechanical circulatory support systems. It may be that many of the subjects addressed are not fully covered and perhaps more questions are raised than answered, but all of this, in our estimation, mirrors the present state of the art in mechanical circulatory support. Our deep gratitude goes to all those who have contributed to the success of the symposium and to the high standard of the presentations included in this book. We hope that readers will experience as much of the excitement as we did during the two days of the symposium in 1995.

Berlin, December 1996   ROLAND HETZER
                                                     EWALD HENNIG
                                                     MATTHIAS LOEBE

Welcome Address

Roland Hetzer

German Heart Institute Berlin, Berlin

Ladies and gentlemen, it is a pleasure and honor for me to welcome you here to Berlin. I must say, quite obviously, we have underestimated the interest in our little meeting. I have to confess that when we planned this meeting and I knew that it was just a few weeks after my friend Reiner Köfer's meeting in Bad Oeynhausen, I thought that probably no one would come to our meeting. This is the reason why we planned everything a bit too small, so, unfortunately, we will be a little crowded. Tomorrow's topics obviously have stirred great interest in advance. This is why for tomorrow we have planned to go to a larger hall, but this was obviously also a miscalculation because unexpectedly there is a lot of interest in the pediatric field as well, which in a way makes me very proud and I think it's very nice, but you probably have to pay for this with some lack of comfort. I apologize and hope that you will take this imposition in stride.

The topic "mechanical circulatory support" has become a field and a topic of many meetings. This is why for this symposium we have selected three topics which are strongly discussed at present, each of which opens a gate for exciting development in the years to come. Tomorrow morning we will discuss the most astounding experience of functional recovery of the hearts of patients with dilated cardiomyopathy who were placed on left ventricular assist devices on an emergency basis, with the prospect of subsequent transplantation. After weeks and months, these hearts returned to their normal size and recovered normal function, prompting us to explant the devices after 5–11 months in four patients to date. None of the patients have experienced subsequent relapse of the disease over an observation period presently at 8 months. This concept has been tried by some surgeons in the past, but without success to our knowledge. We are lucky to have a very competent group of experts entering into this discussion, expert cardiologists and researchers in cardiomyopathy, and we are looking forward to a quite controversial discussion on this field.

Tomorrow afternoon we shall focus on the very pertinent topic of leaving a patient permanently on a supporting left ventricular assist device. Of course the presently available devices were not primarily meant to serve this purpose; however, the longer waiting periods for a donor heart have shown that patients may live with such a device with some mobility and quality of life, which has prompted us to consider the possibility of permanent use. This attempt, of course, opens a wide field of questions as to the psychology, economics, and ethics. In this country, we have begun a dialogue with insurance companies about the spectrum of indications under which such a permanent implant may be acceptable. We are well aware that this will be a continuous discussion during the next years. Our experience involves eight patients with more than 200 days of support: one is at home and one is now 470 days on the device. I was told that this is presently the longest period that a person has been on such a device and I hope that this patient will join us tomorrow afternoon as living proof of the possibility of this concept. He may also answer questions.

This afternoon is dedicated to the collection of experiences with mechanical circulatory assistance in children. In 1991, we placed the first child on a pneumatically driven left ventricular assist device. The child subsequently underwent successful transplantation. Up until now, this concept was used in our hands in 19 children between 2 months and 16 years of age. Meanwhile, pediatric and infant-sized assist pumps were developed, first by the Berlin Heart company, and more recently by the Medos company in Aachen. Of course ECMO, a tool for treating respiratory and cardiac failure, has been used quite extensively for many years. We have used this method alternatively in small infants, in hearts with intracardiac shunts, and for prolonged weaning purposes. Experiences with either method, for cardiac weaning and for bridge-to-transplant, are still scarce. We hope to have a review of at least some institutional experiences and to discuss the important issues of choice of device, indication, and specific pediatric aspects.

We feel very honored that many distinguished researchers and surgeons have accepted our invitations. Unfortunately Dr. Pennington could not come due to unforeseen circumstances and Dr. Glauber from Bergamo just informed me that he did not make his connecting flight in Stuttgart. This will however give us some more time for discussion and more time allowance for the individual speakers. I thank the industrial companies for their support of our meeting, despite the restricted budgedts of today. I sincerly thank my secretaries for their usual good work, and Mr. Jessen of Pro-Berlin Concept for their professional organizing of the meeting.

I would like to ask all the speakers to announce their names and home cities before speaking since we would like to record all contributions for our symposium proceedings volume. Tonight, we will enjoy a traditional variety show in the Friedrichsstadtpalast which will be preceded by a dinner, and I wish you all fun and good entertainment here in Berlin. I hope that this city, which changes rapidly from month to month, will be interesting for you during your time outside of our meeting.

I would like to now turn over the session to our admired mentor and friend, Dr. Aldo Castaneda and to my partner, Peter Lange, with whom I have the good fortune to have a peaceful and long-lasting professional relationship. Thank you.

Contents

Mechanical ventricular assist in children: Experience at the Children's Hospital, Boston (1990 – 1995)

P. J. del Nido, J. E. Mayer, R. A. Jonas

The Department of Cardiac Surgery, Children's Hospital, Harvard Medical School, Boston MA.

Mechanical circulatory support in children with severe cardiac failure is still limited by the availability of devices capable of accommodating the wide range of flows required for pediatric support. In the United States, circulatory assistance for cardiac failure is most commonly achieved by the use of extracorporeal membrane oxygenator circuit (ECMO) (2, 3, 8). The most frequent indication for circulatory support is myocardial dysfunction following cardiac surgery. There is also a growing number of children placed on ECMO for acute decompensation of a chronic cardiomyopathy or a viral myocarditis, where mechanical support is used for temporary support or as a bridge to transplantation.

Although ECMO circuits include the use of an oxygenator, respiratory failure is an infrequent associated complication of cardiac failure requiring mechanical support. Nevertheless, due to the flexibility of roller pumps in generating widely varying flows, the ready availability of ECMO circuits and the necessary support staff in most pediatric centers, ECMO remains the most common mode of cardiac support. There are however an increasing number of reports describing the experience with circulatory support using centrifugal pumps as assist devices (1, 4–7). This paper reports the experience with a centrifugal pump for ventricular assist in severe cardiac failure in pediatric patients at the Children's Hospital of Boston from 1990 to 1995.

Methods

Techniques of support

During the entire period covered by this report, the assist device circuit used for circulatory support consisted of a flexible wire reinforced venous cannula connected to 1/4 inch or 3/8 inch tubing which was connected directly to the pump head of the centrifugal pump (Bio-Medicus Co.). The arterial end of the pump head was then connected directly to the arterial cannula without the use of arterial line filter. More recently a heparin-coated circuit including cannulas, tubing and pump head (Carmeda, Medtronic Co.) have been employed. Minimal systemic heparinization was utilized until mediastinal bleeding was well controlled and subsequently anticoagulation to activated clotting times of 180 to 200 s (230 to 250 s for the mini-tubes) was instituted

Cannulation techniques

In all children, including those requiring support post-cardiotomy and the myocarditis patients cannulation was done through the sternotomy with cannulas inserted directly into the aorta (or pulmonary artery) and left (or right) atrium and exteriorized at the bottom of the sternal skin incision. The incision was covered with a synthetic patch sewn to the skin edges and covered with gauze dressing.

The perfusion technique of circulatory support was similar to that for partial cardiopulmonary bypass where pump flow was gradually increased to 100-125ml/kg/min. Left (or right) atrial pressure was monitored to prevent complete emptying of the atrium and to monitor intravascular volume status.

Results

From January 1990 to September of 1995, at the Children's Hospital in Boston, a total of 22 children were placed on mechanical ventricular assist using a centrifugal pump to treat severe low cardiac output or malignant ventricular arrhythmias. During this same time period a total of 3973 open heart procedures were performed at our institution.

Isolated left ventricular assist with left atrial to aortic cannulation was utilized in 19 of the children. Right ventricular support with right atrial to pulmonary artery bypass was employed in one child with pulmonary hypertension, and single ventricle support with common atrial to aortic bypass was used in three children with single ventricle physiology.

The anatomic diagnoses of the patients are listed in Table 1. Post-cardiotomy myocardial dysfunction with inability to wean from bypass was the most common indication for mechanical support, occurring in 19 of the 22 patients. In one patient, left ventricular support was started 2 days after open-heart surgery to treat severe cardiac dysfunction following cardiac arrest from ventricular tachycardia and fibrillation. The most frequent congenital anatomic defect was anomalous origin of the left coronary artery, accounting for seven of the 22 children.

Table 1. Anatomic Diagnosis and Indications for Mechanical Support

Post-cardiotomy 20 patients	# pts.	alive
Repair Anomalous left coronary artery	7 pts.	5
A-V valve repair/replacement	4 pts.	1
Single ventricle	3 pts.	0*
d-TGA conversion	2 pts.	1*
Post transplant	1 pt.	1
Miscellaneous	3 pts.	1
Myocarditis	2 pts.	2*
Total	22 pts.	11 pts. (Survival –50%)

* – Bridge to transplant – 3 pts. (2 alive)

The average duration of mechanical support was 3.3 ± 2.4 days with a range from 12 h (fibrillatory arrest unable to resuscitate) to 10 days in a non-survivor. Three children were listed for heart transplantation and received an allograft after 5 (2pts.) and 6 days (1pt.) of mechanical support. No child supported for longer than 7 days survived to hospital discharge. Two children were able to be decannulated but died prior to hospital discharge from complications of their original procedure.

The most frequent complication occurring during mechanical support was bleeding requiring multiple transfusions of red cells and coagulation factors (Table 2). Mediastinal reexploration for uncontrolled bleeding or tamponade impeding ventricular filling was required in 8 of the 22 patients. More recently, with the use of heparin-coated circuits and lower levels of systemic anticoagulation, reexploration for bleeding has become less frequent. Thrombus formation in the circuit or at the site of the atrial cannula developed in two children. Mechanical support was promptly discontinued in both patients with one long-term survivor who had no neurologic sequelae.

Table 2. Duration of mechanical circulatory support and complications

Complications:	
Bleeding (reexplored	8/22
Sepsis	2/22
Circuit thrombus	2/22
Duration of VAD support	
All patients (n = 22)	3.3 ± 2.4 days
Anom. LCA (n = 7)	2.3 ± 0.3 days

VAD = ventricular assist device; LCA = left coronary artery

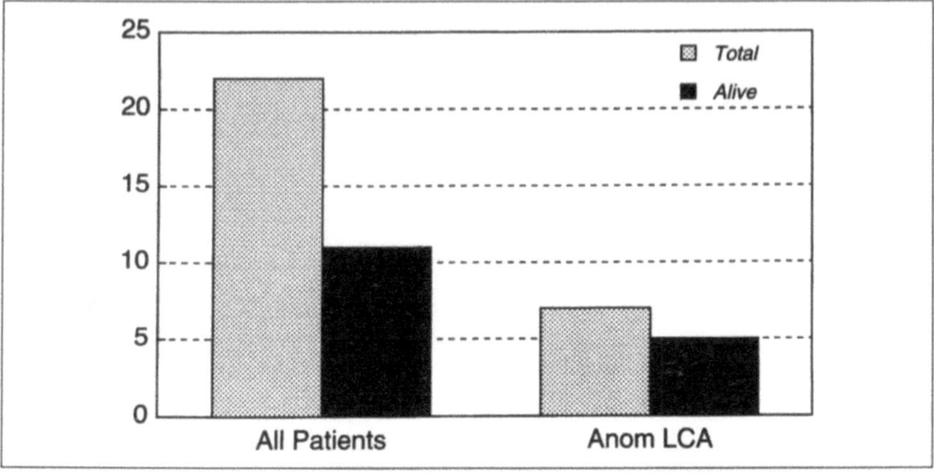

Fig. 1. Hospital survival for all patients requiring ventricular assist (left), and for the subgroup of patients placed on mechanical support following repair of anomalous left coronary artery (anom LCA)

Systemic sepsis occurring during mechanical support or as a consequence of trans-sternal cannulation was seen in two children. Persistent bacteremia leading to multi-organ failure was seen in one patient and fungal mediastinitis leading to systemic candidiasis occurred in the second. Both children died as a consequence of these infections.

Overall survival was 11 patients of the total of 22 (50%), including two children who received an orthotopic heart transplant (Fig. 1). Of all the anatomic diagnoses, the infants with left ventricular failure following repair of anomalous left coronary artery had the best overall result. Duration of mechanical support ranged from 12 h to 3 days (2.3 + 0.3 days) with five of the seven children (71%) being long-term survivors. The indications for mechanical support were the same for this group as for the other 15 patients. These seven children represent 27% (7/26pts) of the total experience with surgical repair of anomalous left coronary artery at The Children's Hospital since 1985.

Conclusions

Overall survival with mechanical circulatory support using a centrifugal pump remains at 50%. This rate is comparable to the larger experience with ECMO for cardiac support reported by the ELSO registry (2, 8). The complication rate with ventricular assist devices is also comparable to that reported with ECMO however, the incidence of sepsis appears to be slightly lower. The significantly better results with the subgroup of patients with anomalous left coronary artery is noteworthy since this group represents a high-risk subset of patients where an aggressive approach with mechanical support may be warranted. For the larger group of patients, however, the lower survival rate probably reflects the irreversible nature of the myocardial injury or anatomic defect. A diligent search for residual correctable anatomic defects, however, must be undertaken in all patients requiring mechanical support. For the group where no reparable defects are found, long term support by mechanical means along with transplantation may be the only alternative to improve their long term outcome.

References

1. Chang AC, Hanley FL, Weindling SN, Wernovsky G, Wessel DL (1992) Left heart support with a ventricular assist device in an infant with acute myocarditis. Crit Care Med 20:712-715
2. Delius RE, Zwischenberger JB, Cilley R, Behrendt DM, Bove EL, Deeb M, Crowley D, Heidelberger KP, Bartlett RH (1990) Prolonged extracorporeal life support of pediatric and adolescent cardiac transplant patients. Ann Thorac Surg 50:791-5
3. del Nido PJ, Armitage JM, Fricker FJ, Shaver M, Cipriani L, Dayal G, Park SC, Siewers RD (1994) Extracorporeal membrane oxygenation support as a bridge to pediatric heart transplantation. Circulation 90:(suppl II) 66-69
4. Jett GK, Picone AL, Clark RE (1987) Circulatory support for right ventricular dysfunction. J Thorac Cardiovasc Surg 94:95-103
5. Karl TR, Sano S, Horton S, Mee RB (1991) Centrifugal pump left heart assist in pediatric cardiac operations; indications, techniques and results. J Thorac Cardiovasc Surg 102:624-30

7. Louis PT, Bricker JT, Frazier OH, Duncan M, Towbin JA, Gelb BD, Macris MA, Radovencavic B, Kearney D, Igo S, Price J, Cooley DA (1992) Nonpulsatile total left ventricular support in pediatric patients. Crit Care Med 20:704-707
8. Meliones JN, Custer JR, Snedecor S, Moler FW,O'Rourke PP, Delius RE (1991) Extracorporeal life support for cardiac assist in pediatric patients. Circ 84:(suppl III)168-172

Author's address:
Pedro J. del Nido, M.D.
Department of Cardiac Surgery
Children's Hospital
300 Longwood Ave.
Boston, MA 02115, USA

Mechanical circulatory support at the Royal Children's Hospital

Tom R. Karl

Victorian Paediatric Cardiac Surgical Unit Royal Children's Hospital, Melbourne, Australia

Introduction

DeBakey reported the first clinical use of a ventricular assist device (VAD) in 1971 (1), and over the ensuing 25 years there has been a gradual evolution and refinement in indications and technique. With an increasingly favourable experience in adults, VAD in various formats has become an accepted treatment option for myocardial failure either with an expectation of recovery or more commonly as a bridge to transplantation. ECMO has had less acceptance in adults due to a generally higher complication rate. This is partially related to the high prevalence of multi organ system (MOS) failure in adults with ARDS and/or cardiac failure, and perhaps a stronger tendency toward thromboembolism.

The value of ECMO in children however is undisputed, with a huge body of evidence supporting its use in various severe neonatal pulmonary problems, persistent foetal circulation, and more recently septic shock (2, 3). There has also been increasing interest in the use of ECMO for postoperative ventricular dysfunction in children of all ages. Conversely, the experience with VAD has been more limited, primarily due to technical factors, but also due to concerns about suitability of children with complex congenital heart disease (CHD) for univentricular support (2, 4, 5). Therefore the great majority of the world experience with extracorporeal life support (ECLS) for cardiac failure in children has been performed with ECMO, as detailed in the annual ELSO reports (6).

ECLS at the Royal Children's Hospital began in 1988, and we now have a combined ECMO/VAD experience of over 100 cases for various pulmonary and cardiac indications in children ages newborn to teenagers. This report provides details of the subgroup of 77 patients who received ECLS for cardiac and cardiopulmonary indications. We have excluded discussion of patients receiving ECMO purely for pulmonary support (7). All of our ECLS experience has been with the centrifugal pump, for short term support (8).

Indications for ECLS

1) Postoperative support: This has been the most frequent indication for cardiac ECLS in our unit and most others. The majority of patients have had reparative open-heart operations (or cardiac transplantation) and could not be weaned from CPB due to severe ventricular dysfunction. A subset have had low cardiac output or cardiac arrest in the intensive care unit following initially successful weaning

from CPB. In such patients, technical failure of the operation should be ruled out. The aim of support is recovery within 10 days followed by separation from the support system, although there may be an option for bridge to transplantation in selected patients. Contraindications include MOS failure, severe coagulopathy, intracranial haemorrhage, neurologic impairment and sepsis. These criteria are of course relative rather than absolute, and often not diagnosable intraoperatively. For example, ECMO has actually been employed in non-cardiac patients specifically for the treatment of MOS with 50% survival (9). We have employed ECMO and VAD in two patients with essentially untreated sepsis due to endocarditis (following emergency aortic valve replacement) with complete recovery (2). One might say that in practise, most children who are surgical candidates would also be ECLS candidates should the occasion arise. Prolonged cardiac arrest is not a contraindication if cardiopulmonary resuscitation has been adequate, which is often the case in a postoperative fully monitored patient (see below).

2) Ventricular dysfunction not associated with cardiac surgery: This group includes children with acute myocarditis, sepsis syndrome, cardiac trauma, and severe post transplantation rejection. The aim is recovery of ventricular function with specific therapy (eg. immunosuppression or antibiotics) within 14 days. There may be a transplantation option in this group as well. Relative contraindications are similar to group 1.

3) Irreversible cardiac dysfunction (planned bridge to transplantation): Patients supported for ECLS for this indication must prospectively meet the institutional criteria for transplantation. Issues such as size, blood group, and donor availability factors must be taken into consideration. For patients < 20 kg, 2 weeks would be considered the maximal projected duration of support in our own unit (using the centrifugal pump). Criteria may vary however, and the duration may ultimately prove to increase using systems such as the Berlin heart which are designed for longer term support (10). Paediatric experience with ECLS for this indication has lagged well behind that in adults.

Melbourne ECMO technique

Our ECMO circuit for cardiac ECLS is the same as that used for neonatal pulmonary support (Fig. 1) (7, 8). We employ a closed venoarterial circuit using the BioMedicus centrifugal pump. We have used both the Avecor membrane oxygenator and more recently the Medtronic Carmeda heparin bonded circuit (Minimax or Maxima oxygenator) in selected cases. Cannulation technique depends on circumstances of initiation of support. For patients who cannot be separated from CPB, the ascending aortic cannula used for CPB can be left in situ, and a second cannula placed in the RA appendage. Both cannulas should support 150 ml/kg flow with a pump inlet pressure of > –20 mmHg and an outlet pressure < 200 mmHg. A second venous cannula can be placed in the left atrial (LA) appendage or right superior pulmonary vein (RSPV) if further decompression is required to cope with the increased collateral return to the left side imposed by ECMO. Direct skin (or PTFE membrane to skin) closure is generally used, with cannulas exiting through the upper and lower poles of the wound. Patients cannulated independent of a transsternal procedure generally undergo right cervical cannulation (11). Permanent ligation of a carotid artery distal to the arterial cannula is unnecessary.

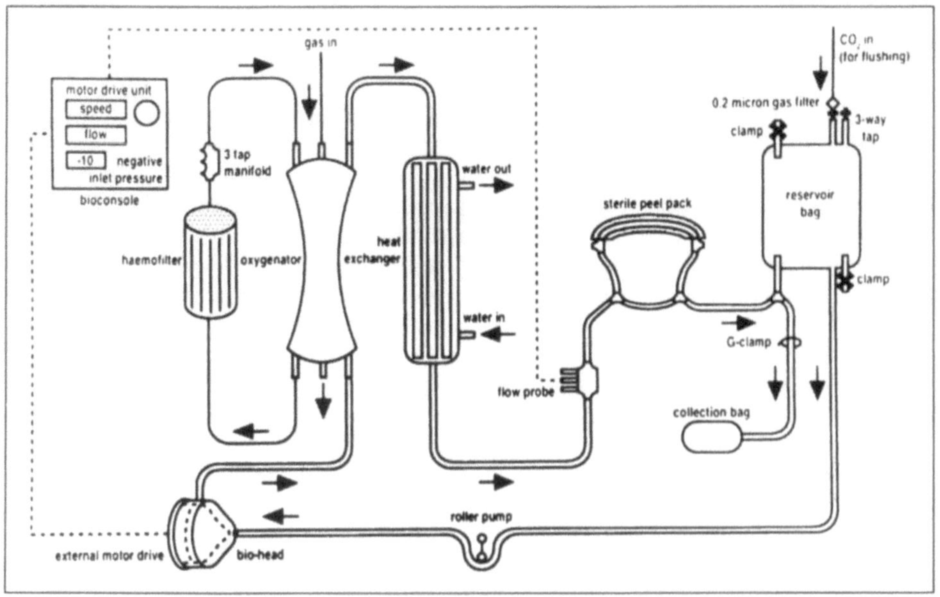

Fig. 1. ECMO circuit used at the Royal Children's Hospital, 1989-1995. Both heparin bonded and non bonded circuits are employed. A haemofilter can be placed in parallel with the oxygenator via a bridge circuit, which can also be used to change an oxygenator without interruption of flow. This circuit is used for cardiac and pulmonary support (8).

With our current technique, reconstruction of the cervical vessels following decannulation has resulted in good long term patency (11).

Patients are managed in our ICU by a specialist team including an ECMO nurse, cardiac surgeons, intensivists and perfusionists. Sedation and paralysis are generally required, along with antibiotics and TPN. Flows on ECMO are initially 120–150 ml/min, but sometimes higher in septic patients. Heparin is infused to maintain the activated clotting time (ACT) between 160–180 s, or 140–150 s for heparin bonded circuits. Inlet pressure should be kept on the positive side of –20 mmHg via appropriate cannula position and attention to patient blood volume status. Excessively negative venous pressures will cause haemolysis to occur. Inotropes are minimised and phenoxybenzamine is employed for vasodilation. Platelet counts are maintained > 100 000/mm³ and epsilon-NH₂ caproic acid is given by continuous infusion as required. We routinely employ haemofiltration via a shunt placed in parallel with the oxygenator, at 10–30 ml/min flow (Fig. 1). The volume of fluid removed can be controlled with an IVAC pump. Ventilator support is reduced to provide the lowest cardiac filling pressures, but must be increased as cardiac ejection improves to prevent coronary hypoxaemia.

Weaning begins when there is evidence of spontaneous ejection at full flow. Minimal flows of 150–400 ml/min can be maintained for several hours prior to decannulation in the operating theatre. Two-dimensional (2D) echo (praecordial or transoesophageal) is quite useful in evaluating cardiac contractility, especially in response to a fluid volume load.

Melbourne VAD technique

The majority of VADs at the Royal Children's Hospital have involved LA-Ao partial assist (LVAD) (4). Support with centrifugal pump LVAD is suitable for almost any size patient (range of survivors 1.9–70 kg in our own experience). The majority of LVAD support has been instituted intraoperatively for patients who could not be weaned from CPB. Cannulation is via ascending aorta and either LA appendage or RSPV, using cannulas designed to carry 150 ml/min flow. If LVAD is instituted for postoperative cardiac arrest, then cardiopulmonary bypass may be required initially, but we have on occasion placed asystolic patients directly on LVAD with successful outcome.

The LVAD circuit consists of a remote BioMedicus pump head mounted on a flexible drive cable (Fig. 2). As with ECMO, we employ inlet and outlet pressure monitoring and an inline flow probe. The tubing length is minimised by mounting the pump head directly onto the patient's bed. LVAD is started at minimum flow and quickly increased to 150ml/kg min. Heparin is reversed with protamine and haemostasis is secured. The skin is closed with cannulas exiting at either pole, or a PTFE membrane is used if required.

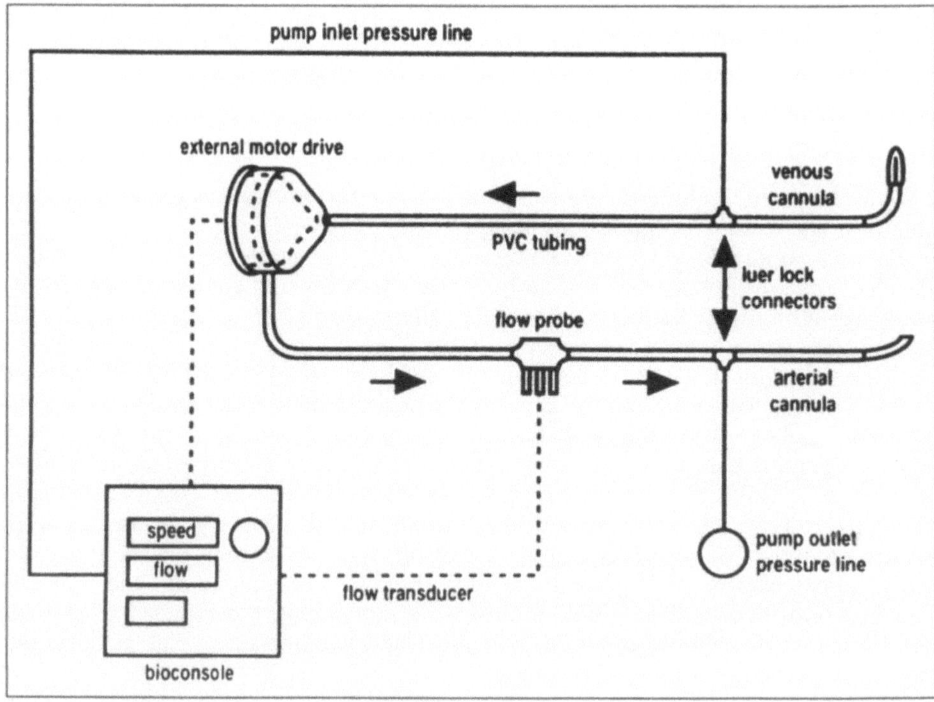

Fig. 2. VAD circuit used at the Royal Children's Hospital, 1989-1995. Both heparin bonded and non bonded versions are currently used. The pump head is mounted on the patient's bed to minimise tubing length, employing a flexible drive cable. Inlet and outlet pressures are monitored, and an inline flow probe is employed (4).

Patients are kept sedated and paralysed in the ICU with full ventilation. Inotropes are minimised to what is required to maintain adequate right heart function. When postoperative bleeding is minimal, systemic heparin anticoagulation is commenced at ACT 140–150 s. The system theoretically can be operated without heparin at high flows in larger patients, although clots may form in this circuit with or without anticoagulation and this must be weighed against the risks of higher dose anticoagulation. Normothermia is maintained with a heating/cooling blanket and the heat generated by the pump head itself. Peritoneal dialysis is used as required for metabolic support. Phenoxybenzamine, TPN, and antibiotics are routinely given. Plasma haemoglobin should remain below 60 mg/decilitre, and haemoglobin above this level, especially in conjunction with noise or vibrations in the pump head, is an indication that mechanical failure may be imminent. Otherwise, the VAD system generally requires little maintenance (as compared to ECMO under similar circumstances). In our own ICU, the patient's nurse also manages the VAD, with cardiac surgeon and perfusionist backup.

Biventricular assist is possible with the centrifugal pump, and we have rarely employed right atrial/pulmonary arterial (in combination with LA/aortic) cannulation, using two pump heads set for identical flows. This set-up is technically cumbersome in a small child, and we would prefer ECMO in this situation if possible.

Decision making for ECLS

1) Should ECLS be used?

In the setting of a patient unweanable from CPB following a cardiac operation, the surgeon must make some difficult decisions. The first, and often most difficult, is whether or not the repair is adequate, leaving (reversible) myocardial dysfunction, usually due to prolonged ischaemic arrest, as the cause of failure to wean. The use of transoesophageal echo and direct cardiac chamber and great vessel pressure and $HbSO_2$ measurements are helpful in this regard. Certainly the chance for recovery on ECLS is greatly reduced when there is a residual cardiac problem (12). The recovery potential must be assessed in context and in some cases suitability for transplantation considered as discussed above. Relative contraindications, family and social factors, and other points must also be weighed. Whether or not conversion of an intraoperative death to an ICU death several days later is a positive or negative step for the family is another question to be considered.

2) Which type of support system is most appropriate?

Univentricular support (VAD) is not adequate when global RV and LV failure are present, and ECMO (or biVAD) will be required in such cases. This is also true if severe pulmonary hypertension complicates the clinical picture. It should be borne in mind, however, that the decrease in left atrial pressure usually seen with LVAD may dramatically improve PHT and RV dysfunction in borderline cases. In our unit, we prefer to use VAD rather than ECMO whenever possible, providing that an adequate level of cardiac and organ support can be maintained. In order to assess the prospects for VAD rather than ECMO support intraoperatively, a venous cannula is placed in the LA, and the RA or caval cannulas used for CPB are clamped. Using the CPB system, pRA, pPA and RV function are assessed at 150ml/ kg min pump flow (as partial left heart assist). If all are adequate (pRA <12 mm, pPA < 1/2 systemic, no RV dilation), the patient is ventilated normally while gas exchange in the CPB oxygenator is temporarily interrupted. If pCO_2 and pO_2 are acceptable, the patient is recannulated for VAD as described above. Otherwise, ECMO is established. During support there is an option for conversion of VAD to ECMO and vice versa, if conditions should change for cardiac support in the non-operative setting, we generally prefer cervical ECMO.

3) What are the relative benefits of centrifugal pump VAD vs ECMO for short term cardiac support?

a) *Simplicity:* VAD using the centrifugal pump is straight forward in concept and design. Little technical attention is required to maintain the system after insertion. Only a few minutes are needed to set up the circuit, providing a great advantage in the cardiac arrest situation. ECMO is more complex in terms of set-up, requiring 30 min to 1 h to assemble, prime and debubble. This renders it less useful for the cardiac arrest situation. A major advantage of ECMO, however, is that in many patients total cardiac support can be established with peripheral (closed chest) cannulation, which is currently not possible using LVAD in small children.

b) *Oxygenation:* ECMO potentially provides total cardiac and pulmonary support, although as mentioned above during periods of cardiac ejection the coronaries may be perfused with blood having HbSO2 close to the LA level rather than oxygenator outlet level. Patients supported with VAD are totally dependent on the lungs for gas exchange, but pO2 tends to remain uniform throughout the arterial circulation, barring residual intracardiac shunts at ventricular level in patients having significant cardiac ejection. If an interatrial communication is present, significant right to left shunting consequent to low pLA can cause significant uniform arterial desaturation.

c) *Anticoagulation:* Centrifugal pump VAD, especially with a heparin bonded circuit, requires significantly less anticoagulation than ECMO (see above). The oxygenator and heat exchanger in the ECMO circuit result in more platelet consumption and dysfunction, as well as more haemolysis. The heparin requirements for ECMO, even with a heparin bonded circuit, are greater than for VAD. Data from the pre-Carmeda circuit era in our own institution would suggest that there was a significantly lower blood and platelet transfusion requirement for VAD (vs ECMO) patients ($p < 0.06$). The exact safe level of anticoagulation for either circuit may be difficult to establish, and an approach based on individual patient and circuit factors will be required.

d) *Long term support:* Neither centrifugal pump VAD nor ECMO is suitable for long term support, although other currently available paediatric devices may be better (10). Our longest ECMO and VAD supports for cardiac indications in surviving patients have been 120 and 144 h respectively. Non survivors have been well supported for 384 and 428 h respectively for cardiac indications, and longer for pulmonary indications. The limiting factor for both systems is development of sepsis. This experience is in contrast to VAD use in adults, in whom sedation and paralysis are not required due to more durable and sepsis resistant cannulation techniques and for whom chronic support is possible, either for recovery or bridge to transplant.

e) Cost: At the Royal Children's Hospital, LVAD adds A\$234.00/day to the patients hospital costs, vs A\$ 1050.00/day for ECMO. We currently employ two nurses per patient (i.e. an ECMO specialist and the patient's regular nurse) during ECMO support, but only one for VAD management.

RCH results of ECLS for cardiac indications

To September 1995, 77 patients have been supported with either ECMO or VAD for cardiac failure or combined cardiac and pulmonary failure at the Royal Children's Hospital. The age range was newborn to 19 years (median 4 months). Weight varied from 1.6 to 70 kg (median 6.9 kg), and was similar for VAD and ECMO patients (p = 0.32). The indications for support and patient diagnoses are outlined in Table 1. Anatomic diagnosis of postoperative patients is outlined in Table 2. For the entire series, the mean duration of support was 83 h in survivors vs 141 h in non-survivors (p = 0.05) Since December 1993 the support duration in survivors and non survivors has been similar 78.8 h (SD 29 h) vs 89.9 h (SD 65 h) (p = 0.5925). Duration of VAD support tended to be shorter throughout the series (91 vs 155 h, p = 0.03). Long duration of ECMO for pulmonary support was not predictive of poor outcome (13) in pooled ELSO data, although ECMO performed specifically for cardiac indications has not been subjected to this analysis. In the Toronto experience (12) recovery tended to occur within 6 days or not at all for cardiac ECMO patients.

The outcome for all our patients, stratified according to support type, is presented in Figure 3. In interpreting these results it should be borne in mind that our LVAD survivors would likely all have been supportable with ECMO, although the reverse is not necessarily true, imposing some unfavourable selection bias on the ECMO group. The proportion of patients weaned from support was higher for VAD than ECMO (0.75 vs 0.45, p = 0.02), although this result was neutralised by post weaning (in hospital) deaths in the VAD group, all related to continued cardiac problems. For patients supported prior to 1994, actuarial survival at 1 year (from time of initiation of ECLS) was 0.30 (CL = 0.18 – 0.43), and was similar for VAD and ECMO at 6 months follow-up (0.45, CL = 0.26 – 0.64 vs 0.32, CL = 0.13 – 0.52). Also, there was no difference in survival for ECLS used as postoperative support versus ECLS for non-operative support. Perhaps most importantly,

Table 1. Indications for initiation of paediatric ECLS at the Royal Children's Hospital

Indications	VAD	ECMO	VAD & ECMO	Total
Failure to wean patients from CPB	28	7	5	40
Sepsi syndrome (nonoperated patients)	–	9	–	9
Trauma, cardiomyopathy or myocarditis (nonoperated patients)	–	4	2	6
Cardiopulmonary dysfunction (nonoperated patients)	–	6	–	6
Cardiac arest or low CO following operation	9	6	1	16
Total	37	32	8	77

Table 2. Anatomic diagnoses and surgical procedures for which children received ECLS following cardiac operations at the Royal Children's Hospital. Support was possible in univentricular as well as biventricular hearts.

Diagnosis	Operation
Aortic arch obstruction with DORV, multiple VSDs	Arch Repair and PA band
Anomalous LCA from PA	Takeuchi procedure Coronary reimplantation
AV septal defect	Complete repair Repair & LAVVR
AV septal defect & hypoplastic arch	Repair of AV septal defect and arch
AV septal defect and tetralogy of Fallot	Repair
Complex cyanotic lesion	Heart lung transplant
Complex UVH	BCPS Fontan DKS & central shunt Fontan revision
Discordant TGA with VSD	Senning & switch
DORV	Repair
Endocarditis	AVR & mitral repair Aortic root replacement
HLHS	Norwood Heart transplant
Hypoplastic arch	VSD closure & arch repair
Mitral stenosis	MVR
Pulmonary atresia & sinusoids	BCPS
RV failure after Mustard operation	Switch conversion
Shone's Complex	Redo arch repair VSD closure & MVR CoA repair, MVR, aortic valvotomy Konno operation Aortic root replacement
Subaortic stenosis following IAA repair	Konno operation
Subaortic stenosis & multiple VSDs	Subaortic resection VSD closure & PA band
Tetralogy of Fallot	Repair
TGA.IVS	Arterial switch
TGA.VSD	Arterial switch & VSD closure
VSD (probable cardiomyopathy)	VSD repair
William's syndrome, supravalvar AS	Repair of supravalvar AS

Abbreviations: LCA, left coronary artery; PA, pulmonary artery; AV, atrioventricular; LAVVR, left atrioventricular valve replacement; CHD, congenital heart disease; UVH, univentricular heart; BCPS, bidirectional cavopulmonary shunt; DKS, Damus-Kaye-Stansel; TGA, transposition of the great arteries; DORV, double-outlet right ventricle; AVR, aortic valve replacement; HLHS, hypoplastic left heart syndrome; VSD, ventricular septal defect; MVR, mitral valve replacement; CoA, coarctation of the aorta; IAA, interrupted aortic arch; TGA.IVS, transposition of the great arteries-intact ventricular septum; AS, aortic stenosis.

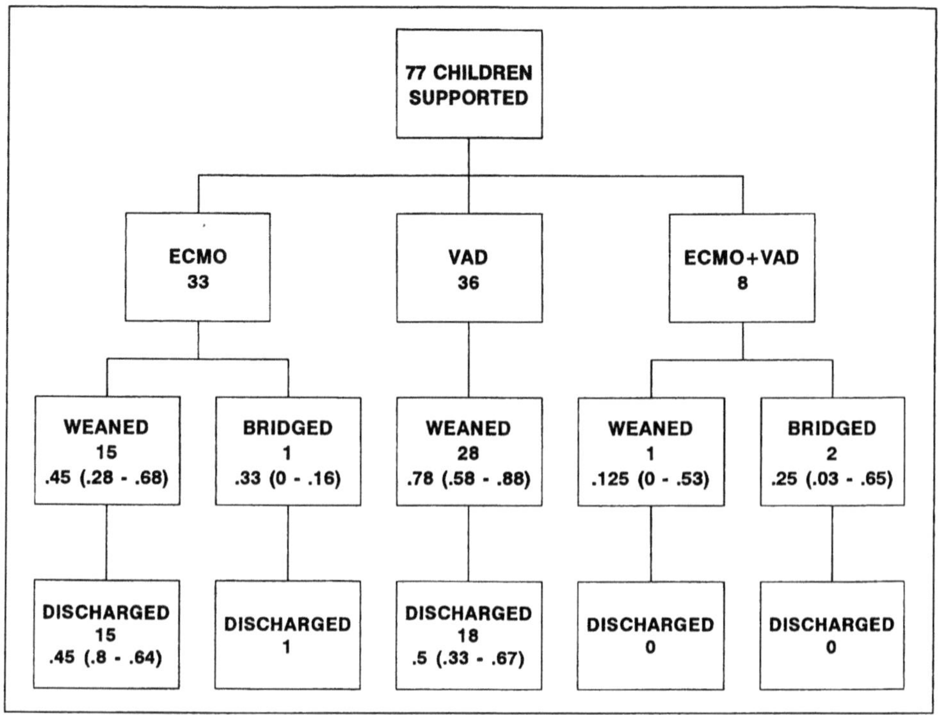

Fig. 3. Outcome of ECLS for cardiac indications at the Royal Children's Hospital. Proportions are expressed with 95% confidence limits. There was a significant difference in the proportion weaned from VAD vs ECMO (p = 0.007), but not in the proportion discharged from hospital (p > 0.05).

over a total follow-up time of 1159 patient months, the general clinical status of survivors has been very good, with no permanent neurologic or vascular sequelae. The main ongoing morbidity has been related to the patients' residual cardiac problems.

Our results are similar to those recorded for cardiac ECMO in the most recent ELSO report (44% survival for neonatal and paediatric cardiac indications) (5) as well as several other published series (12, 14), suggesting that the patient population probably exerts more influence than the technique of support. Pooled data from many centres would predict a 0.4 – 0.6 chance of survival for cardiac ECLS in centres already using ECMO on a routine basis. In an earlier ELSO report, most deaths on ECMO for cardiac support were related to irreversible cardiac or brain injury (15). It was concluded that results could be improved by earlier identification of high risk patients and earlier institution of ECLS.

Comment

There are really 2 issues to be considered when analysing results of ECLS:
– Does ECLS (ECMO and VAD) support patients adequately when cardiac function is severely compromised?

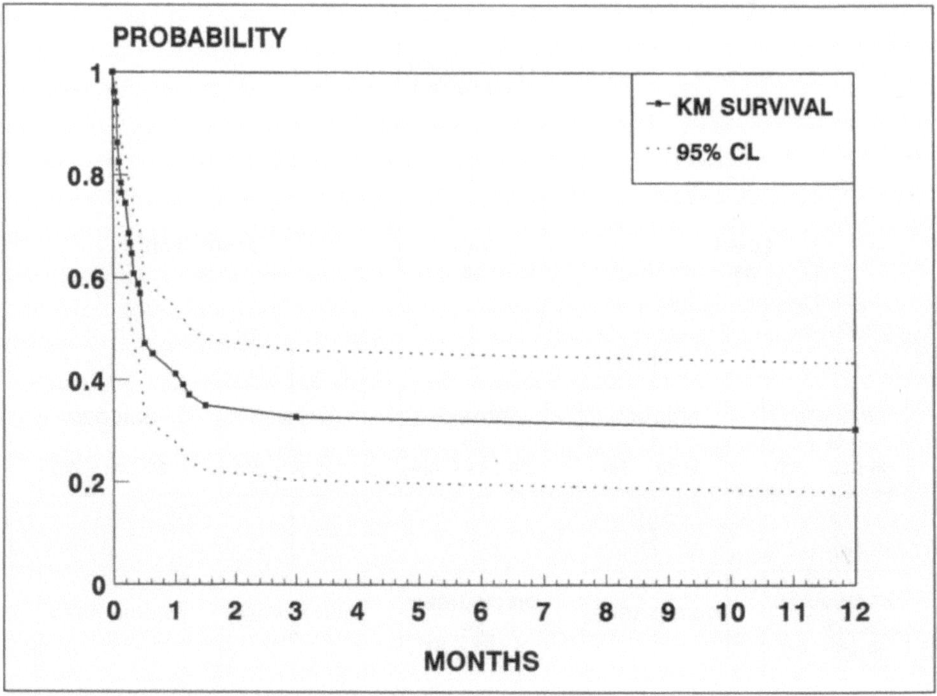

Fig. 4. The actuarial survival for the first 51 patients undergoing extracorporeal circulatory support at the Royal Children's Hospital. At 1 month, there was no significant difference for mode of support (ECMO vs VAD vs Both) or intraoperative versus non-intraoperative initiation of support ($p > 0.05$ for both). As with most congenital heart lesions, there is an initial (rapidly declining) hazard followed by a flatter (but not horizontal) curve.

– Does the use of ECLS allow cardiac improvement to occur if it would not have done so otherwise?

The answer to the first issue is clearly yes, but the second is not as clear. Because most patients can be well supported with a centrifugal pump system, the results will be profoundly influenced by patient selection. Numerous risk factors have been identified in published reports mainly dealing with ECMO for paediatric cardiac support. The results in our own unit (and in most others) reflect a policy of expanding the indications to include nearly all cardiac surgical patients who are not expected to survive without ECLS. Whether this strategy is appropriate or not is a decision to be taken by each team in the context of local resources and philosophy. To most of us, a 30-40% long-term survival probability would immediately justify the effort and expense, especially if the child would have minimal or no disability. One would expect a steady improvement in the technical side of ECLS perhaps obscured somewhat by expansion of indications.

The best cardiac ECLS candidates are patients who have rapidly reversible problems, usually consequent to a long intraoperative ischaemic time or other preoperative factors, but a relatively normal heart from a structural point of view. Examples in our own experience include children with ALCAPA syndrome, patients undergoing arterial switch in the context of "deconditioned" LV (ie, low pLV in an older child), and transplant recipients who have graft dysfunction related to long ischaemic time. Certainly the availability of ECLS has influenced surgeons' willingness to accept donor hearts with projected long ischaemic times, a common problem for our team due to the distances involved in Australia. The routine use of nitric oxide will probably reduce the need for perioperative ECLS in transplant recipients.

In our own experience the worst candidates are those who have a poor outlook even if ECLS is not required, eg. Shone's syndrome, hypoplastic left heart syndrome (HLHS), complex univentricular hearts (UVH) etc, as well as patients who have significant bleeding when support is initiated. In the Toronto experience (12) the strongest correlate of ECMO failure was the presence of a residual cardiac defect, and our own experience supports the importance of this finding. Pennington (16) noted the need for dialysis or ultrafiltration as well as sepsis to be risk factors for death. In our own unit, dialysis and/or ultrafiltration are used routinely during both VAD and ECMO and have not emerged as independent risk factors.

Is ECLS possible for patients with a univentricular circulation? This is currently a controversial point. We have supported patients with VAD following the Norwood operation for HLHS, as well as following BCPS for other complex UVH variants. In such cases, higher than normal flows may be required, as the assist device provides both pulmonary and systemic output. Blalock shunts have been left open in ECMO patients as well during ECLS.

Patients who have mechanical valves in mitral or aortic position may be at increased risk for valve thrombosis during ECMO or VAD, (especially with minimal anticoagulation) due to low flow through the valve orifice, and as such may be higher risk candidates.

We have experience with only three bridge to transplant cases to date, although other centres are reporting larger and more favourable experience (14, 17), even for postoperative patients whose initial plan was intracardiac repair. The question of when transplantation is a better option than continued ECLS support in a postoperative patient continues to challenge our judgement. In using ECMO for such patients, (and others with minimal LV ejection) LA or LV decompression may be necessary to prevent haemorrhagic pulmonary oedema (17, 18). This can be accomplished via balloon or blade septostomy in some patients (18, 19). We do not clinically employ ECLS for bridging purposes in smaller children and infants due to the donor availability problem in Australia, but there is no technical reason to prevent this strategy being successful in other centres having better access to small donor hearts. We await improvements with pneumatic or implantable devices for longer term support in children, and it would be fair to say that at present the majority of cardiac ECLS in children is performed with a view to myocardial recovery.

Is ECLS appropriate for resuscitation during or following a cardiac arrest? This is a complex question, the main worry of course being neurologic outcome. Pre arrest status is a critical factor, both for the brain and the heart, although recovery of cardiac function can occur well beyond the point of severe brain damage. We have employed ECMO (via peripheral cannulation) after $1\frac{1}{2}$ hours of asystolic normothermic arrest in a 7-year-old transplant patient with severe late rejection. The result was apparent full cardiac and neurologic recovery following intense immunosuppression on ECMO. We have also initiated LVAD and ECMO support during cardiac arrests of shorter duration with good quality survival. In the Pittsburgh experience 11/17 patients with cardiac arrest (6/11 who had > 15 min cardiac massage) survived to discharge following ECMO support (14). Use of ECLS under such circumstances is certainly justified in our view, but the philosophy will vary from one centre to another.

Which type of pump is best for ECLS? The majority of paediatric VAD support worldwide has been accomplished using the centrifugal pump system. We also use this pump in our ECMO circuit, although most centres employ a roller pump for this purpose. The centrifugal pump is simple in concept, and is designed to run at a constant (but operator varied) speed. The constrained vortex design results in subatmospheric pressure at the tip of the cone, generating suction in the venous cannula. Care must be taken to keep this pressure above –20 mmHg, or excessive haemolysis may occur. This particular problem is not encountered in roller pumps, which generate constant flow at a given speed, but have a potential for haemolysis for other reasons. Studies in our own unit suggest that haemolysis is lower in the properly managed centrifugal pump circuit than in the roller pump circuit (8). More importantly, the centrifugal pump allows fine tuning of the peripheral circulation prior to weaning, as it is responsive to the patient's intravascular volume and resistance. There is also less chance of accidental line disruption and air embolus. The battery backup in the system makes the pump convenient for transport. For these reasons, we currently favour the use of the centrifugal pump for all of our ECLS. Other electrical or pneumatic systems are available, with limited clinical experience in small children.

Is the Carmeda system likely to improve the results of the cardiac ECLS? The Carmeda process involves endpoint covalent bonding of fragmented heparin molecules to the circuit components, including oxygenator, tubing, pump head, cannulas and all connectors (20). Consequently the heparin dose given systemically can be reduced or perhaps eliminated altogether. This system is especially attractive for intraoperative conversion of CPB to ECMO or VAD. Accumulating experience in our own unit and elsewhere would suggest that postoperative bleeding is less with the heparin bonded Carmeda system for cardiac ECLS. Thus, the indications for ECMO and VAD may ultimately be extended to patients with haemorrhage, coagulopathy, ARDS from trauma, etc (21). We have successfully supported two children with severe intrapulmonary haemorrhage using Carmeda components. However, even with a fully bonded circuit and moderate heparin doses, the problem of thrombus formation in the tubing and pump head has not been completely eliminated (22, RCH unpublished data).

The heparin bonded circuit may have the added advantage of improved biocompatibility (23, 24, 25). Recent studies in humans would suggest that serum concentrations of various inflammatory mediators on ECLS are reduced with Carmeda circuits (using low dose heparin) as compared to non-Carmeda circuits with higher dose heparin. Also, in animals, CPB induced pulmonary injury appears to be less severe with heparin bonded than non-bonded circuits (25). The main disadvantage of commercially available Carmeda oxygenators is that because heparin cannot be bonded to the silicone polymers used in true membranes (eg. Avecor), a hollow fibre oxygenator is required. This latter type of oxygenator is subject to serum leakage with prolonged usage and therefore is less suitable for long-term support. Whether or not the improved biocompatibility and decreased lung injury can offset this disadvantage is currently under study in our unit and elsewhere. In clinical practise, we have employed Carmeda circuits for up to 8 days, although the median time span is closer to 48 h. This is in contrast to the Avecor non-heparin bonded membrane, which has a median ECMO life of approximately 5 days. Our current protocol is to employ Carmeda circuits for all VAD patients and all ECMO patients requiring intraoperative or early postoperative support, or for patients who have significant bleeding/coagulopathy for other reasons, or who will require surgical procedures on ECMO. Other patients are supported with an Avecor membrane oxygenator. Detailed analysis will be possible after more patients have been supported with heparin bonded circuits.

Conclusions

Centrifugal pump VAD and ECMO are extremely useful short-term treatment modalities for children with no other survival options. We await further improvements in support systems which may provide a chance for longer term assistance with a view to either myocardial recovery or bridge to transplantation. In preparing this manuscript, I gratefully acknowledge the critical role of the RCH perfusionists in the development and management of our ECLS program.

Proposal for Paediatric VAD Registry

Data collection for infants and children receiving VAD support is not included in the ELSO report. Even the data for ECMO as a cardiac assist device is not presented in a format that provides adequate detail for cardiac surgical decision making. A main problem is that the cardiac support patients in most reports tend to be grouped together as a "post cardiotomy" cohort, a term which is nebulous at best. An attempt to prospectively identify candidates for myocardial recovery on ECLS will require a breakdown of anatomic subgroups, details of CPB events, myocardial protection, repair technique, and other factors. In Melbourne, we are initiating the International Paediatric VAD Registry. The aim is to encourage detailed reporting of VAD results in infants and children, involving all centres and all types of devices, worldwide. The Registry will be announced in the Annals of Thoracic Surgery in 1996. All centres are invited to participate and data collection will be facilitated by the use of electronic mail with direct transfer from each institute's existing data base. Detailed statistical analysis will be performed in our unit on a yearly basis and reported periodically in an international cardiac surgical journal. Results will also be made available continuously on an Internet forum. All centres are invited to participate, irrespective of patient numbers.

References

1. DeBakey ME (1971) Left ventricular bypass for cardiac assistance: Clinical experience. Am J Cardiol 27:3
2. Karl TR (1994) Extracorporeal circulatory support in infants and children. Seminars in Thoracic Cardiovascular Surgery 6:154–60
3. Butt WW, Karl TR, Horton AM, et al. (1992) Experience with extracorporeal membrane oxygenation in children more than one month old. Anasth Intensive Care 20:308-310
4. Karl TR, Horton SB, Sano S, Mee RBB (1991) Centrifugal pump left heart assist in Pediatric cardiac surgery: Indications, technique and results. J Thorac Cardiovasc Surg 102:624-30
5. Karl TR, Horton SB, Mee RBB (1989) Left heart assist for ischaemic postoperative ventricular dysfunction in an infant with anomalous left coronary artery. J Card Surg 4:352-4
6. Tracy TF Jr, DeLosh T, Bartlett RH (1994) Extracorporeal Life Support Organisation 1994. ASAIO Journal 40:1017-9

7. Cochrane AD, Horton AM, Butt WW, Skillington PD, Karl TR, Mee RBB (1992) Neonatal and paediatric extracorporeal membrane oxygenation. AustAs J Cardiac Thorac Surg 1:17-22

8. Horton SB, Horton AM, Mullaly RJ, et al. (1993) Extracorporeal membrane oxygenation life support: a new approach. Perfusion 8:239-247

9. Farmer DL, Cullen ML, Philippart AI, Rector FE, Klein MD (1995) Extracorporeal membrane oxygenation as salvage in pediatric surgical emergencies. J Ped Surg 30:345-7; discussion 347-8

10. Warnecke H, Berdjis F, Hennig E, Lange P, Schmitt D, Hummel M, Hetzer R (1991) Mechanical left ventricular support as a bridge to cardiac transplantation in childhood. Eur J Card Thorac Surg 5:330-3

11. Karl TR, Iyer KS, Mee RBB (1990) Infant ECMO cannulation technique allowing preservation of carotid and jugular vessels. Ann Thorac Surg 50:105-109

12. Black MD, Coles JG, Williams WG, Rebeyka IM, Trusler GA, Bohn D, Gruenwald C, Freedom RM (1995) Determinants of success in pediatric cardiac patients undergoing extracorporeal membrane oxygenation. Ann Thorac Surg 60:133-8

13. Green TP, Moler FW, Goodman DM (1995) Probability of survival after prolonged extracorporeal membrane oxygenation in pediatric patients with acute respiratory failure. Critical Care Medicine 23:1132-9

14. Dalton HJ, Siewers RD, Fuhrman BP, del Nido P, Thompson AE, Shaver MG, Dowhy M (1993) Extracorporeal membrane oxygenation for cardiac rescue in children with sever myocardial dysfunction. Critical Care Medicine 21:1020-8

15. Meliones JN, Custer JR, Snedecor S, Moler FW, O'Rourke PP, Delius RE (1991) Extracorporeal life support for cardiac assist in pediatric patients. Review of ELSO Registry data. Circulation 84:168-72

16. Pennington DG, Swartz MT (1993) Circulatory support in infants and children. Ann Thorac Surg 55:233-7

17. del Nido PJ, Armitage JM, Fricker FJ, Shave M, Cipriani L, Dayal G, Park SC, Siewers RD (1994) Extracorporeal membrane oxygenation support as a bridge to pediatric heart transplantation. Circulation 90:1166-9

18. Hausdorf G, Loebe M (1994) Treatment of low cardiac output syndrome in newborn infants and children. Zeitschrift fur Kardiologie 83:91-100

19. Alexi-Meskishvili V, Weng Y, Uhlemann F, Lange PE, Hetzer R (1995) Prolonged open sternotomy after pediatric open heart operation: experience with 1134 patients. Ann Thorac Surg 59:379-83

20. Bindslev L, Bohm C, Jolin A, Hambraeus Jonzon K, Olsson P, Ryniak S (1991) Extracorporeal carbon dioxide removal performed with surface-heparinized equipment in patients with ARDS. Acta Anaesthesiologica Scandinavica 95:125-30; discussion 130-1

21. Rossaint R, Slama K, Lewandowski K, Streich R, Henin P, Hopfe T, Barth H, Nienhaus M, Weidemann H, Lemmens P, et al. (1992) Extracorporeal lung assist with heparin-coated systems. Int J Artificial Organs 15:29-34

22. Bianchi JJ, Swartz MT, Raithel SC, Braun PR, Illes MZ, Barnett MG, Pennington DG (1992) Initial clinical experience with centrifugal pumps coated with the Carmeda process. ASAIO Journal 38:143-6

23. Shigemitsu O, Hadama T, Takasaki H, Mori Y, Kimura T, Miyamoto S, Sako H Soeda T, Kawawaki Y, Uchida Y (1994) Biocompatibility of a heparin-bonded membrane oxygenator (Carmeda MAXIMA) during the first 90 minutes of cardiopulmonary bypass: clinical comparison with the conventional system. Artificial Organs 18:963-41

24. Fosse E, Moen O, Johnson E, Semb G, Brockmeier V, Mollnes TE, Fagerhol MK, Venge P (1994) Reduced complement and granulocyte activation with heparin-coated cardiopulmonary bypass. Ann Thorac Surg 58:472-7

25. Redmond JM, Gillinov Am, Stuart RS, Zehr KJ, Winkelstein JA, Herskowitz A, Cameron DE, Baumgartner WA (1993) Heparin-coated bypass circuits reduce pulmonary injury. Ann Thorac Surg 56:474-8; discussion 479

Author's address:
Dr Tom R. Karl
Victorian Paediatric Cardiac Surgical Unit
Royal Children's Hospital
Flemington Road
Parkville, 3052, Melbourne, Australia

The MEDOS assist device was developed at the Helmholtz Institute for Biomedical Engineering at the RWTH Aachen, Germany. It is available for infants and children with pumping chambers for the left heart of 10 and 25 ml (Fig. 1). For biventricular assist the right chambers have a stroke volume 10% less (9 and 22.5 ml) to prevent hyperperfusion of the lungs. The MEDOS assist device has undergone various in vitro and in vivo studies with consecutive refinements of the different components (3, 19, 20, 28). The final pump is made of polyurethane and consists of a housing and a multi-layer diaphragm with a seamless D-H junction. Both are completely transparent. The chamber geometry has been optimized by various experimental techniques such as flow visualization, wash-out methods and Laser-Doppler-Anemometry (Fig. 2). Main purpose of this optimization procedure was the elimination of stagnation areas and regions of poor wash-out (12). Therefore, and in contrast to some similar devices, in- and outlets of the pump are widely separated and arranged in such a way that laminar in-and outflow of the pump chamber is provided. The angle between the connectors and the membrane plane is as flat as possible (20 °C) (Fig. 3). The membrane has a spherical geometry, whereas the housing is elliptical. These combined features provide a circular laminar flow and assure an optimized wash-out of blood. Three-leaflet polyurethane valves, size 12 and 16 mm respectively, are utilized with a pressure drop lower than the best commercial valves of respective size (11, 21). These valves have no leakage and their in vitro durability is much higher than the required 20 million load cycles. The leaflets are integrated into a sinus-shaped housing in order to provide a proper wash-out of the space behind the leaflets and to avoid stasis in this critical region (Fig. 4). The transition between the leaflets and the housing is again seamless. Both

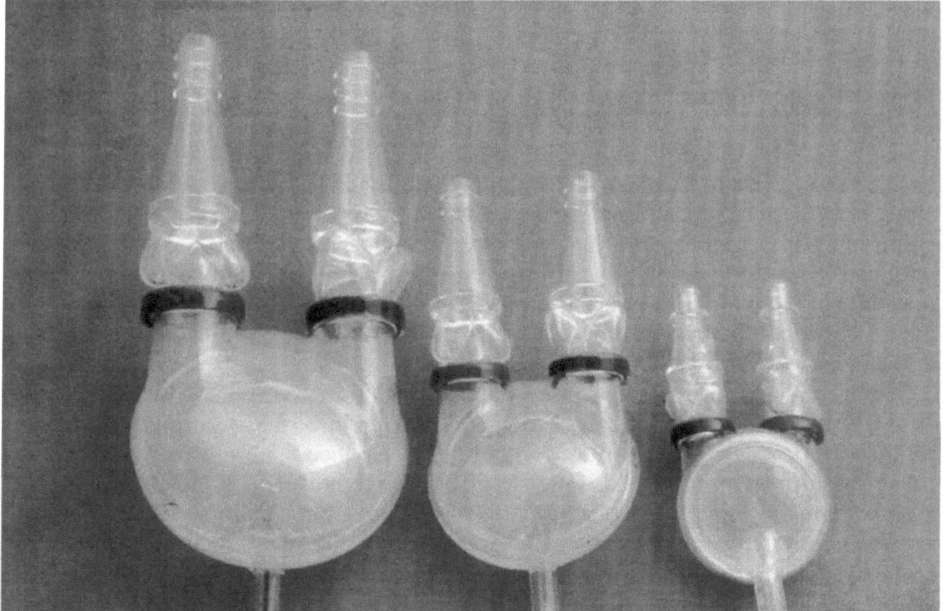

Fig. 1. Three different sizes of the left prosthetic ventricles of the MEDOS assist device: 10 ml, 25 ml and 60 ml.

Individual center experiences in pediatric mechanical circulatory support for bridge-to-transplant and myocardial recovery

S. Däbritz, B. J. Messmer

Department of Thoracic and Cardiovascular Surgery, Klinikum RWTH, Aachen

For more than two decades mechanical circulatory support (MCS) has been applied to sustain patients with low cardiac output refractory to pharmacological treatment. The aim is to convert terminal heart failure into treatable heart disease or to bridge the patient to transplantation. As the less invasive possibility of partial circulatory support the intraaortic balloon pump (IABP) has been used extensively and successfully (7). However, its use is mainly limited to the improvement of left ventricular function. More effective support can be achieved with left ventricular (LVAD), right ventricular (RVAD) or biventricular assist devices (BVAD). The impact of these devices rises with the increasing number of patients waiting for heart transplantation as bridge-to-transplant. Therefore paracorporeal or intracorporeal mechanical ventricular assistance is frequently applied in adults either for temporary myocardial decompression or for bridge-to-transplant mostly after surgical treatment of aquired heart disease. The mode of pumping is either nonpulsatile or pulsatile. In the nonpulsatile group the greatest experience is gained with the paracorporeal centrifugal pump with overall survival rates of 25-39% (15, 16, 22). In the pulsatile group the systems of the currently inserted pumps are either pneumatic or electromechanic. Some of them are used as implantable LVADs, others as total artificial heart (TAH). The overall survival rates range from 25 to 69% (2, 4, 9, 13–16, 17, 22, 27). The duration of circulatory assistance is extending continuously with the ultimate goal of total mechanical replacement of the heart. In contrast cardiomyoplasty or muscular pumps for biomechanical support are under investigation, but need further improvement prior to wide application (1).

Even though there has been a vaste increase in knowledge concerning mechanical circulatory support in adults, there is only little experience with assist devices in children. With exception of the extracorporeal membrane oxygenation (ECMO) with centrifugal pumps mainly for respiratory problems, only few centers have done mechanical circulatory support for ventricular failure in children (6, 8, 10, 13, 24, 25). Also in contrast to adults, the effect of the IABP in children is controversial and not convincing (18, 26).

Therefore the need for parallel mechanical circulatory support is increasing, particularly because more and more demanding operations are performed in early infancy and cardiac transplantation in children has become an alternative therapy for terminal heart failure and noncorrectable congenital defects, respectively.

Apart from the centrifugal pump, most of the pulsatile pumping systems are not applicable in children because of the lack of small chambers. Recently, two pneumatic systems were developed with special regard to pediatric cardiac surgery with pumping chambers as small as 10 ml: the Berlin heart and the MEDOS assist device. Both have shown convincing results in adults for bridging-to-transplant as well as for myocardial recovery with overall survival rates of 44 to 60% (2, 13, 23).

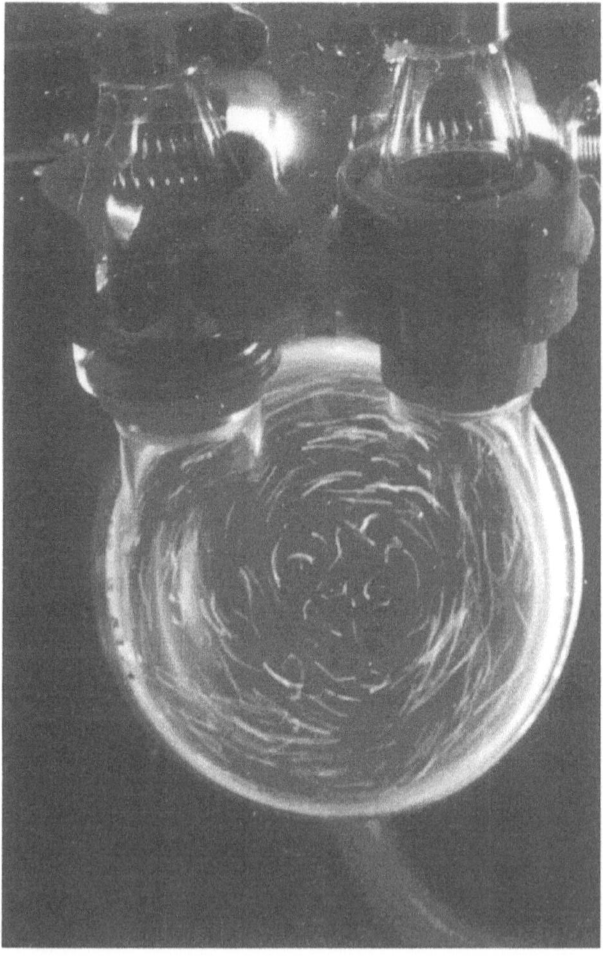

Fig. 2. Flow visualization of the laminar circular flow in the prosthetic ventricle of the MEDOS assist device.

components, the valves and the prosthetic chamber, have been investigated with regard to hemolysis and thrombosis under different conditions (19, 20, 21, 27). The driving system consists of a control and pressure unit and can work on external or internal pressure and vacuum supply (5). A smooth systolic and diastolic operation mode (physiologic dp/dt) is provided by linear servo valves. Handling is easy by a touch screen monitor. The VAD can operate under different control modes: asynchronous, fixed rate mode and synchronous EKG-triggered mode equivalent to R-wave counterpulsation. Systolic and diastolic times are variable over a wide range. A full-to-empty actuation is desired and controlled by setting the parameter limits for pump output accordingly. This is of great importance in order to minimize thromboembolic complications. Therefore it is more advantageous to have a lower heart rate with complete filling of the chamber compared to higher heart rates without full-empty operation.

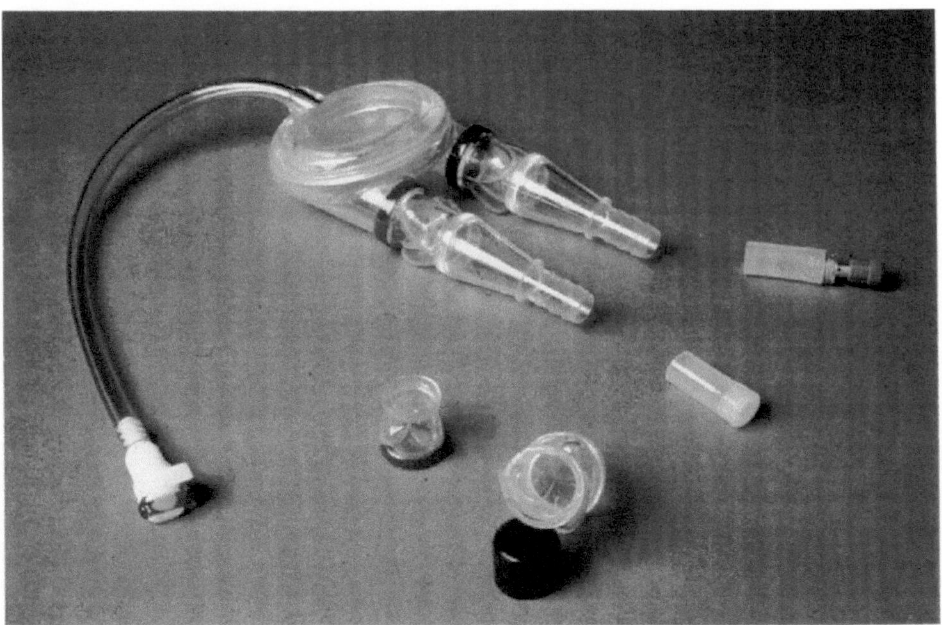

Fig. 3. Prosthetic ventricle of the MEDOS assist device with wide separation and flat angle of the in- and outlets (20°).

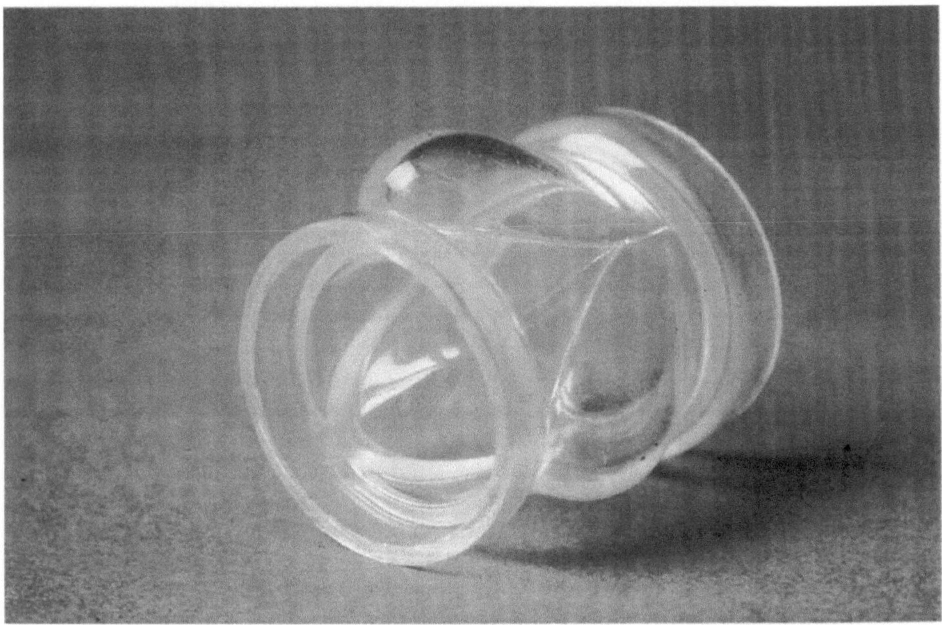

Fig. 4. Sinus-shaped housing of the three leaflet polyurethane valves of the MEDOS assist device.

Indications for assist devices in children

The range of indication for assisted circulation in pediatric cardiac surgery encloses all states of cardiac failure which are presumably reversible within a certain period of time or which imply the indication for cardiac transplantation. Different situations for implantation of a VAD can be distinguished according to whether an operation has been performed or not, how the ventricular function was before an intervention and what kind of operation has been done:

Indications without operation:
- myocarditis
- endocarditis
- neoplasm
- temporary respiratory insufficiency particularly in neonates (ECMO)
- Eisenmenger

Indications postoperatively
- deteriorated preoperative ventricular function exacerbating after the operation
- Bland-White-Garland-Syndrome
- hypoplystic left heart, neoplasm etc
- change in hemodynamic situation postoperatively with good preoperative status
- arterial switch in simple Transposition of the great arteries (TGA) after the neonatal period
- secondary arterial switch after atrial switch or in congenitally corrected TGA
- Fontan or Fontan-type procedures with postoperative left ventricular deterioration
- pulmonary hypertensive crisis refractory to prostacyclin or NO treatment
- right ventricular failure of any other source (Fallot etc.)
- myocardial failure due to prolonged cross-clamp and CPB time or unsatisfactory operative outcome with good preoperative status
- Kawasaki-disease
- procedures with intraoperative complications
- impossibility of planed correction

All indications are either for myocardial or pulmonary recovery or as bridge-to-transplant. In contrast to adults, some special considerations have to be taken into account in infants and children. Pathophysiology in congenital heart disease is different from aquired heart disease. An isolated left ventricular assist device can be unsatisfactory. Besides, it has to be considered that a LVAD can only be inserted if intracardiac shunts are closed. Right ventricular assist device (RVAD) requires at least some kind of pulmonary valve. In mechanical mitral valve replacement aggressive anticoagulation is recommended because LVAD leads to a stagnation of the flow across the valve. Infection is generally not considered an absolute contraindication for MCS (10).

In adults certain directives have been noted to determine the need for mechanical support concerning hemodynamic parameters and oxygen saturation (2). In children this is much more difficult and guidelines are not yet existing. Inability of weaning from CPB is an evident indication. Postoperative low cardiac output, however, has to be recognized early, as hesitation may be followed by multiorgan failure. Careful observation with detection of early signs of low output such as centralization (body temperature to toe temperature gradient of more than 5 °C), beginning metabolic acidosis, and decreasing urine output is necessary. The better the patient's condition is prior to mechanical circulatory support, the better the clinical outcome will be.

Insertion technique

Insertion is easier in patients, who were weaned from cardiopulmonary bypass (CPB) or didnot have an operation at all. Still most of the candidates for VAD in pediatric surgery are those whose circulation is dependent on CPB, so that the VAD has to be inserted simultaneously.

First, the ascending aorta is cannulated for LVAD proximally to the CPB cannula with a small, commercially available, right-angled wirewound cannula which is fixed with two purse-string sutures. This might be difficult in small infants or after a Lecompte maneuver. In such patients a distal cannulation may be preferable. If CPB support can be interrupted for a few minutes, the CPB aortic cannula can also be used for the assist device. Heparin coating of the cannulas is not necessary, but might be advantageous. The chamber is deaired by filling it with 20% human albumin from inflow to outflow and by tilting. It is then connected to the aortic cannula first. A venous wirewound cannula of adequate size is inserted through a thoracic intercostal space from the right side. Most children requiring a LVAD have already a left atrial vent. This is removed and replaced by the venous cannula which is preferably right angled. It is fixed with two pursestring sutures; rubber tourniquets are not useful in children. After attachment to the chamber CPB can be stopped and the assist device is activated simultaneously with 2.5 l/min/m^2. There is no need of starting the VAD at minimal flow. If additional RVAD is requested, it can be inserted before CPB is stopped by cannulation of the pulmonary trunc and the right atrial appendage in the same way as described above for the LVAD. In small children it is advantageous to place one of the RVAD cannulas (preferably the pulmonary one) into the chest through an intercostal space at the left side to avoid too many tubes exiting the sternotomy wound in terms of avoiding infections. Thus in BVAD the right outflow catheter crosses the left inflow tube outside the chest. It is of great importance to keep the circuit as short as possible to minimize contact surface area of blood and to reduce cooling of the patient. Insulation of the VAD lines against heat loss is usually not necessary. Closure of the sternum or even the skin is not recommended in infants, as there is not enough space and the cannulas may compress the heart. Besides, closure of the skin with a PTFE-patch has advantages of early recognition of bleeding, as any bulging of the patch is a sign for it. In this way pericardial tamponade can be avoided or treated easily by incision of the patch. Nevertheless, additional insertion of pericardial and pleural drainages is useful. The wound is finally covered by a transparent surgical dressing which is left untouched (Fig. 5).

Intensive care management

Intensive care management implies sedation without relaxation, reduction of inotropic support to the level required for adequate function of the right ventricle in LVAD or the left in RVAD. Vasodilatators may be used. Antibiotics are given

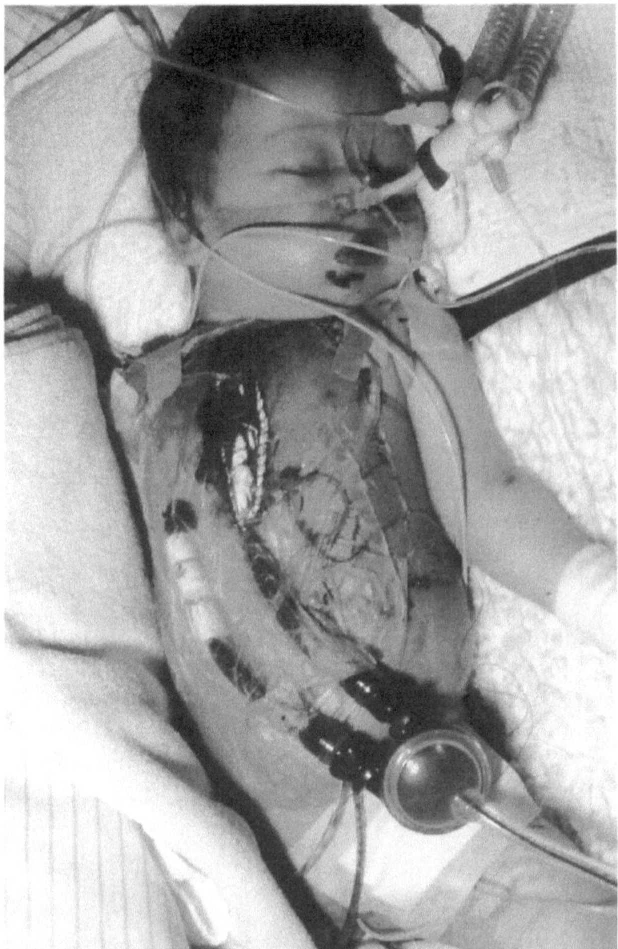

Fig. 5. MEDOS - LVAD (10 ml chamber) implanted in an infant. The circuit is kept as short as possible. The skin is closed with a PTFE-patch and a transparent wound dressing is used.

routinely. Parenteral nutrition is started early to avoid catabolism. Platelets, fresh frozen plasma and blood is substituted if necessary. The active coagulation time (ACT) is titrated to a level of about 150 s with heparin. Laboratory tests are done according to intensive care standards controlling liver and kidney function as well as hematologic and coagulation parameters. Peritoneal dialysis is performed if required.

Complications

There are several complications in connection with MCS described in literature:
– clotting disorders (bleeding into the chest, cerebral hemorrhage etc.)

- infections
- capillary leakage
- thromboembolism
- hemolysis

Some of the complications are due to wrong adjustment or performance of the assist device, but some are connected to the mechanical support itself and are therefore unavoidable. Generally complications occur more frequently if the patient's condition was bad at the beginning of MCS. The treatment of the complications is always symptomatic, except if bleeding is due to surgical problems of the insertion of the device.

Weaning-off

The weaning from MCS in small children implies some special aspects. Even if the support rate is reduced to 1/3 of the heart rate in EKG-triggered control mode or down to 40/min in fix rate driving (lowest frequency), the device is able to produce an almost normal cardiac output (CO). Thus the capability of the own ventricle is difficult to assess by echocardiography. In non-pulsatile mechanical support the appearance of pulsatile ejection on the arterial pressure trace is a good indicator, but this does not apply for pulsatile systems. The definite decision for removal of the device is therefore made in the operation theater when the MCS is stopped. Medical support is usually started a few hours before. In case of recurrent low output, a new prosthetic ventricle needs to be used. Some authors recommend increase of heparin dosage before weaning-off. Yet, thromboembolic risk is lower, the longer the device has been inserted.

Case report

A 10-week-old infant, weight 4.2 kg, body surface 0.26 m^2, was referred to our institution with the diagnosis of Bland-White Garland-Syndrome, made by EKG (myocardial infarction with Q-wave) and echocardiography (LV-failure and mitral insufficiency (MI)). Cardiac catheterization proved the diagnosis and showed impaired LV function with severe MI. The operative correction was performed urgently by direct transposition of the left coronary artery ostium from the pulmonary artery into the ascending aorta. Additionally, the mitral valve was reconstructed by Kay-Wooler-plasty and an atrial septal defect was closed. The correction was performed under deep hypothermia and circulatory arrest with cardioplegic cardiac arrest (Bretschneider, 30 ml/kg KG). The patient was weaned from CPB with moderate medical support. Shortly before closure of the chest LV failure with dilatation and concomitant ischemic changes in EKG occurred. Emergent connection of CPB was performed. EKG returned to normal at once after decompression of the LV by insertion of a left atrial vent. Revision of the left coronary artery revealed tension on the anastomosis under LV dilatation. Therefore the left mammary artery was dissected and anastomosed to the LAD in deep hypothermic circulatory arrest. Again clamping of the left atrial vent lead to LV dilatation.

Under these circumstances decision for application of LVAD with the MEDOS device with the 10 ml ventricle was made. Connection was performed according to the above description. An 8F catheter was chosen for the inflow, and an 18F heparin-coated one for the outflow. Hemodynamic situation stayed stable after turning from the CPB to the LVAD with only low cathecholamine dosage and without the need of a RVAD.

Postoperative-course:

ACT ranged between 144 and 212 s, but increased to unmeasurable values on the 2nd postoperative day with a PTT of > 150 s. due to a heparine-overdose. A hematoma occurred between the PTFE-patch and the wound dressing without any signs of pericardial tamponade. To minimize the risk of infection, the dressing was changed, the hematoma and the patch removed and skin was closed. Fresh frozen plasma and blood was supplied according to the consumption and the loss; platelets had to be substituted once. Cathecholamines were reduced to a minimal dosage to support the right ventricle. Enoximone therapy, started while still on CPB, was gradually reduced to zero, nitroprusside medication was continued. Suprarenine and enoximone therapy were started again 2 h before explantation of the device, which could be done on the fourth postoperative day without complications.

The LVAD was active for 4 days with a frequency of 80 to 85/min resembling an output of 800 to 850 ml. Core temperature ranged from 35.8 to 37.8 °C without insulation of the tubes. Urine output, creatine and urea were normal without diuretics. There was a slight reversal increase of transaninases, which is frequently recognized after CPB. The highest LDH was 556 U/l with the peak level on the first day. Signs of myocardial infarction were not found in EKG nor in laboratory tests. Under antibiotic cover with a cephalosporine and gentamicin no symptoms of infection occurred; antithrombin III stayed in the range usually found after CPB. Oxygen saturation was $> 90\%$ with an FiO_2 of 30–40%.

The clinical course was also uneventful. There were no signs of thromboembolic complications, focal seizures or convulsion. Important to notice, capillary leakage did not occur.

The day after removal of the LVAD (5th p.o. day), the infant was referred to the pediatric intensive care unit. Enoximone was given for another day, suprarenine for 3 and dopamine for 6 days. Digitalisation was started overlapping with reduction of catecholamines. Mechanical ventilatory support was continued to the 11th postoperative day. Altogether the infant stayed in the intensive care unit for 14 days and was discharged from hospital in good clinical condition on the 29th day. Echocardiography showed a mild mitral insufficiency and good LV-function. Follow-up for 1 year is uneventful with a good clinical development and unchanged echocardiographic findings of cardiac function.

Conclusion

The MEDOS assist device is applicable for infants and even neonates. Due to the technical refinements with optimized fluid dynamics and biocompatibility, risk of thromboembolic complications and hemolysis is low. Implantation is feasable and operation of the device is simple and safe. The device provides a good back-up for several surgical interventions in pediatric cardiac surgery and can be used as bridge-to-transplant, too. Early implantation is a prerequisite for successful application.

References

1. Chachques JC, Grandjean P, Serraf A, Latremouille C, Jebara VA, Ponzi O, Mihaileanu S, Chauvaud S, Bourgeois I, Carpentier A (1990) Atrial cardiomyoplasty after Fontan-type procedures. Circulation 82 (suppl IV): IV-183–IV-189
2. Duveau D, Baron O, Meilhan E, Soulard D, Commin PL, Chevalier JC, Trochu JN, Tirouvanziam A, Al Habash O, Despins P, Michaud JL (1995) What about total artificial heart as a bridge to transplant?. Fifth International Symposium Bad Oeynhausen September 7–9, p 15 (abstr)
3. Eilers R, Harbott P, Reul H, Rakhordt G, Rau G (1994) Design improvement of the HIA-VAD based on animal experiments. Artificial Organs 18(7):473–478
4. Everts PAM, Schönberger JPAM, Peels CH (1995) The Abiomed BVS 5000 for Treatment of Postcardiotomy Cardiogenic Shock. In: Unger F (4th eds) Assisted Circulation, Springer-Verlag Berlin Heidelberg New York, pp 87–100
5. Farrar DJ, Compton PG, Lawson JH, Hershorn JJ, Hill JD (1986) Control modes of a clinical ventricular assist device. IEEE Engineering in Medicine and Biology Magazine 3:19–25
6. Ferrazzi P, Glauber M, Domenico AD, Fiocchi R, Mamprin F, Gamba A, Crupi G, Cossolini M, Parenzan L (1991) Assisted circulation for myocardial recovery after repair of congenital heart disease. Eur J Cardio-thorac Surg 5:419–424
7. Frazier OH; Cooley DA (1989) Use of cardiac assist devices as bridges to cardiac transplantation: Review of Current Status and Report of the Texas Heart Institute's Experience. In: Unger F (3rd eds) Assisted Circulation, Springer-Verlag Heidelberg, 247–259
8. Hausdorf G, Loebe M (1994) Behandlung des Low-cardiac-output-Syndroms bei Neugeborenen und Kindern. Z. Kardiol. 83:Suppl 2:91–100
9. Icenogle T, Copeland JG (1989) Experience with the total artificial heart as a bridge to transplantation. In: Unger F (3rd eds) Assisted Circulation, Berlin Heidelberg New York, pp 260–268
10. Karl TR, Sano S, Horton S, Mee RBB (1991) Centrifugal pump left heart assist in pediatric cardiac operations. J Thorac Cardiovasc Surg 102:624–30
11. Knierbein B, Rosarius N, Unger A, Reul H, Rau G (1992) CAD-design, stress analysis and in vitro evaluation of three leaflet blood-pump valves. J Biomed Eng 14:275–285
12. Knierbein B, Rosarius N, Reul H, Rau G (1990) New methods for the development of pneumatic displacement pumps for cardiac assist. The International Journal of Artificial Organs 13,11:751–759
13. Konertz W, Laube H, Herwig V, Waldenberger F, Redlin M, Kleber FX, Hausdorf G (1994) NOVACOR and HIA/MEDOS: Two different devices for different indications, The Third International Conference on Circulatory Support Devices for Severe Cardiac Failure, Pittsburgh USA
14. Lawson JH, Cederwall G (1989) Clinical Experience with the Thoratec Ventricular Assist Device. In: Unger F (3rd eds) Assisted Circulation, Springer-Verlag Berlin Heidelberg New York, pp 191–196
15. Minami K, Körner MM, Posival H, El-Banayosy A, Körfer R (1995) Mechanical ventricular support in postcardiotomy cardiac failure. Transplantforum 1:16–20
16. Minami K, Posival H, El-Bynayosy A, Körner MM, Schrofel H, Murray E, Körfer R: Mechanical ventricular support using pulsatile Abiomed BVS 5000 and centrifugal Biomedicus-pump in postcardiotomy shock.
17. Poirier V, Dasse K (1995) Clinical Results of the Heart Mate Implantable Blood Pump. In: Unger F (4th eds) Assisted Circulation. Springer-Verlag, Berlin Heidelberg New York, pp 77–86
18. Pollock JC, Charlton RN, Williams WG, Edmonds JF, Trusler GA (1980): Intraaortic balloon pumping in children. Ann Thorac Surg 29:522–528
19. Rakhorst G, Hensens AG, Blanksma PK, Bom VJJ, Elstrodt J, van der Meer J, Schakenraad JM, Verkerke GJ, Reul H (1992) Evaluation of a Protocol for Animal Experiments with Helmholtz Left Ventricular Assist Devices. Cor Europ 4:155–159
20. Rakhorst G, Hensens AG, Verkerke GJ, Blanksma PK, Bom VJJ, Elstrodt J, Magielse CPE, van der Meer J, Eilers R, Reul H (1994) In-vivo Evaluation of the 'HIA-VAD': a New German Ventricular Assist Device. Thorac cardiovasc. Surgeon 42:136–40
21. Reul H, Taguchi K, Herold M, Lo HB, Reck B, Mückter H, Messmer BJ, Rau G (1988) Comparative evaluation of disk- and trileaflet valves in left-ventricular assist devices (LVAD). The International J Artific Organs 11:127–130

22. Richenbacher EW, Myers JL, Waldhausen JA (1989) Current Status of Cardiac Surgery: A 40 Year Review. JACC 14, 3:535–544
23. Schiessler A, Friedel N, Weng Y, Heinz U, Hummel M, Hetzer R (1994) Mechanical Circulatory Support and Heart Transplantation. Pre-Operative Status and Outsome. ASAIO Journal 40,3 :476–481
24. Taenaka Y, Takano H, Noda H, Kinoshita M, Tatsumi E, Yagura A, Sekii H, Sasaki E, Akutsu T (1989) Experimental Evaluation and Clinical Application of a Pediatric Ventricular Assist Device. ASAIO-Trans 35(3):606–608
25. Taenaka Y, Takano H, Noda H, Kinoshita M (1990) A pediatric ventricular assist device: ist development and experimental evaluation of hemodynamic effects on postoperative heart failure of congenital heart disease. Artif-Organs 14(1):49–56
26. Veasy LG, Blalock RC, Orth JL, Boucek MM (1983) Intra-aortic balloon pumping in infants and children. Circulation 68:1095–110
27. de Vivo F, Galdieri N, Livi U, Martinelli L, Munoretto C, Pagani F, Quaini E, Villa L, Casarotto D, Cotrufo M, Pellegrini A, Vigano M, Scuri S (1995) Novacor LVAS as bridge to heart transplant: Italian multicenter study. Fifth International Symposium Bad Oeynhausen, September 7–9, p 19 (abstr)
28. Waldenberger FR (1995) Novel Cardiac Assist Devices with different unloading capacities. An experimental study. Acta Biomedica Loveniensa 107

Appendix

The 5 ml and 4,5 ml pumping chambers with 10 mm polyurethane valves for MCS in neonates are currently developed and will be available soon.

Author's address:
Dr. Sabine Däbritz
Dept. of Thoracic and Cardiovascular Surgery
Klinikum RWTH
Pauwelsstraße
D-52057 Aachen
Germany

Extracorporeal circulatory support in pediatric cardiac patients - The Berlin Experience

V. Alexi-Meskishvili, R. Hetzer, Y. Weng, K. Ishino, E. Potapov, M. Loebe,
E. Hennig, F. Uhlemann, P.E. Lange

Department of Cardiothoracic and Vascular Surgery, German Heart Institute Berlin, Berlin,
Germany

Introduction

The institution of extracorporeal circulatory support in the pediatric population
has been limited due to the scarcity of suitable devices. Although the successful use
of miniaturized intra-aortic balloon pumps in children has been reported occasion-
ally (23, 34), providing intra-aortic balloon pump support in this cohort has been
hampered by difficulties associated with inserting cannulas into small vessels and
synchronizing the device to a rapid heart rate. Its efficacy has further been ques-
tioned in small children because of increased aortic compliance. Over the last decade circulatory support in pediatric surgery has most commonly been provided
through extracorporeal membrane oxygenation (ECMO)(14, 17, 25, 36). The capability of ECMO to provide biventricular as well as respiratory support may be
beneficial in maintaining circulation in children, especially those with congenital
heart defects. Some recent reports have described the successful use of a centrifugal
ventricular assist device (VAD) in children for cardiogenic shock after cardiac surgery (6, 15), for donor heart failure, and as a bridge to cardiac transplantation
(26). However, the impossibility of mobilizing the patient, generating a pulseless
flow, and the short durability of the components are critical disadvantages for long-
term support with ECMO or centrifugal VADs.

Altogether the experience with extracorporeal circulatory support with mechan-
ically-driven ventricles in children is very limited. In this chapter we analyze our
experience in the use of two types of support, extracorporeal membrane oxygenation and Berlin Heart ventricular assist device (BVAD) support, for myocardial
recovery or as a bridge to transplantation in 40 infants and children at the German
Heart Institute Berlin since 1990 (Fig. 1).

Patients and Methods

ECMO group
Twenty-six patients (2.2%) who had undergone complex surgical correction of congenital heart defects were connected to an ECMO system after postoperatively
developing severe myocardial insufficiency which failed to respond to maximum
treatment with inotropic agents and vasodilators (Table 1): two preoperatively, 17
in the operating room, and seven in the intensive care unit. The patients ranged in

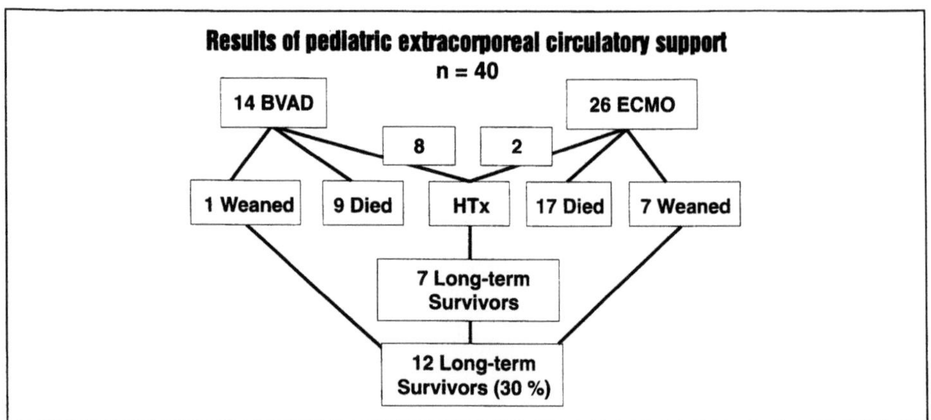

Fig. 1. Results of pediatric extracorporeal circulatory support at the German Heart Institute Berlin. Abbreviations: BVAD – Berlin Heart ventricular assist device, ECMO – extracorporeal membrane oxygenation, HTx – heart transplantation

Table 1. Diagnosis and number of patients supported with ECMO

Diagnosis	Number of patients undergoing ECMO
Transposition of the great arteries with/without ventricular septal defects	7 (1)
Total anomalous pulmonary venous drainage	4 (1)*
Tetralogy of Fallot	3 (0)
Aortic/mitral valve reconstruction	2 (0)
Anomalous origin of the left coronary artery from the pulmonary artery	2 (2)
Pulmonary atresia with/without ventricular septal defects	1 (0)
Complete atrioventricular septal defect	1 (1)
Double outlet right ventricle	3 (0)
Variants of a single ventricle	3 (1)
Total	26 (6)

* 2 patients underwent ECMO preoperatively. ( ) Number of survivors

Table 2. Patient characteristics and type of VAD support

Patient Nr.	Age	Weight (kg)	Diagnosis	Etiology	CPR	Type of Support	Pump SV r/l (ml)	Outcome
bridge group								
1	12 yrs	52	cardio-myopathy	idiopathic	–	biventricular	50/60	
2	8 yrs	27	cardio-myopathy	AS, CoAo	–	left ventricular	50	
3	13 yrs	51	cardio-myopathy	Op. TGA (Mustard)	+	left ventricular	60	
4	9 yrs	35	cardio-myopathy	idiopathic, Op. AR, endocarditis	–	biventricular	50/60	
5	2 weeks	3.2	myocardial infarction	PA + IVS BT-shunt	+	left ventricular	15	
6	15 yrs	43	cardio-myopathy	Op. Wilms' tumor s/o adri-amycin	–	left ventricular	60	
7	15 yrs	39	cardio-myopathy	idiopathic	–	biventricular	50/60	
8	3 yrs	14	cardio-myopathy	myocarditis	–	biventricular	50/60	
9	12 yrs	36	cardio-myopathy	idiopathic	–	biventricular	50/60	
10	10 yrs	35	cardio-myopathic	idiopathic	–	biventricular	50/60	
11	14 yrs	49	cardio-myopathy	myocarditis	–	biventricular	50/60	
Recovery group								
1	6 mos	7.0	cardiac arrest	Op. VSD	+	biventricular	12/12	
2	10 mos	7.8	allograft failure	transplanta-tion	–	biventricular	12/12	
3	4 yrs	16	cardiac arrest	acute myocarditits	+	biventricular	25/30	

AR – aortic regurgitation; BT – Blalock-Taussig; CPR – cardiopulmonary resuscitation; r/l – right/left; TGA – transposition of the great arteris; AS – aortic stenosis; CoAo – coarctation of the aorta; PA + IVS – pulmonary atresia with intact ventricular spetum; SV – stroke volume; VSD – ventricular septal defect

age from 2 days to 17 years (median = 3.4 years), whereby the percentage of newborns was 54%. Body weight ranged from 2.3–83 kg (median = 8 kg). The duration of ECMO ranged from 4–401 h (median = 104 hours). The patients were divided into two groups. The criterion for this division was the initiation of ECMO as a consequence of insufficient weaning from extracorporeal circulation despite prolonged reperfusion (more than 3 h) and maximal medicamentous therapy in the operating room (Group I, 19 patients) or postoperatively for cardiopulmonary instability in the intensive care unit as a final attempt to rescue the patient (Group II, seven patients).

VAD Group

Fourteen patients under 16 years of age were supported with the Berlin Heart VAD as a bridge to cardiac transplantation (bridging group) or for recovery of myocardial function (recovery group). Patient data and type of support are listed in Table 2.

Bridging Group

Six girls and five boys with an average age of 10.1 years (range: 2 weeks to 15 years) and an average weight of 34.9 kg (range: 3.2 to 52 kg) were implanted with an LVAD or a BVAD. Nine of the 11 patients manifested cardiomyopathy (five idiopathic, two myocarditis, two secondary), one case of which was induced through adriamycin. A 2-week-old baby with pulmonary atresia and an intact ventricular septum suffered from massive myocardial infarction 10 days after a modified Blalock-Taussig shunt. Patients 3 and 5 required emergency VAD implantation under cardiopulmonary resuscitation (CPR). Due to the unavailability of a suitably sized pump, patient 8 received a pump which was too large for her body weight.

Recovery Group

Three patients were supported with pediatric VADs for cardiogenic shock. Patient 1 suffered sudden cardiac arrest 32 hours after the closure of a ventricular septal defect. Biventricular support was initiated under CPR. Patient 2, who had undergone left internal thoracic artery to left anterior descending artery bypass for ostium atresia of the left coronary artery at the age of 8 months, underwent heart transplantation. She developed severe cardiac allograft failure and could only be weaned from cardiopulmonary bypass with BVAD support after 7 h of reperfusion. Patient 3, displaying acute myocarditis, was admitted under emergency conditions caused by progressive dyspnea and hypotension. He suffered cardiac arrest in the intensive care unit, necessitating the initiation of BVAD support under CPR.

ECMO and VAD Techniques

In the two patients treated preoperatively with ECMO (8%), the right carotid and the internal jugular vein were primarily cannulated, with this cannulation being maintained after surgery. Twenty-three patients (89%) were cannulated over the right atrium and the ascending aorta either while in the operating room or after a stay in the intensive care unit. Cannula sizes varied from 12 to 24 Fr for the venous side and from 8 to 14 Fr for the arterial (dlp, Jostra, Polystan). The sternum was left open and the skin either closed directly or with an Ethi-Touch Patch (Ethicon Norderstedt, Germany). Veno-venous ECMO was initiated via the femoral vein in one patient with postoperative pulmonary embolism, while a left ventricular assist device was used in a patient with extensive myocardial dysfunction. In two cases a left ventricular vent was inserted in order to prevent left ventricular dilatation. Due to the lower flow rates during perfusion in infants, particularly during the weaning phase, roller pumps were indicated rather than centrifugal pumps, as the former operated independent of afterload. Systemic anticoagulation was accomplished through continuous infusion of heparin. Heparinization was monitored hourly by measuring the activated clotting time (ACT). The ACT was maintained between 160 and 200 s.

If necessary, platelet and blood transfusions were administered to keep platelet counts and hemoglobin above $50\,000/mm^3$ and 10 g/dl, respectively. ECMO flow rate was set at 150 ml/kg/min in patients weighing less than 10 kg and at 110 ml/kg/min in those weighing more. Inotropic agents and vasodilators were reduced or eliminated. To minimize barotrauma to the lungs while patients were on ECMO, the ventilatory settings were maintained at a rate of 10 cycles/min, inspired oxygen fraction at 0.21 to 0.30, and positive end-expiratory pressure at 4 to 8 cm H_2O.

Description of BVAD devices

The Berlin Heart VAD (Berlin Heart GmbH, Berlin, Germany) is a paracorpore-ally-placed air-driven blood pump consisting of a polyurethane housing with an integrated diaphragm which forms a continuous blood contact interior (Fig. 2). Two drive diaphragms connected to a circular base plate form the air chamber. Because of the multilaminar construction of the diaphragm, the single membrane can be very thin, thus providing high flexibility, even at the diaphragm-housing junction (12). The adult-sized VAD has #21 Björk-Shiley tilting disc valves, metal connectors at the inlet and outlet ports with diameters of 12 mm, and stroke volumes of 50 and 60 ml. Several different types of special silicon inlet cannulas for the atria and outlet cannulas for the aorta or pulmonary artery are available. The atrial cannulas have various tip lengths (22, 26, 30 mm) with a small screen to prevent occlusion by the atrial wall. Arterial cannulas are bent at angles of 45°, 60°, or 85° with a Dacron ring at the end for the end-to-side anastomosis with the vessel. The newly-developed pediatric VAD incorporates polyurethane tri-leaflet valves with a diameter of 12 mm in the inflow and outflow positions and has stroke volumes of 12, 15, 25, or 30 ml. Custom-made aortic and venous cannulas for cardiopulmonary bypass (CPB) can be used for implantation.

The electro-pneumatic console/drive unit (Heimes HD-7, Vetschauer, Germany) is capable of operating two blood pumps in an alternate left-right fixed-rate mode (Fig. 3). Two computer disk drives, for a program and data diskette, respectively, together with a built-in computer and keyboard, allow for easy analysis and super-vision of the system. All important values such as drive pressure, left and right pump flow, left and right stroke volume, and calculated hemodynamic parameters are displayed on the screen. The unit has a completely redundant backup system and an internal energy source enabling independent operation for more than 6 h. This semi-portable drive unit weighs less than 10 kg.

Implantation and management of BVADs

With the exception of three patients implanted with a left ventricular assist device (LVAD), VAD implantation was accomplished under CPB. For the implantation of an adult-sized LVAD, a purse-string suture was placed immediately posterior to the interatrial groove near the origin of the right upper pulmonary vein and the inflow cannula inserted through this into the left atrium and secured by mattress

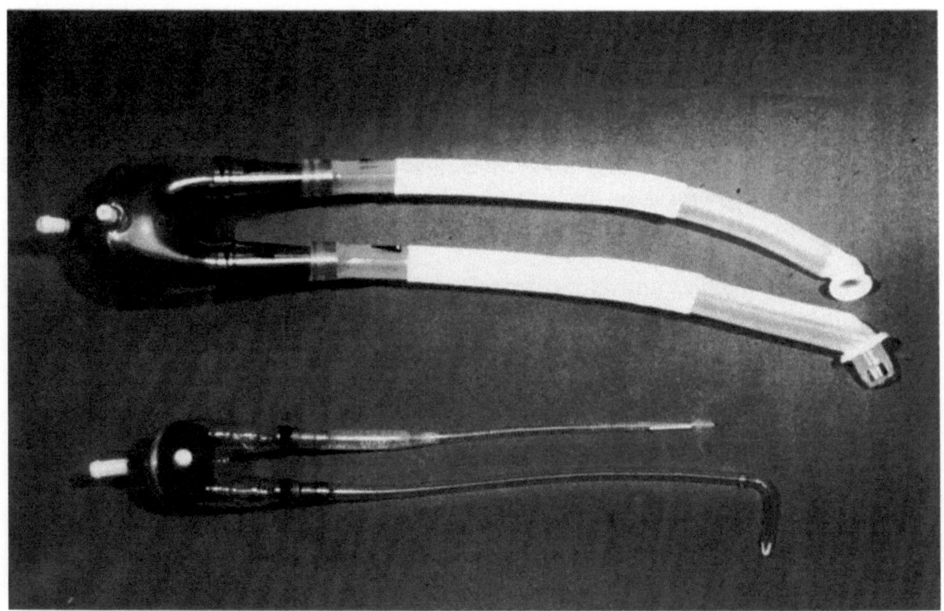

Fig. 2. The Berlin Heart adult-sized ventricular assist device (stroke volume: 50 ml) with special silicon inlet and outlet cannulas (above), and the pediatric ventricular assist device (stroke volume: 15 ml) with a right-angle venous cannula and straight-tip aortic cannula (below)

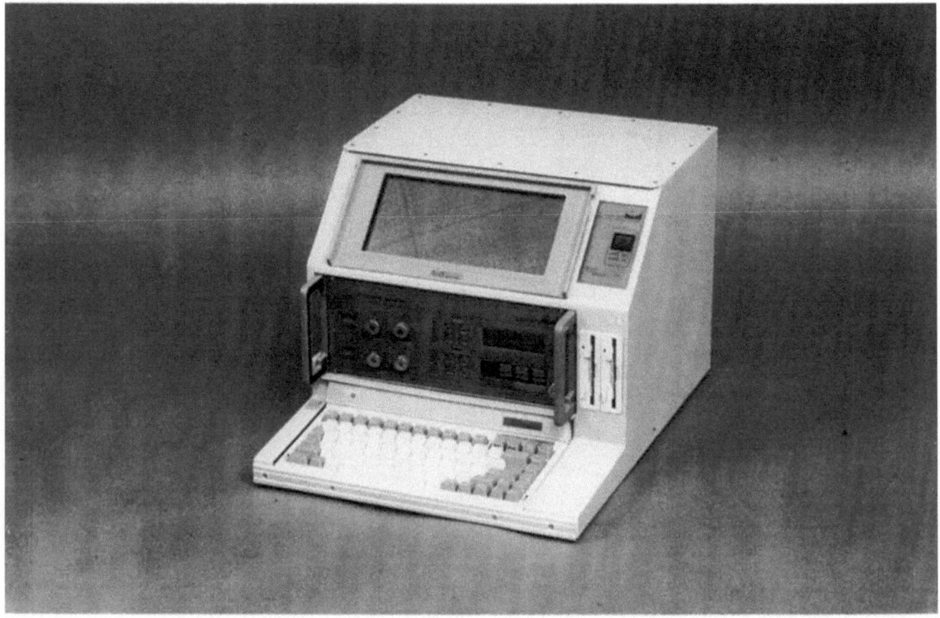

Fig. 3. "Heimes HD-7" electro-pneumatic console/drive unit.

sutures. The outflow cannula was anastomosed to the ascending aorta with mattress sutures. In cases requiring both-sided VAD (BVAD), an additional VAD was installed between the right atrium and the main pulmonary artery in a similar fashion. In order to implant a pediatric VAD, a right-angle atrial cannula (Polystan, Varlose, Denmark) and a straight-tip aortic cannula (Jostra Medizintechnik GmbH, Hirrlingen, Germany) were inserted through two purse-string sutures and secured with silicon rubber tourniquets. The transcutaneous course of the cannulas was established by tunneling through the abdominal wall in the epigastrium. The sternum was subsequently closed in all patients.

Anticoagulation was maintained with continuous heparin infusion to keep an activated clotting time of 160 to 180 s. Pump operation was monitored daily and, if necessary, readjusted to achieve full diaphragm movement. Patients who could be extubated were transferred to an intermediate ward to promote rehabilitation.

Results of ECMO and VAD treatment

Six patients (23%) were released, an improvement in myocardial function was observed in eight (31%), and seven (27%) were successfully weaned from ECMO. Five patients (26%) in Group I survived, one patient (14%) from Group II survived after undergoing heart transplantation. The age of the survivors varied between 2 days and 13 years. There was no significant difference in age between the groups or between survivors and non-survivors.

Both of the two patients who underwent surgery for anomalous origin of the left coronary artery from the pulmonary artery (ALCAPA) and the two who were

Table 3. Patient survival after circulatory support with extracorporeal membrane oxygenation

Nr.	Age	Diagnosis	Operation	Type of Support	ECMO duration	Outcome
1	7 days	TGA Intramural correction	Switch	ECMO	163.0	survived
2	2 days	TAPVD	Total correction	ECMO pre- and postop	193.0	survived
3´	9.5 months	ALCAPA	Coronary reimplantation	LVAD	190.5	survived
4	8.5 years	ALCAPA	Coronary reimplantation	ECMO	120.0	survived
5	7 years	CAVSD small LV	Partial correction	ECMO	401.0	HTx
6	13 years	SV, MVI, CAVSD, PA	Fontan type	ECMO	216.0	HTx

operated for complete AVSD (one of the latter pair having undergone heart transplantation) survived. One of the six patients who underwent a switch operation also survived, as did one of the four with total anomalous pulmonary venous drainage (TAPVD), and one of three patients with variants of the single ventricle (after heart transplantation) (Table 3). Median ECMO duration was significantly longer in survivors (179 h/range 112–401 hours) than in non-survivors (79 h/range 4–235 h) (p = 0.0042) while it was not significantly different between Group I (median 112 hours / range 4–401 hours) and Group II (median 58 h/4–140 h) (p = 0.27).

The courses of several hepatic parameters, such as aspartatamine transferase (GOT), alaninaminotransferase (GPT), gamma glutamyltransferase (γ-GT), and total bilirubin of 22 patients in this study cohort were analyzed. In 86% of the cases analyzed it was observed that 30 h after the initiation of ECMO the median activity of the GPT increased significantly by almost three times the value before ECMO (median 8 vs. 21.5, p = 0.0006, normal range 0–22 U/L). Beginning on the third day, the activity began to decrease slightly. A constant decrease in median GPT activity was observed in only three patients who preoperatively had excessively high (over 500 U/L) transaminase activity levels. GOT activity exhibited a similar course with a significant increase after 30 h (median, range 18–54 h) after the initiation of ECMO to six times the previous levels (median 30 vs. 177, p = 0.0004, normal range 0–18 U/L) and a subsequent slow decrease, albeit of smaller magnitude. The three patients with excessively high transaminase activity levels before ECMO initiation did not survive the ECMO therapy. These patients were excluded from the analysis. No significant difference in the transaminase courses were observed between the groups or between survivors and non-survivors.

Until the third day, the median γ-GT activity remained unchanged (median 6 U/L, normal range 4–28 U/L). Beginning on the third day, the median γ-GT activity increased slowly and reached 14 U/L. The preoperative excessively high γ-GT activity in three patients decreased during ECMO to a normal level. The γ-GT course exhibited no significant differences between the groups or between survivors and non-survivors.

The activity of cholinesterase (normal range 2800–8500 U/L) was low immediately after the initiation of ECMO (median 1355 U/L, range 164–3405). On the first day the median activity increased to 2385 U/L, (range 1575–3246). Afterwards it remained virtually unchanged. No significant difference in the course of cholinesterase was noted between the groups or between survivors and non-survivors.

In 95% of the cases analyzed, the median concentration of total bilirubin increased after 30 h (median, range 12–72 h) almost threefold (median 1.5 vs. 5.1, p = 0.0002, normal range 0–1.0 mg/dL) and subsequently decreased continuously. In 70% of the cases analyzed, hyperbilirubinemia (> 1.1 mg/dL) was observed immediately after surgery. After 12 h of ECMO therapy, total bilirubin levels in all of the patients analyzed increased by over 1.1 mg/dL. The median bilirubin concentration directly after the initiation of ECMO (1.2 vs. 1.6, p = 0.12), as well as after 36 h (2.5 vs. 4.3 p = 0.37), was not significantly lower in survivors as in non-survivors. Beginning on the 14th day the courses began to converge.

Peritoneal dialysis was begun in two patients before the initiation of ECMO and accomplished parallel to ECMO therapy in the other patients. Hemofiltration was primarily initiated in two patients. After ECMO initiation, a third patient was switched from hemodialysis to hemofiltration. The median urea concentration in patients without renal failure remained under 70 mg/dL (normal range 10–50 mg/dL).

Complications

The complications which occurred during ECMO included bleeding, neurologic deficits, and mechanical complications.

Bleeding: On the average, the patients bled at a rate of 18.6 ml/kg/h during ECMO (range 0–294, median = 4.2). In most of the cases the bleeding could be controlled either after repeat thoracotomy (necessary twice in two cases) or through retransfusion and the administration of blood products. One patient died due to pulmonary bleeding. Platelet substitution was accomplished in every patient at 50 000/μl and the hemoglobin level maintained at 10 g/dl. Therapy was ceased in three cases due to uncontrollable bleeding. The average thrombocyte count was 51 600/mm^3 (range 2.8–11.5 × 10^4). The median thrombocyte count was not significantly lower in the survivors compared to the non-survivors (41 vs. 48 000 /mm^3, p = 0.096). The average Hb concentration was 9.1 ± 2.4 g/dl.

Neurologic complications occurred in for cases (15%) either during or immediately after ECMO therapy. Intracerebral hemorrhaging was observed in two cases in Group I; one patient survived. In Group II brain death and hypoxemic defects with advanced seizures were observed. A total of two patients died of these neurologic complications.

Mechanical complications occurred in 28 cases. Thrombus formation in the reservoir accounted for 50%, centrifugal pump failure for 29%, oxygenator failure for 18%, and thrombus formation in the filter in 3.5% of the cases (one patient). These complications affected 35% of the patients, whereby 43% of the complications were observed in one patient who underwent ECMO for 401 h. There were altogether one complication per 4.4 ECMO therapy days and 1.1 complications per patient. None of the mechanical complications proved to be fatal.

Other complications: Renal failure was observed in six children and controlled either by peritoneal dialysis (two patients) or continuous hemofiltration provided by the ECMO system.

Severe mediastinitis without systemic reaction developed in one case after ECMO and was successfully treated.

The most common cause of death in both groups (a total of 45%) was persistent myocardial insufficiency, affecting six patients in Group I and 3 patients in Group II. Next in frequency of occurrence was bleeding with 12%. One patient in Group I died of intracranial bleeding, one patient in Group II of brain death. ECMO was not effective in two patients in Group II, each of whom were supported for 4 h, due to circulatory collapse which was unresponsive to therapeutic decrease in peripheral resistance. One weaned patient died after 10 days due to multi-organ failure with indications of ileus, a second patient due to bleeding, and a third due to pulmonary hypertonia.

Bleeding as a cause of death was only observed in Group I (three patients / 12%). Another patient in this group died of pulmonary hemorrhaging.

Creatinine levels also stayed within tolerable limits (normal range = 0.5–1.1 mg/dL). In patients in whom hemofiltration or dialysis were used, the median urea concentration increased constantly and after 60 h (median) reached a level of 70 mg/dL. At the end of therapy the median urea levels of these patients increased to 120 mg/dL.

The median creatinine levels in these patients were primarily within tolerable limits and at the end of therapy reached a value of over 2 mg/dL. In 50% of the cases, hemofiltration or dialysis were initiated simultaneously with ECMO. In the other cases the average time between the initiation of ECMO and that of hemofiltration or dialysis was 26 h. The course of urea concentration in survivors and non-survivors was approximately the same. Survivors and non-survivors had the same initial creatinine values. In non-survivors the median creatinine concentration levels increased on the third day of ECMO (after 60 h) and reached values up to 1.8 mg/dL, whereby the median creatinine concentration in survivors remained within a normal range until the 16th day of ECMO. The median of the values from 60–126 h did not differ significantly (1.1 vs. 0.7, p = 0.13).

Five of twenty-six patients were scheduled for heart transplantation and one for heart-lung transplantation. The mean duration of ECMO in these six patients was 260.5 h, ranging from 101 to 402 h (Table 4). ECMO was successful as a bridge to cardiac transplantation in three patients. Patients 1 and 3 survived transplantation and were discharged from the hospital. Patient 2 suffered immediate cardiac allograft failure and died intraoperatively. The other three patients, who incidentally were also the smallest, did not develop contraindications to transplantation until the last day on ECMO, when, despite good ECMO flow, support was electively terminated due to progressive hypotension caused by profound capillary leak syndrome (Table 4).

Major complications were encountered in four patients in this subgroup during ECMO. Bleeding was observed in two patients, necessitating re-exploration. Patient 3 had a focal seizure, but no recurrence after transplantation. Three patients re-

Table 4. Results of ECMO as a bridge to cardiac transplantation

Patient Nr.	Age	Sex	Weight (kg)	Diagnosis	Operation	Duration of ECMO (hrs)	Heart Tx	Complications	Outcome
1	6 yrs	M	18.0	Complete AVSD	Two-patch repair ↓ take down	402	yes	Blleding, renal failure	Survived (3 yrs 9 mos)
2	22 mos	M	10.5	DORV, PS, BT shunt × 2	VSD enlargement, PS release	101	yes	None	Died after HTx
3	14 yrs	F	28.5	Tricuspid atresia, mitral insufficiency, endocarditis	RA-RV homograft, VSD closure, mitral repair	178	yes	Renal failure, seizure	Survived (2 yrs 8 mos)
4	9 mos	M	6.8	d-TGA, VSD, PA banding	Switch, VSD closure	230	no	None	Died
5	2 mos	F	2.7	IAA type B, VSD	Arch repair, VSD closure	268	no	Bleeding	Died
6	13 mos	M	8.4	DORV, multiple VSD, SAS, PS	Switch, VSD closure, SAS, PS release	384	no	Renal failure	Died

AVSD – atrioventricular septal defect; DORV – double outlet right ventricle; PA – pulmonary artery; RA-RV – right atrium-right ventricle; TGA – transposition of the great arteries; TX – transplantation; BT – Blalock-Taussig; IAA – interrupted aortic arch; PS – pulmonary stenosis; SAS – subaortic stenosis; VSD – ventricle septal defect

quired hemodialysis after developing renal failure. In two of these, both transplant recipients, renal function recovered and hemodialyses was discontinued on the 13th and 25th days, respectively, after transplantation. Although leukocytosis (> 10 000/ mm^3) was observed in three patients, neither local nor systemic infection was noted in any of the six patients. Two patients exhibited evidence of liver dysfunction (glutamic-oxaloacetic transaminase and glutamic-pyruvic transaminase values > 50 IU/L). Both, however, recovered before transplantation.

VAD Bridging Group

Eight of the eleven patients subsequently underwent heart transplantation after a mean bridge duration of 32 days (range: 6 to 98 days); five were later discharged from the hospital. Thus, post-transplantation survival was 62.5% and survival from device implantation to patient discharge 45.5%. Three patients died while receiving ventricular support: due to sudden massive bleeding as a result of systemic (right) ventricular perforation in patient 3, respiratory failure in patient 4, and severe hypoxemia in patient 5. Three patients did not survive cardiac transplantation. Patient 1 suffered severe allograft failure of the right ventricle and thus required right-sided VAD. Double bridge procedure was successful 2 days later, but she again suffered from donor heart failure during the second transplantation. Patient 9 could not be weaned from CPB due to critical pulmonary hypertension, was placed on ECMO, yet subsequently died due to uncontrollable bleeding. Severe adhesion developed in the mediastinum of patient 11 after 72 days of support, which made establishing CPB difficult. After aortic cannulation was performed, a massive amount of air was recognized in the cannula and the aorta immediately clamped. An atrial septal defect with a diameter of 1.5 cm was found in the ex-

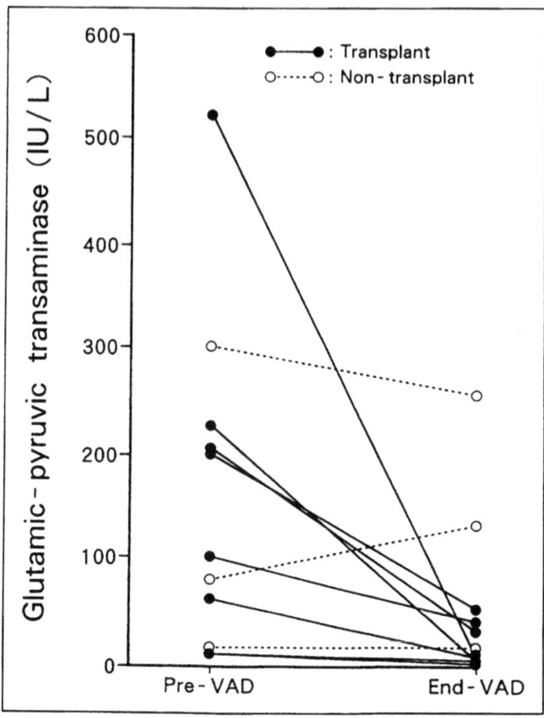

Fig. 4. Recovery of hepatic function during bridge to transplantation. VAD – ventricular assist device

planted heart. Although transplantation was performed without incident, brain death was diagnosed 2 days later.

Significant complications were encountered in seven of the 11 patients. Bleeding was the most common problem necessitating re-exploration in six patients. With the exception of patient 3, however, bleeding was not directly related to the outcome in any patient. Despite meticulous anticoagulation monitoring, thrombus formation in the blood chamber or on the mechanical valves necessitated exchanging the pumps in three patients; twice in patient 6, five times in patient 7, and three times in patient 8. Computed tomography confirmed cerebral infarction in two of these patients. Although seven patients had leukocytosis (> 12 000/mm^3) before device implantation, neither local nor systemic infection was noted in any of the 11 patients.

The recovery of major organ function was evaluated by comparing pre-implant data with those measured immediately before device explantation, i.e. upon transplantation or death. Six patients had liver dysfunction (glutamic-pyruvic transaminase > 100 IU/L) before ventricular support (Fig. 4). However, this improved in all but one of them and they subsequently underwent transplantation. Pre-implant renal dysfunction (serum creatinine > 1.5 mg/dl) was observed in three patients (Fig. 5). One who developed renal failure requiring hemodialysis died before transplantation, but the other two underwent transplantation after recovering of renal function. Four patients had been intubated prior to VAD implantation (Fig. 6). Only one could be extubated and subsequently undergo transplantation; another died on VAD within 1 week of its initiation. Seven patients without pre-implant respiratory failure were all transplanted. Two of them underwent transplantation without extubation and both were long-term survivors.

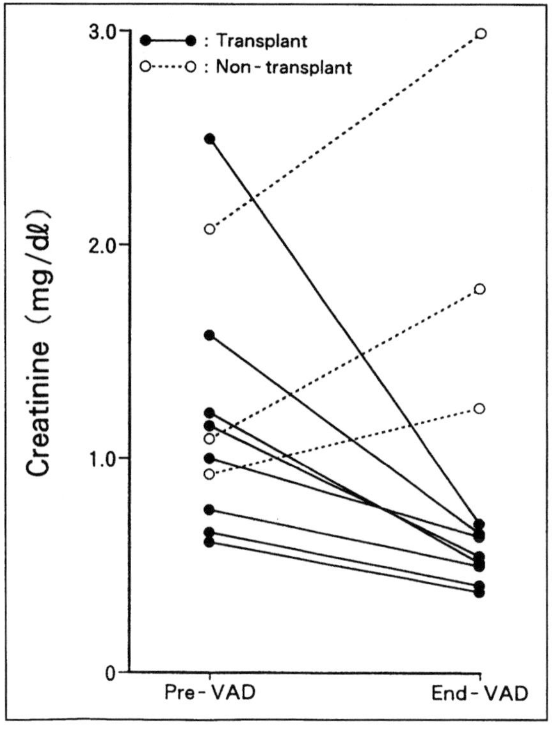

Fig. 5. Recovery of renal function during bridge to transplantation

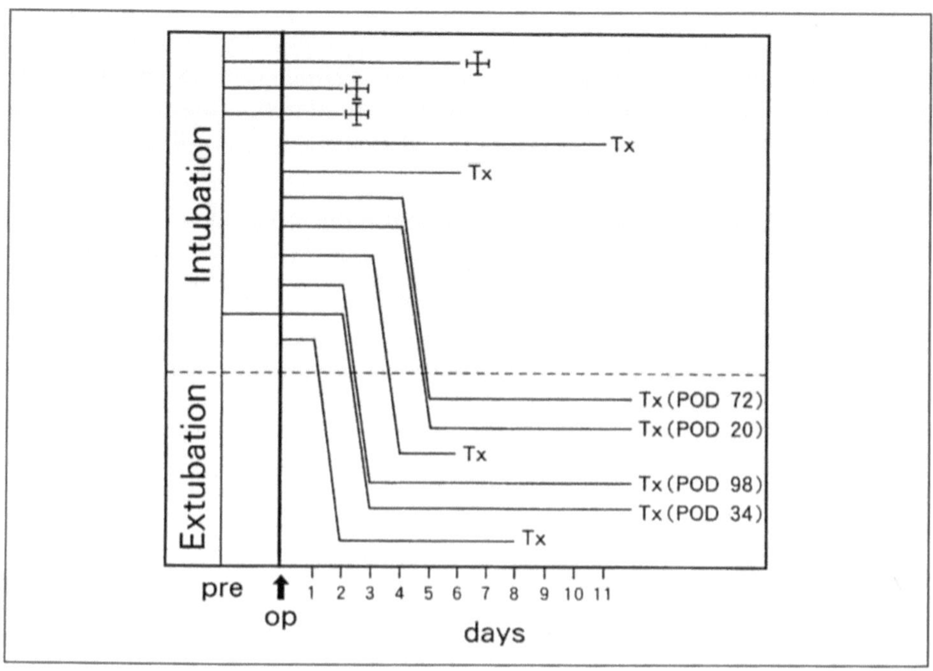

Fig. 6. Recovery of respiratory function during bridge to transplantation. Tx = transplantation, POD – postoperative day

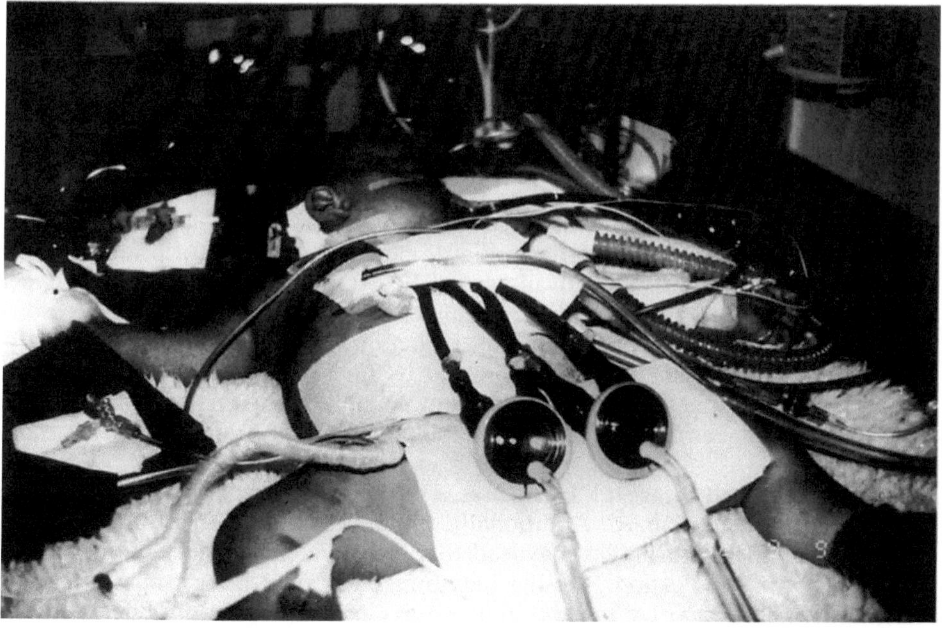

Fig. 7. A 6-month-old infant (7 kg) undergoing biventricular support with the Berlin Heart pediatric ventricular assist device (12 ml stroke volume)

As of August 1995, the average follow-up time of the five survivors was 35 months (range: 25 to 58 months). Patient 2 underwent repair for coarctation of the aorta 18 months after cardiac transplantation. Neurological deficits which developed in two patients who had suffered cerebral infarction during bridging resolved, and thus all five children currently enjoy an active daily life.

VAD Recovery Group

In Patient 1 the thorax could be closed without influencing pump operation. The VADs were placed paracorporeally, as shown in Fig. 7. Although the patient had anuria before support, excellent pulsatile blood pressure was produced by a 12 ml VAD and renal function recovered immediately. Despite normal hemodynamics, brain death, which may have developed during an episode of cardiac arrest, was diagnosed and biventricular support subsequently discontinued on the second postoperative day (POD).

Patient 2 initially received biventricular support at a maximum pump rate of 110 beats/min after transplantation. One day after support was initiated, transesophageal echocardiography indicated an improvement in cardiac allograft function. However, re-exploration was necessary due to bleeding. On the 3rd POD the BVAD flow was reduced to 75% and further to 50% the next day. On the 8th POD the patient could be weaned from the BVAD. Ten hours later, however, left ventricular function had deteriorated and the thorax was reopened. Despite receiving maximal inotropic support, the patient died from recurrent donor heart failure 2 days after weaning.

Myocardial function in patient 3 did not recover during the first 2 weeks of biventricular support, but thereafter serial echocardiographic evaluation indicated a gradual recovery in cardiac function. Difficulty with weaning, however, necessitated exchanging ECMO for biventricular support on the 21st POD. Although the patient required re-exploration once due to bleeding, he ultimately could be weaned from ECMO after 5 days. Upon discharge echocardiography revealed good biventricular function with a left ventricular ejection fraction of 64%.

Discussion

For some time now, ECMO has been recognized as beneficial for supporting patients with failed circulation after pediatric cardiac surgery or for bridging others to heart transplantation. The advantages of ECMO therapy are total relief (when coupled with a vent) of the previously damaged ventricle, more sufficient cardiac output, normal blood oxygenation, and reduction of the oxygen consumption of the myocardium, which is heavily increased by high-dose catecholamine therapy. When sufficiently functional correction is not possible due to an anatomic situation first noted during surgery, ECMO offers the possibility of bridging to heart transplantation.

A distinct disadvantage of ECMO as a bridge to transplantation is that the patient cannot be mobilized. Additionally, prolonged intubation with transsternal placement of ECMO cannulas may lead to a life-threatening infection (14, 30).

The following indications for the initiation of ECMO after pediatric cardiac surgery have been reported in medical literature: low cardiac output due to univentricular or biventricular myocardial insufficiency (18), a pulmonary-vasoreactive crisis (13), bridging to heart transplantation (11), and post-heart transplantation support (9, 13,).

Several authors (2, 31) consider surgically uncorrectable heart defects, as well as sepsis, renal insufficiency with anuria and agonal neurologic deficits as direct contraindications. In contrast, Hunkeler (13) considers the above-mentioned heart defects only relative contraindications. Del Nido (12) excludes patients whose heart defects cannot be adequately corrected.

Bleeding is one of the main complications in patients after cardiotomy support with ECMO (2, 18, 30, 31, 37) and was common in our patients. Patients who were connected to an ECMO system in the operating room immediately after surgery involving a heart-lung machine tended to bleed more and longer than those in Group II (median 2.96 ml/kg/hr ECMO / range: 0–23 compared to 4.7 ml/kg/h ECMO / range 0.6–292). That this difference was not statistically significant may have been mainly due to the low number of patients. Regarding patients in this study with hemodynamically relevant residual deficits, the two patients who were weaned due to increasing complications died shortly after weaning.

The effects of ECMO on the pediatric organism are enormous, yet barely researched. These are caused primarily by altered perfusion relationships, extensive, long-term contact with a foreign surface, the creation of a new compartment with fluid displacement, long-term changes in the coagulation system, and many other factors. These effects are reflected by changes in various organ functions. An attempt was made to measure several such changes by analyzing the most important hepatic and renal functions. Renal failure developed in 26% (6 of 26) of the patients. All of the patients were successfully treated, half with dialysis and half with hemofiltration. Hemofiltration was employed due to the development of edema and/or electrolyte displacement as a result of renal failure (10, 11). Since large molecules, such as creatinine and urea, tend to accumulate more often in patients with catabolic metabolism after surgery (11) and in those evidencing low energy quotient due to restriction of fluids, retention values increased in patients treated with hemofiltration, as this method is less effective in filtering such molecules. The results in this present study support and supplement those of Heney et al. (11). They observed a similar increase in retention values in patients treated with hemofiltration, although these were newborns undergoing ECMO for respiratory insufficiency.

The courses of several hepatic parameters, such as transaminase, cholinesterase, and total bilirubin, are appropriate parameters for evaluating the adequacy of organ perfusion (21). The phenomena observed in this present series, such as an increase in GPT (within the normal range), hyperbilirubinemia, and decreased hepatic synthesis function, could have been brought about by hypothermic, hepatocellular, and/or canalicular damage caused during surgery involving the heart-lung machine. The undeveloped liver of the newborns, massive transfusions, hemolysis activated through the compliment cascade (28, 29), constant mechanical alteration of the erythrocytes through contact with the membranes in the ECMO system (24, 28), and additionally (if present) in the ultrafilter (28), all contribute to hyperbilirubinemia. The hepatic parenchyma can further be damaged through microthrombi (28).

It is unknown what effect a continuous circulatory flow has on the hepatic parenchyma. In this context the toxic effects of aluminum (b1) and di-(2-ethylhexyl) phthalate (DEHP) (28), whose effects are said to increase with the duration of ECMO, are also discussed. This increase, however, was not noted in this present study, as aluminum-free oxygenators (Jostra, SciMed Kolobow) were used. With the exception of cholinesterase, a decrease in the hepatic parameters measured was observed on the second day of ECMO therapy, which could be explained by an improvement in hepatic function through prolonged ECMO support (28). The patients who did not survive were transfused more often due to excessive bleeding, which could have fostered the high increase in total bilirubin observed. GPT and γ-GT activity, which both remained within normal range, and slightly decreased hepatic synthesis function indicated a hemolytic genesis for hyperbilirubinemia. Evaluating hyperbilirubinemia is generally difficult due to numerous transfusions.

Because of previous damage caused by the heart-lung machine during surgery, its course cannot be compared to that in patients with respiratory insufficiency. To this end, evaluating free hemoglobin in serum to monitor the course of hemolysis during ECMO for respiratory insufficiency in newborns and to determine the necessity of switching to a different ECMO system (33) has been suggested. The increase in GOT activity, and at least partially that of GPT, at this point is considered an expression of myocardial damage. Microthrombi with damage to hepatic and renal parenchymal with subsequently excessive transaminase activity and renal insufficiency may be considered a sign of multi-organ failure.

Generally, the lower increase in retention values and more promising course of total bilirubin in survivors, the higher probability of survival in patients who did not undergo hemofiltration (5 of 20 vs. 1 of 6), and the fact that in this present study no patient with excessive initial transaminase activity survived may indicate that renal and hepatic functions restricted by beginning or advanced multi-organ failure may worsen the probability of successful ECMO therapy.

Survivability in the two youngest age groups (up to 1 month, between 1 month and 1 year) was the same (29%) while it was 17% in the older patients. The percentage of patients in whom ECMO was effective, i.e. leading to weaning or heart transplantation, was 43%, 29%, and 42%, respectively for the three ages groups. From this it was concluded that patient age does not have a significant influence on the effectiveness of ECMO therapy.

The median duration of ECMO therapy was approximately the same in both groups. Nevertheless, a significantly longer duration of ECMO was noted in survivors compared to non-survivors. Dalton (11) observed similar results in his series. This could mean that longer periods of ECMO therapy improves the probability of patient survival and that ECMO should be initiated earlier before brain damage caused by cerebral hypoperfusion occurs (11). Long-term treatment with high doses of catecholamines leads to circulatory collapse and ineffectiveness of subsequent ECMO therapy. The grave difference in survivability (26% versus 14%) between both groups could be explained in that, although the patients in Group I had more problems with bleeding, their myocardium were not so irreversibly damaged by extreme stress during the postoperative period such that recovery would have been impossible. An improvement in myocardial function during ECMO therapy, as evaluated by transesophageal echocardiography, was observed in 42% of the patients in Group I. No improvement in myocardial function was noted in Group II. Conventional and transesophageal echocardiography are effective methods for monitoring myocardial contractility, ejection fraction, cannula placement, and cardiac hemodynamics (26). The stabilization in blood pressure which occurred during a reduction in ECMO flow was regarded as a sign of stability and was also used as a guideline during weaning.

Altogether, ECMO therapy exhibited positive effects on the myocardial contractility in eight patients. In seven patients the myocardium recovered to the extent that the patients could be weaned from the ECMO system. Accordingly, the expectations of ECMO therapy were fulfilled in 42% of the cases. Further developments for ECMO systems exist in the use of fully heparin-coated systems, in particular heparin-coated oxygenators (4, 21). The danger of bleeding would be reduced thus making prolonged ECMO therapy with low ACT possible. This and other considerations, such as controlling bleeding and criteria for discontinuing ECMO therapy in hopeless cases, require further study.

Regarding the last point, determining just when to discontinue ECMO is very difficult. While weaning, heart transplantation, and brain death are clear indications, this decision is not otherwise as easily made after adequate surgery has been performed. ECMO duration of more than 3 to 5 days (33) as well as the development of contraindications to heart transplantation during ECMO therapy (multi-organ failure, sepsis) (5) are indications for decannulation. Regardless of ECMO duration, which in some cases remained complication-free for 5 to 17 days, excessive bleeding and ineffective ECMO therapy due to circulatory collapse were further indications in this present series.

The results from 14 patients supported with ventricular assist devices indicate that the Berlin Heart VAD can maintain circulation in infants and children threatened by imminent heart failure. However, the unfavorable outcome of the treatment of the 2-week-old baby in this study suggests that the type of mechanical circulatory support in pediatric patients must be carefully selected according to the cardiac anatomy. Although circulatory support with a VAD in the univentricular heart and shunt-dependent pulmonary perfusion may be possible (14), Matsuda et al. reported difficulties with VAD support in this setting (20). Therefore, we believe that common atrium/univentricular circulation is an absolute indication for ECMO.

Left ventricular support with a centrifugal pump has proven effective for cardiogenic shock after pediatric cardiac surgery and was feasible even in a 1.9-kg baby (16). On the other hand, due to the lack of suitable devices, ECMO has still been the first choice for biventricular support in small children, regardless of the existence or not of respiratory failure. Although overall the patients undergoing ECMO therapy for acute cardiac support attained a survival rate of 45% (30), the particular shortage of pediatric donor hearts and the tendency of increasing bridging time in adults (mean: 35 days in 75 transplanted patients in our institution (27), suggest that the use of ECMO for bridging in children may be hazardous. Undoubtedly, pneumatic VADs are preferable to ECMO for long-term circulatory support. The problem of limited pericardial space is the major surgical concern for VAD implantation in children, especially in cases requiring biventricular support, which necessitates the employment of four cannulas. However the observation that older children awaiting cardiac transplantation often suffer heart failure with resulting dilatation of the cardiac chambers, thus requiring adult-sized VAD equipment, appears to be valid as this was the case for most of the patients in the bridge group. The results of the recovery group also suggest the possibility of chronic biventricular support in infants and small children.

The Berlin Heart pneumatic VAD has proven to be feasible and effective in promoting the recovery of the failing myocardium or in acting as a bridge to cardiac transplantation in selected infants and children. It appears that the best candidates for its application may be patients with biventricular hearts without intracardiac shunts who suffer from severe biventricular failure.

Increasing experience with mechanical support as a bridge to cardiac transplantation in adults has shown that the recovery from endstage organ failure (5, 8) and an improvement in patient mobilization (19, 32) during bridging are the most important parameters for the ultimate success of transplantation. In this series, more than half of the patients had pre-implant major organ dysfunctions. Although all eight patients underwent heart transplantation after recovering hepatic and renal functions, respiratory failure requiring mechanical ventilation seems to have a negative impact on the outcome of mechanical circulatory support.

Cerebral infarction clearly related to thrombus formation in the VAD was a complication in two patients. Both of the patients were implanted with VADs too large for their body size, necessitating a reduction in pump rate to achieve adequate pump filling. This, however, resulted in poor wash-out of the blood contacting surface. Therefore, selecting the appropriate pump for the patient's body size may be essential to successful VAD support in children.

Although ECMO was associated with substantial, and unfortunately, commonly occurring complications, none of the six surviving patients would have survived without ECMO therapy. ECMO support significantly reduced the early mortality associated with excessively severe myocardial insufficiency. This is accomplished through two means: through recovery of the myocardium during ECMO therapy and through bridging to heart transplantation as a consequence of persistent myocardial insufficiency.

Options for mechanical circulatory support in pediatric patients awaiting heart transplantation are limited, mainly owing to the reduced anatomical space available, which explains the prevalence of univentricular support. Frazier et al. reported using a centrifugal LVAD (7) to support a 9-year-old boy. We have used an adult-sized pneumatic LVAD in an 8-year-old boy (35). Both of these aforementioned patients underwent successful transplantation. The results of Karl et al. (15) from a series of postcardiotomy support showed the feasibility of the centrifugal LVAD in small infants. However, in cases involving biventricular failure, ECMO has generally been the first choice for circulatory support in children (3, 9). Because of its high complication rate, ECMO should be carefully considered and restricted to patients requiring biventricular support. Specific criteria for ECMO as a bridge to transplantation have not yet been established at our institution. Nevertheless, irreversible postcardiotomy myocardial failure with intracardiac shunt or imbalanced ventricles is considered an absolute indication for ECMO.

Overall, our evaluation of the feasibility of ECMO as a bridge to cardiac transplantation in six pediatric patients who suffered irreversible myocardial failure after open-heart surgery was positive. ECMO sustained all patients by preserving their organ functions for up to 17 days. Three patients were successfully transplanted with two long-term survivors. Our results indicate that ECMO can safely keep some critically ill pediatric transplant candidates alive for more than 1 week.

Pneumatic BVAD, if available, is clearly ideal for biventricular support in selected patients. Taenaka et al. first developed a miniaturized pneumatic VAD with a stroke volume of 20 ml which was applied as a LVAD for postcardiotomic shock in two children with univentricular hearts (20) and two with biventricular hearts (32). As observed in the recovery group in this study, pneumatic BVAD can be implanted with excellent function in the smallest patient (7 kg). Because the Berlin Heart GmbH has recently developed smaller VADs with stroke volumes of 8 and 10 ml, we believe that biventricular support using pneumatic VADs is now possible without lower limitations in patient body size.

We conclude that ECMO is suitable for prolonged recovery after open-heart surgery in infants and children. The best results were obtained when ECMO was begun immediately after the initial procedure. However, circulatory support with a BVAD is more successful for long-term support when subsequent heart transplantation is planned. ECMO is indispensable in patients with intracardiac shunts and presently may be easier to use in small infants.

Further studies are necessary to determine more precise indications for extracorporeal circulatory support and to further perfect the systems available for pediatric patients for the purpose of myocardial recovery and as a bridge to heart transplantation.

Acknowledgments

This study was supported in part by Deutsche Forschungsgemeinschaft grant number DFG He 1669-2/1. We thank Jonathan Davis and Dr. Larry Thompson for their assistance in the preparation of the manuscript.

References

1. Dalton H, Siewers R, Fuhrman B, del Nido P, Tompson A, Shaver M, Dowhy M (1993) Extracorporeal membrane oxygenation for cardiac rescue in children with severe myocardial dysfunction. Crit Care Medicine Vol. 21 No 7:1020–1028
2. del Nido PJ, Dalton HJ, Thompson AE, Siewers RD (1992) Extracorporeal membrane oxygenation rescue in children during cardiac arrest after cardiac surgery. Circulation 86 suppl II:300–304
3. del Nido PJ, Armitage JM, Fricker FJ, Shaver M, Cipriani L, Dayal G, Park SC, Siewers RD (1994) Extracorporeal membrane oxygenation support as a bridge to pediatric heart transplantation. Circulation 90[part 2]: II-66–69
4. Delius R, Bove E, Meliones J, Custer J, Moler F, Crowly D, Amirikia A, Behrendt D, Bartlett R (1992) Use of extracorporeal life support in patients with congenital heart disease. Crit Care Med 20:1216–1222
5. Farrar DJ, Hill JD (1994) Recovery of major organ function in patients awaiting heart transplantation with Thoratec Ventricular Assist Device. J Heart Lung Transplant 13:1125–1132
6. Ferrazzi P, Glauber M, Di Domenico A, Fiocchi R, Mamprin F, Gamba A, Crupi G, Cossolini M, Parenzan L (1991) Assisted circulation for myocardial recovery after repair of congenital heart disease. Eur J Cardio-thorac Surg 5:419–424
7. Frazier OH, Bricker JT, Macris MP, Cooley DA (1989) Use of a left ventricular assist device as a bridge to transplantation in a pediatric patient. Tex Heart Inst J 16:46–50
8. Friedel N, Viazis P, Schiessler A, Warnecke H, Hennig E, Trittin A, Böttner W, Hetzer R (1992) Recovery of end-organ failure during mechanical circulatory support. Eur J Cardiothorac Surg 6: 519–523
9. Galantowicz ME, Stolar CJH (1991) Extracorporeal membrane oxygenation for perioperative support in pediatric heart transplantation. J Thorac Cardiovasc Surg 102: 148–152
10. Heiss KF, Petit B, Hirschl RB, Cilley RC, Chapman R, Barlett RH (1987) Renal Insufficiency and volume overload in neonatal ECMO managed by continuous ultrafiltration. Trans Am Soc Artif Intern Organs 23:557–560
11. Heney D, Brocklebank JT, Wilson N (1989) Continuous arteriovenous haemofiltration in the newlyborn with acute renal failure and congenital heart disease. Nephrol Dial Transplant 4:870–876
12. Hennig E, Bücherl ES (1989) The "Berlin artificial heart" system. In: D'Alessandro LC (ed) Heart Surgery, C.E.S.I., Rome, pp 167–179
13. Hunkeler N, Canter, Donze A, Sray T (1992) Extracorporeal life support in cyanotic congenital Heart Disease Before Cardiovascular Operation. Am J Cardiol 69:790–793
14. Kanter KR, Pennington DG, Weber TR, Zambie MA, Braun P, Martychenko V (1987) Extracorporeal membrane oxygenation for postoperative cardiac support in children. J Thorac Cardiovasc Surg 93:27–35
15. Karl TR, Sano S, Horton S, Mee RBB (1991) Centrifugal pump left heart assist in pediatric cardiac operations. J Thorac Cardiovasc Surg 102:624–630
16. Karl TR (1994) Extracorporeal circulatory support in infants and children. Seminars in Thorac and Cardiovasc Surg 6:154–160

17. Klein MD, Shaheen KW, Whittlesy GC, Pinsky WW, Arciniegas E (1990) Extracorporeal membrane oxygenation for the circulatory support after repair of congenital heart disease. J Thorac Cardiovasc Surg 100:498–505
18. Klein MD, Withlesey GC (1994) Extracorporeal membrane oxygenation. Pediatric Clinics of North America. Vol. 41 No 2:365–384
19. Loebe M, Weng Y, Hennig E, Alexi-Meskishvili V, Uhlemann F, Schiessler A, Lange PE, Kopitz M, Hetzer R (1995) Mechanische Kreislaufunterstützung bei Kindern und Jugendlichen mit pulsatilem und non-pulsatilem Fluß. Z. Herz-, Thorax-, Gefäßchirur 9:85–93
20. Matsuda H, Taenaka Y, Obkubo N, Ohtani M, Nishigaki K, Ohtake S, Miura T, Taenaka N, Takano H, Hirose H, Kawashima Y (1988) Use of a paracorporeal pneumatic ventricular assist device for postoperative cardiogenic shock in two children with complex cardiac lesions. Artif Organs 12:423–430
21. Pavie A, Muneretto C, Aupart M, Rabago G, Leger P, Tedy G, Bors V, Gandjbakhch I, Cabrol C (1991) Prognostic indices of survival in patients supported with temporary devices (TAH, VAD). International Journal of Artificial Organs 14(5):280–285
22. Pennington DG, Kanter KR, McBride LR, Kaiser GC, Barner HB, Miller LW, Naunheim KS, Fiore AC, Willman V (1988) Seven years' experience with the Pierce-Donachy ventricular assist device. J Thorac Cardiovasc Surg 96:901–911
23. Pollock JC, Charlton MC, Williams WG, Edmonds JF, Trusler GA (1980) Intraaortic balloon pumping in children. Ann Thorac Surg 29:522–528
24. Robinson TM, Kickler TS, Walker LK, Ness P, Bell W (1993) Effect of extracorporeal membrane oxygenation on platelets in newborns. Crit Care Med 21:1029–1034
25. Rogers AJ, Trento A, Siewers RD, Griffith BP, Hardesty RL, Pahl E, Beerman LB, Fricker FJ, Fischer DR (1989) Extracorporeal membrane oxygenation for postcardiotomy cardiogenic shock in children. Ann Thorac Surg 47:903–906
26. Scheinin SA, Radovancevic B, Parnis SM, Ott DA, Bricker JT, Twobin JA, Abou-Awdi NL, Frazier OH (1994) Mechanical circulatory support in children. Eur J Cardio-thorac Surg 8:537–540
27. Schiessler A, Friedel N, Weng Y, Heinz U, Hummel M, Hetzer R (1994) Mechanical circulatory support and heart transplantation. ASAIO J 40:M476–M481
28. Schneider B, Cronin J, Van Marter L, Maller E, Truog R, Jacobson M, Kevy S (1991) A prospective analysis of cholestasis in infants supported with extracorporeal membrane oxygenation. Journal of Pediatric Gastroenterology & Nutrition 13(3):285–289
29. Steinhorn R, Isham-Schopf B, Smith C, Green T (1989) Hemolysis during long-term extracorporeal membrane oxygenation. J Pediatr 115:625–630
30. Stolar CJH, Delosh T, Bartlett RH (1993) Extracorporeal Life Support Organization Registry Report. ASAIO J 39:976–979
31. Suddaby E, O'Brien A (1993) ECMO in cardiac support in children. Heart Lung 22:401–407
32. Taenaka N, Takano H, Noda H, Kinoshita M, Tatsumi E, Yagura A, Sekii H, Sasaki E, Akutsu T (1989) Experimental evaluation and clinical application of a pediatric ventricular assist device. ASAIO Trans 35:606–608
33. Ungerleider R (1994) Current application of neonatal ECMO. Presented at the 14th Annual San Diego Cardiothoracic surgery symposium. San Diego, USA. P. 119–130
34. Veasy LG, Blalock RC, Orth JL, Boucek MM (1983) Intra-aortic balloon pumping in infants and children. Circulation 68:1095–1100
35. Warnecke H, Berdjis F, Hennig E, Lange P, Schmitt D, Hummel M, Hetzer R (1991) Mechanical left ventricular support as a bridge to cardiac transplantation in childhood. Eur J Cardio-thorac Surg 5:330–333
36. Weinhous L, Canter C, Noetzel M, McAlister W, Spray TL (1989) Extracorporeal membrane oxygenation for circulatory support after repair of congenital heart defects. Ann Thorac Surg 48:206–212
37. Zwischenberger J, Cox C (1992) ECMO in the management of cardiac failure. ASAIO Journal 38:751–753

Authors' address:
V. Alexi-Meskishvili, M.D.
German Heart Institute Berlin
Augustenburger Platz 1
D-13353 Berlin/Germany

Mechanical circulatory support in pediatric age: Experience of Bergamo

M. Glauber, P. Ferrazzi

Department of Cardiac Surgery, Bergamo, Italy

Introduction

Postcardiotomy ventricular failure is a potentially clinical reversible condition where recovery of myocardial function (3, 11, 12, 17) is generally attempted with pharmacological treatment. However, when full inotropic and vasodilator support fails to restore a satisfactory cardiac output, some type of mechanical support becomes lifesaving. Extra-Corporeal Membrane Oxygenator (ECMO) which has provided excellent results in the management of respiratory failure (1, 2, 7, 9) has also been employed in the treatment of postcardiotomy cardiogenic shock in children (3, 8, 17, 18, 21, 23). In this setting the use of a Mono- or Bi-Ventricular Assist Device (BVAD) might have the theoretical advantage to avoid, when possible, the use of an oxygenator.

The clinical use of implantable artificial ventricles to support the failing heart in case of end-stage cardiomyopathies is proven to be a real alternative to medical therapy in adult patients as bridge to tansplant. Different isolated bridged pediatric cases has been reported with different devices, centrifugal pumps or pulsatile pumps, but in most of them the size of the device was suboptimal.

Yet, the most important limit for the use of circulatory support in children is the lack of a system which is adequate for size and pumping capabilities.

In this paper, we analyze the results of postoperative circulatory support employed in 25 children with congenital heart lesions, and in 3 children as bridge to transplantation.

Materials and methods

Among a series of 52 patients who underwent circulatory support between January 1987 and September 1995, there were 28 patients in pediatric age (under 14 years). Twenty-five with congenital cardiac lesions who had severe postoperative low cardiac output, while three had end-stage dilated cardiomyopathies. Their age ranged from 15 days to 14 years, the weight ranged from 2.2 to 36 kg while circulatory support averaged 6.0 ± 2.4 days. The different diagnoses of the patients are reported in Table 1 while in Table 2 are presented the characteristics of the patients assisted as bridge to transplantation.

One or two centrifugal pumps (BioMedicus, Eden Praire, MN, USA) were used for mono or biventricular support. A single centrifugal pump with a 0.8 to 2.5 m^2

Tab. 1. Demographics

Sex:	12 females, 16 males	
Age:	15 days – 14 yrs	(mean 4.3 yrs)
Weight:	2.2–44 kg	(mean 16.1 kg)

Table 2. Postcardiotomy: Diagnosis

Tetralogy of Fallot:	9	
VSD:	5	(2 swiss cheese)
AVSD:	4	
TGA:	2	
PA:	1	
Ebstein:	1	
Post Htx RVF:	1	
Complex:	2	

SciMed Kolobow spiral-coil silicone membrane oxygenator (SciMed, Life System, Inc., MN, USA) was employed for ECMO. Polyviny chloride tubing, 1/4 or 3/8 inches in diameter, provided continuity between the cannulae and the circuit. "Right angle" cannulae, ranging in size from 16 to 34 F were used for the venous drainage. Aortic return was achieved using straight cannulae ranging in size from 12 to 24 F. Right atrial drainage was always achieved by cannulation of the appendage in patients supported with transthoracic ECMO or BVAD. Left atrial drainage in patients with Left Ventricular Assist Device (LVAD) or BVAD was obtained by cannulation through the interatrial groove near the orifice of the right superior pulmonary vein. In four ECMO cases a neck (jugular vein and carotid artery) cannulation with Biomedicus cannulae (10–14 F) was performed. Pump flow rate was initially set at 2.4 l/min/m^2 (1.22–3.60 l/min) and the flow was gradually increased during the first 24 h to about 20% of the initial flow to prevent extravascular leakage due to continuous flow (23). Right pump blood flow was kept about 20% lower than left pump flow in the single patient who received BVAD.

Systemic anticoagulation was performed using a continuous infusion of heparin (4) in a first series of 17 patients. The initial heparin dose was 30 I.U./kg/h which was then adjusted to obtain an Activated Clotting Time (ACT) ranging from 120 to 220 s, depending on the type of circuit (ECMO or BVAD) and on the presence of bleeding disorders. The coagulation status of the system was assessed hourly at the beginning of heparin infusion and at intervals of 4 h, when the desired ACT was obtained. Hemolysis was monitored by measuring the plasma free hemoglobin levels daily or more frequently, if necessary. In a second series of 11 patients a multi-system protocol was employed. The goal of this protocol was the stabilization of coagulation system by the simultaneous administration of dipiridamole (15–25 mg/kg/day), heparin at low doses (1 mg/kg/day), aspirin (1 mg/kg/day) and aprotinine (10 000 KIU/kg/day).

Inotropic support was discontinued as soon as possible in postcardiotomy and bridge to transplant patients, but a mild dose of dopamine was maintained to improve renal flow. Fluid overload was avoided with furosemide infusion and only three patients needed hemofiltration. All patients received total parenteral nutrition with high dosages of glucose and insulin.

All patients were not systematically isolated in intensive care units, the use of a large spectrum prophylactic antibiotic therapy was avoided, but blood and urine cultures and bronchial aspirates were performed routinely and specific antibiotic therapy was initiated with guidance of antibiograms. A low frequency, low pressure ventilation was maintained in ECMO patients.

Color-Doppler echocardiography was performed twice a day to evaluate cardiac function and this was used as the most reliable means for weaning. Echocardiography was also useful to rule out the presence of clots and to reassess the proper position of the venous and arterial cannulae.

Patients who showed an improvement in cardiac function and recovery of contractility underwent attempted weaning from device with a progressive decrease of pump flow. Flow was reduced on the basis of hemodynamic parameters, metabolic parameters (like mixed venous saturation) and echocardiographic results. At the achievement of 25–30% of estimated flow a inotropic support was added before a new flow reduction and device explantation.

Results

Bridge to transplant

Patient # 1: a 14-years-old female with severe rheumatic valvular disease who was operated for a combined aortic and mitral replacement. Three days after operation she developed a low output syndrome with cardiogenic shock. A BVAD support was implanted and maintained for 17 days until a donor heart became available. During support she recovered organ function except for a complete spontaneous ventilation which required continuous intubation. After succesful transplantation extubation was performed 24 h later, but a massive bronchial bleeding caused death.

Patient # 2: an 8-year-old male with a dilated cardiomiopathy; LVAD was implanted because of unresponsive medical treatment; after 48 h the patient was extubated and in good clinical condition. While waiting a donor heart, on the 7th day a sudden cannula leakage prompted a unsuccessful cardio-pulmonary resuscitation.

Patient # 3: a 7-year-old female operated 3 months before mechanical support for a severe mitral incompetence; prior to surgery (mitral repair) the left ventricular function was depressed with an ejection fraction (EF) of 45%. A rapid deterioration was observed after surgery and with 3 month the patient was adrenaline and enoximone dependent with an EF of 10%. LVAD was implanted for a duration for 7 days and transplantation was performed succesfully.

Postcardiotomy recovery

Twenty-five patients were supported for recovery of myocardial function after correction of congenital heart defects. The indications were right ventricular failure (11 pts), isolated left ventricular failure (6 pts) or biventricular failure (8 pts). Right ventricular failure was present in 9 of the 13 patients who underwent circulatory support by ECMO and in whom surgical repair included the use of a transannular patch. The choice of ECMO as opposed to BVAD was made in these patients to

Table 3. Bridge to transplant

14 yrs, female	8 yrs, male	7 yrs, female
Rheumatic disease	DCM	Mitral repair
MVR + AVR	LVAD 7 days	3 months before
BVAD 17 days	Extubated 2 nd p.o.d.	CMD
Died after Tx for bronchial bleeding	(drainage problem due to left atrium pressure too low?)	LVAD 7 days Tx

avoid overloading of the failing right ventricle due to pulmonary incompetence caused by the transannular patch. ECMO was implanted in another four cases because of combined biventricular failure and respiratory disease.

Circulatory support was begun in the operating room in 13 patients who were unable to be weaned from cardiopulmonary bypass (CPBP); in 12 patients mechanical support was implanted because of a progressive hemodynamic deterioration in Intensive Care Unit; the mean time from CPBP was 26.5 h.

Table 4 shows the different types of support and corresponding outcome. Weaning was attempted in 18 of 25 (72%) patients and was followed by long-term survival in 13 (52%) of all cases. All patient surviving are in good clinical condition and in NYHA class I. Mean duration of support was 6.0 ± 2.8 days while mean duration of weaning was 34 ± 11 hours.

Table 4. Postcardiotomy. Type of support and outcome

	N	Weaned	Survived
LVAD	6	6 (100%)	6 (100%)
BVAD	4	4 (100%)	3 (75%)
RVAD	2	2 (100%)	1 (50%)
ECMO	13	6 (46%)	3 (23%)
	25	18 (72%)	13 (52%)

mean duration 6,0 days (2,8)

Table 5. Postcardiotomy. Complications (28 pts)

	Tot.	ECMO'S pts
Bleeding	13	10
Reexploration	9	7
Infection	6	5
Renal	6	4
MOF	3	3
Seizures	3	3
Thromboembolic	2	2
Hemolysis	3	1

Table 6. Postcardiotomy. Cause of deaths

	On Device	Post weaning
Low output syndrome	2	2
Bronchial bleeding	2	1
Untreatable bleeding	1	–
Multiorgan failure	–	2
Brain deaths	3	–
Sepsis	–	1
Drainage problem	1	–
	9	9

Complications included hemorrhage (13) requiring reentry (9). Positive blood cultures (6), renal failure (3), multi-organ-failure (3), seizures (3), thromboembolic events (2) and hemolysis (3) were the most important complications. Most of these complications were observed in patients on ECMO support (Table 5). The causes of death were multi-organ failure due to low output (6), bleeding (4), brain death (3), sepsis (1) and an acute cannula leakage. Table 6 shows the different causes of death on device and after device removal.

While in the group of patients in which only heparin infusion was used as anti-coagulation the incidence of bleeding was very high (11 of 17), in the group in which the multi-system therapy protocol was used the incidence of bleeding complication was much lower (2 of 11). In this series all patients were weaned from device.

Discussion

Refractory heart failure is the most important cause of death after open-heart surgery. Conventional medical therapy is usually employed to achieve adequate circulatory support in patients with a persistent postoperative low cardiac output despite an apparently satisfactory surgical correction. However, when pharmacological therapy becomes ineffective the use of circulatory mechanical support should be considered in the attempt to decrease myocardial oxygen consumption and work and to achieve recovery of the failing myocardium (14, 15, 19).

Following the good results achieved in the management of neonatal respiratory disease (1, 2, 7), ECMO has been employed as a form of ventricular support (8,13, 14, 19, 20, 23). Indeed, ECMO does have the great advantage of achieving a complete bypass of the heart using only two cannulae which can be quite easily placed even in small infants. ECMO is also useful when pulmonary incompetence is inevitable for achieving correction of congenital cardiac lesions such as tetralogy of Fallot or when a Fontan-type operation has been performed. In contrast, the use of a BVAD should be considered to avoid the problems related to the use of an oxygenator when an "anatomic correction" has been performed. Undoubt, arterial and venous cannulations are technically more demanding when BVAD is employed, particularly in small children. However, this was successfully done in a 5 kg child. A larger mediastinal space is obtained by keeping the sternum splinted open and by using a pericardial patch sutured to the skin edges. As a consequence, cardiac tamponade is less likely to occur and much easier to recognize. Indeed, bulging of patch is a clear sign of increased pericardial pressure and any fluid accumulation can be easily evacuated through a small incision in the patch.

Extravascular leakage is known to be a major drawback of circulatory support when a continuous flow is used. Yet, experimental studies have shown that this complication can be avoided by maintaining a flow in excess of 20% from a basal flow of 2.4 l/min/m^2 (11, 21). We have strictly followed this policy and, when necessary, the infusion of renal doses of dopamine or the use of furosemide infusion have avoided fluid retention in most of our cases.

Bleeding due to clotting disorders was, in our experience, a major complication. To overcome this problem in the first series of patients, heparin infusion was discontinued in five of 17 patients without any sign of thrombi formation. Yet, discontinuation of heparin infusion might induce the production of thrombi, particularly in the oxygenator. Worsening of the capacity of gas exchange and the increase of pressure flow between the inflow and the outflow of the oxygenator in excess of 300 mmHg were considered indications for replacement of the oxygenator. With the use of the multi-system protocol we never had the necessity to modify heparin infusion also in the two patients with prolonged bleeding; in these patients bleeding was significant in the first hours but controlled within the first postoperative 12 hours.

Thrombi generally develops either in the areas of turbulent flow or in those of low flow velocity (5). The formation of thrombi induce further vorticosity with consequent hemolysis. Plasma free hemoglobin levels were measured daily to rule out this possibility. Indeed, sudden increase of free hemoglobin levels was the only parameter which we considered as an indication to replace the head pump. As a consequence, the head pump was not replaced every 2 to 3 days, as suggested by others (5, 6). Following this policy, we were able to use the same head pump for as long as 7 days without any evidence of thrombi formation at the discontinuation of the VAD. No patient required head pump replacement.

The use of mechanical circulatory support in children is still controversial because of the relatively undefined indications and contraindications (23, 24). Weinhaus et al. (24), reviewing the literature dedicated to the use of ECMO in children, have reported an overall survival of approximately 45%. Survival can be possibly enhanced by a careful evaluation of the timing of commencement of circulatory support. According to Weinhaus (24), no survival was achieved in children when ECMO was begun in the operating room. However, we believe that an even a more precocious use of circulatory support could be more successful to achieve myocardial recovery. Indeed, in our experience, survival was achieved only in the two patients in whom a circulatory support was implanted in the operating room.

In conclusion, we believe that early use of mechanical circulatory support may beneficial and life-saving in children with postcardiotomy low cardiac output. We are fully aware that hemorrhage remains a serious complication especially when an ECMO is used. However, further developments in non-thrombogenic surfaces and preheparinized circuits could decrease the incidence of bleeding problems encountered with the use of ECMO.

VAD, mono or biventricular, is technically feasible even in small children. Results are more encouraging and the general management is facilitated by the absence of the oxygenator. VAD should be considered whenever a normal cardiac anatomy is restored after repair.

In conclusion, both ECMO and centrifugal pump VAD are extremely useful treatment modalities for children with no other options for survival. While currently unsuitable for long-term use in small patients, these devices could be considered essential for acute support for postcardiotomy shock and for bridge to transplant.

References

1. Andrews AF, Nixon CA, Ciley RF (1986) One to three-year outcome for 14 neonatal survivors of extracorporeal membrane oxygenation. Pediatrics 78:692-298
2. Bartlett RH, Gazzaniga AB, Fong SW (1977) Extracorporeal membrane oxygenator support for cardiopulmonary failure. Experience in 28 cases. J Thorac Cardiovasc Surg 73:375-386
3. Bartlett RH, Gazzaniga AB, Wetmore NE (1980) Extracorporeal membrane oxygenation (ECMO) in the treatment of caridac and respiratory failure in children. Trans ASAIO 26:578-581
4. Copeland JG (1989) Bleeding and anticoagulation. Ann Thorac Surg 47: 88-95
5. Didisheim P, Olsen Don B, Farrar DJ, Portner PM, Griffith BP, Pennington DG, Joist JH, Schoen FJ, Gristina AG, Anderson JM (1989) Infections and thromboembolism with implantable cardiovascular devices. Trans ASAIO 35:54-70
6. Dixon CM, Magovern GJ (1982) Evaluation of the Bio Pump for long cardiac support without heparinization. J Extra Corp Tech 14:331-336
7. Hill JD, de Leval MR, Fallat RJ (1972) Acute respiratory insufficiency: treatment with prolonged extracorporeal oxygenation. J Thorac Cardiovasc Surg 64:551
8. Kanter KR, Pennington DG, Weber TR (1987) Extracorporeal membrane oxygenation for postoperative cardiac support in children. J Thorac Cardiovasc Surg 93:27-35
9. Lantos JD, Frader (1989) Extracorporeal membrane oxygenation and the ethics of clinical research in pediatrics. Letter to Editor, N Engl J Med 323:409-413
10. McBridge LR, Ruzevich SA, Pennington DG, Kennedy DJ, Kanter KR, Miller LW, Swartz MT, Termuhlen DF (1987) Infectious complications associated with ventricular assist device. Trans ASAIO 33:201-202
11. NosÇ Y, (1990) My life with the National Institutes of Health Artificial Heart Program. Artif Organs, 14:174-190
12. Pennington DG, Merjavy JP, Codd JE (1984) Extracorporeal membrane oxygenation for patients with cardiogenic shock. Circulation 70 (Suppl 1):130-137
13. Pennington DG, Bernhard WF, Golding LR, Berger RL, Khuri SF, Watson JT (1985) Long-term follow-up postcardiotomy patients with profound cardiogenic shock treated with ventricular assist devices. Circulation 72:II-216
14. Pennington DH, Samuels LD, Wiliam G (1985) Experience with the Pierce-Donachy ventricular assist device in postcardiotomy patients with cardiogenic shock. World J Surg Surg 9:37-46
15. Pennington DG, Meriavy JP, Swartz MT, Codd JE, Barner HB, Lagunoff D, Bashiti H, Kaiser GC, Willman VL (1985) The importance of biventricular failure in patients with postoperative cardiogenic shock. Ann Thorac Surg 39:13-26
16. Pennington DG, Codd JE, Merray JP (1984) The expanded use of ventricular bypass systems for severe cardiac failure and as a bridge to cardiac transplantation. J Heart Transplant 3:170-178
17. Redmond CR, Graves ED, Falterman KW, Ochsneer JL, Arensman RM (1987) Extracorporeal membrane oxygenation for respiratory and cardiac failure in infants and children. J Thorac Cardiovasc Surg 93:199-204
18. Rogers AJ, Trento T, Siewers RD, Griffith BP, Hardesty RL, Pahl E, Beerman LB, Fricker FJ, Fisher DR (1989) Extracorporeal membrane oxygenation for postcardiotomy cardiogenic shock in children. Ann Thorac Surg 47:903-906
19. Ruzevich SA, Kanter KR, Pennington DG, Swartz MT, McBride LR, Termuhlen DF (1988) Long-term follow-up of survivors of postcardiotomy circulatory support. ASAIO Transactions 34:116-124
20. Soeter JR, Mamiya RT, Sprague AY, McNamara JJ (1973) Prolonged extracorporeal oxygenation for cardiorespiratory failure after tetralogy correctioin. J Thorac Cardiovasc Surg 66:214-218
21. Trento A, Thompson AA, Siewers R (1988) Extracorporeal membrane oxygenation in children. New trends. J Thorac Cardiovasc Surg 96:542-547

22. Tutsui T, Sutton C, Harasaki G, Jacobs G, Golding L, NosÇ Y (1986) Idioperipheral pulsation during nonpulsatile biventricular bypass experiments. Trans ASAIO, 22:263–268
23. Zumbro Jr. GL, Shearer G, Kitchens WR, Galloway RF (1985) Extracorporeal membrane oxygenation for circulatory support after repair of congenital heart defects. Heart Transplantation IV: 348–352
24. Weinhaus L, Canter C, Noetzel M, McAlister W, Spray TL (1989) Extracorporeal membrane oxygenation for circulatory support after repair of congenital heart defects. Ann Thorac Surg 48:206–212
25. Cohrane A, Horton A, Butt W, Skillington P, Karl T, Mee R. Neonatal and Pediatric Membrane Oxygenation. AustraAs J Cardiac Thorac Surg 1992; 1:17–22

Authors' address:
M. Glauber
Department of Cardiac Surgery
Azienda Ospedaliera
24100 Bergamo (Italy)

Discussion Session, October 21, 1995

Castaneda: Perhaps before we open up the discussion to questions from the audience, let me just ask the panel, because there might be a little bit of confusion, at least I had some, about indications, and sometimes speakers used the terms ECMO and ventricular assist device interchangeably. I mean, why don't we try to concentrate on the young child, because I mean, once they are older it is about the same as with an adult. There's no longer that much of a difference. So let's say the first 2 years of life, babies in particular. Dr. Del Nido, succinctly, would you still make a difference or have a preference between one and the other system, i.e. a ventricular assist device of whatever type and/or ECMO, or do you think that in the baby ECMO is usually preferable under all circumstances?

Del Nido: No, I don't think so. In the children who come in with cardiomyopathy, at least in my view, without question I would go with the simplest system that we have the most experience with, which is ECMO. In the children who are post-cardiotomy, I think you can be more selective. If you think you have a single ventricle problem and you've corrected the defect, then you should probably use a ventricular assist device (LVAD, RVAD, or BVAD). If you have a residual shunt, you can't do that because you'll decompress the left ventricle, you'll get desaturated blood into the circuit, and you'll pump desaturated blood systemically and there you're stuck with ECMO.

Castaneda: Dr. Karl, what do you think?

Karl: I think we'd like to use ventricular assist devices whenever we can. It's a simpler system. It's safer. It's cheaper and the device doesn't hurt the patient as much as ECMO does. It's just really a question of whether the patient can be supported with the lower level. I mean as far as intracardiac shunts go, we've used ventricular assist in a number of cases.

Castaneda: Excuse me, let's say there is a kid after surgery. We had difficulties with this kid who was on cardiopulmonary bypass longer than he should have been. So are you telling me that the lungs are normal in those kids?

Karl: No, I'm not. But they may get worse initially when you place the patient on ECMO because you're exposing the baby to another oxygenator at a time when the lungs are quite vulnerable to new injury. So the lungs aren't normal, but if they are good enough to oxygenate the patient, I think that it's still better to use the patient's lungs.

Castaneda: Dr. Däbritz, do you agree?

Däbritz: Yes, we do not have any experience with ECMO because we can't do that. But I'm also of the same opinion. I think it's better to have a less inflammatory reaction. Such a reaction would appear if an oxygenator is inserted, too. If it's not necessary, it's better to leave it out. You can try and then if it doesn't work, you can use an ECMO.

Castaneda: Dr. Alexi, I suppose you have the same opinion. If I understood the slides, you had a lot of biventricular assist devices in surgery. You would do that in a 2-week-old baby.

Alexi: No. For a two-week-old baby we have no appropriate assist device.

Castaneda: So what do you do?

Alexi: But it's also the technical problems. For example, in a 2-month-old child we used a ventricular assist device and had a homograft in the pulmonary position. It's very difficult too.

Castaneda: But I'm asking about a 2-week-old baby right now. Tomorrow you'll have one. Tomorrow is Sunday. Well let's say Monday you'll have one.

Alexi: I think we would use ECMO.

Hetzer: In the smallest baby we've treated to date, a 2-month-old, we used a biventricular assist device. But the problem with the small ones is cannulation. With ECMO you can handle cannulation much better. The driving pressures you need for an artificial ventricular systems are much higher. This is an unsolved problem. I think it needs to be elucidated how to construct a cannula for the assist devices for the smaller ones. But if you have those, I think the assist devices are better than the ECMO because they give you a longer range of assistance.

Del Nido: May I ask one question, why do you want to insert the cannulas in the atrium? In the adult ventricular assist devices, you use the ventricle to fill the bladder and therefore you insert your cannula in the ventricle. So why not do the same thing with the child's?

Hetzer: That's what we do. You see the one child that Dr. Alexi has shown, the child with myocarditis, had a transmitral angled cannula which emptied the left ventricle. I think it's very important to have the ventricle completely emptied.

Del Nido: True, but I'm saying through the apex. So you don't leave the mitral valve incompetent.

Hetzer: Not through the apex.

Del Nido: But why not do it that way? Why not do it through the apex?

Hetzer: I think we always have the hesitation to sacrifice myocardium. But it works. You know, we thought it wouldn't work because of possible mitral incompetence with the transmitral cannula. But this child, for instance, resuscitated his left ventricle completely just by draining through a transmitral cannula. I think you can do this very well in small babies also.

Castaneda: Could we focus on one of your questions, namely about bleeding? If we forget the past history and focus on now, October 1995, in which there are better cannulas, there are better heparin-bonded circuits. Five or six years ago you would hear in conferences such as this that you cannot do ECMO immediately post-op because of bleeding. I think that is not true any more.

Del Nido: I would certainly agree with that. In fact, having been one of the people who used to say we shouldn't do it, I've reversed my opinion 180 degrees. I think it's much worse to try to force the ventricle to stay off bypass with inotropic agents. In my experience the thing that has made the greatest difference has been the use of antifibrinolytic agents. It used to be taboo. We now have a child who had a mitral valve prosthesis in place who was placed on ECMO on antifibrinolytics, kept on ACTs of about 200-220, and was supported for 5 days. This is for viral pneumonia that he encountered. He had no problems with the prosthesis and came off. So, I've changed my opinion and I think it's made a large difference in the immediate post-bypass cannulation.

Castaneda: My experience is much smaller, but nevertheless we've had a few cases and I must say I find for the management of those babies, I'm talking about small babies, primarily neonates, I think that ECMO is a very simple way of dealing with these children. With biventricular assistance with all these cannulas sticking out, I get nervous. We use ECMO and I must repeat we have a very small series, but nevertheless I think the picture in 1995 is very different than 5, 6, or 7 years ago.
  As to indications, I was a little bit concerned to see in your slide that you had, if I remember correctly, 14 patients who you put on ventricular assist devices with uncorrected residual defects. Do you mean that? Why, isn't it important to fix the defects? I don't mean to be flippant about it.

Alexi: There were many patients in whom palliation was performed under cardiopulmonary bypass. This was not correction but palliation.

Castaneda: Now I see. It's a matter of semantics.

Alexi: And there was a problem with weaning these patients from bypass, despite that, for example, the pulmonary valve was reconstructed and a new shunt was put on.

Castaneda: No, no, I'm sorry. I understand. I think we all understand. I was concerned there was a residual VSD or something that hadn't been taken care of. It led itself to this conclusion. I'll ask one more question and then I'll shut up. Dr. Däbritz, you said a number of indications, one of them including Fontan patients. What experience do you have with Fontan patients?

Däbritz: I mentioned that we are happy to have the LVAD as a back-up when left ventricular function is not particularly good and when problems may occur because of left ventricular function deteoriation postoperatively. Of course there have been investigations involving right ventricular assist devices in dogs, I think, where pulmonary resistance was too high. But we are afraid of performing total correction in such patients and therefore use two steps with a bidirectional shunt in the first place.

Castaneda: But what is the experience of the panel with Fontan operations of whatever sort and assist devices and postoperative management?

Alexi: We had one case. It was unsuccessful because of bad myocardial function.

Karl: We've never used it after a Fontan. When I was a junior resident I heard you speaking at a conference, Dr. Castaneda, and you said that we shouldn't be afraid to dismantle the Fontan early on if we're unhappy with hemodynamics. I'd be thinking about that long before I'd be thinking about an assist device. I doubt very much that you'd get a good Fontan at the end of it, even if the patient got through it.

Castaneda: That was our experience. I think the experience with the Fontan-type circulation was very poor with assist devices.

Del Nido: I think they are a good group that you can bridge to transplant. But I think I would use just ECMO. They are a very good group to do ECMO with and you can support them for a long time.

Castenda: I would like to invite the audience to ask questions also.

Stellin (University of Padua, Italy):   From the speakers I haven't heard anything about the use of ECMO as a rescue for patients in the ICU after cardiac arrest. I think there is a paper from Dr. Del Nido, if I'm not mistaken, which mentioned something about a number of patients who were resuscitated, then put on ECMO, and that some of them survived. I would like to know something about this. Another question, no one has mentioned anything about the technical details of ECMO, for instance, how to switch from cardiopulmonary bypass with a roller pump to the Bio-Medicus to keep the patient with a full flow, or half flow if the heart is ejecting, obviously. I would like to know something about this.

Del Nido: Well, to answer your first question, the experience that we had with resuscitation was just with ECMO, simply because it was the fastest way that you could cannulate. I believe we reported on 11 or 12 children in that group. They all had experienced arrest and I think that's critical. I think it has to be a witnessed arrest so that typically it's in the intensive care unit. The resuscitation lasted anywhere from 30 min up to, I think we had one child who went 95 min with open-chest massage, who was successfully cannulated and successfully transplanted. That child could not be weaned from bypass. I think you have to remember that the patient population that typically arrests unexpectedly is different from the patient population in whom you have high inotrope and you know that you have either problems with myocardial function or problems with your correction. If you have a patient in whom you are having problems with your correction, the best thing you can do for him is to look very thoroughly for something you can do technically to improve your correction. The ones that are unexpected arrests, digoxin toxicity, arrhythmias, or simply totally unexplainable arrests, in that group we actually had probably the best results, about 65% long-term survival with those children. It typically was because they started off with relatively good cardiac function. These are children who were doing well and arrested for unexpected reasons. The best example are children who were suctioned 2 or 3 days after a bypass procedure and suffered an acute unexpected arrest. Resuscitating those children with mechanical support for

1 day or 2, in most cases, led to a very good result. So I think it's important to be aggressive, but I think there are some criteria you need to follow.

Castaneda: How long does it take you in the intensive care unit to put the child on an assist device?

Del Nido: That's a good question. I think from the time you decide that your standard resuscitation measures are not going to work, which typically should be no more than 10 or 15 min after beginning to the time that all the phone calls are over, the perfusionist, or whoever the person is, has arrived and the pump primed, it shouldn't be much more than 30 to 40 min. If you can do that, then you should undertake that kind of program. If you cannot do that, if it takes you 1 h or 1.5 h, then you shouldn't be trying it.

Stellin: So you are telling me that you can wean a patient from a ECMO after 1 h of external massage.

Del Nido: Up to 1.5 h in one case, yes.

Castaneda: In small children, would you always use bi-atrial cannulation?

Del Nido: No, I think for ECMO I'd certainly just go right atrial to aortic and only decompress the left atrium if you had a problem later. You can always do it in the intensive care unit. It's not very difficult to do.

Castaneda: Yes, it is. You have to reopen the chest, you have to cannulate it.

Del Nido: No, but that really shouldn't be a problem. You should have the facilities to be able to reexplore someone in the intensive care unit, to remove clot, or whatever, and also to put a purse string in, and put in another cannula.

Castaneda: For whatever it's worth, we would place a left atrial line, a small one, just to keep the left side decompressed. We have found that to be very important. We do that routinely.

Lange: Do you keep the patient on full flow while the patient is recovering?

Del Nido: I am guided quite a bit by the echocardiogram. If the echo shows that the left ventricle is not dilated, then I would certainly wean them down, and let them eject. If you have a very dilated left atrium or left ventricle, then I think you want to take as much flow as possible. In that situation you should be guided either by echo or by left atrial pressure.

Karl: I think the best way to do that is with echo, not just looking at the baseline state of dilation of the ventricle, but response to fluid volume load, whether you have a Starling response or anti-Starling and if the fluid load results in more ejection and so on in the context of the same or better ventricular function, then you're well on the way to weaning the device. We do it in our unit by reducing flow. There is some risk in going to very low flows, and of course, how low you can go on a baby is not as much of an increment as to how low you can go on an older child. We've augmented our anticoagulation while we're running at low flows and so on trying to take care of that. But that's how we do it.

Castaneda: Could one use the need for assist devices as an index of an institutional standard of pediatric cardiac surgery?

Karl: I hope not.

Castaneda: I'm not talking about cardiomyopathy, I'm talking about postoperative need because of a failing ventricle, because of long bypass, whatever. Should it be more than 1% in a unit?

Karl: No, much less. It should be much less.

Castaneda: Well, I'm talking about a full-fledged, broad-based unit which does everything.

Alexi: Yes, I think about 1%.

Castaneda: About 1%, is that a fair assessment?

Karl: Well, I think you'd have to look at the survival rates for the various lesions, with and without the support device.

Castaneda: I'm sure that pretty much everybody could show that they've had at least 50% mortality, if I remember the slides correctly.

Karl: No, I don't mean for the device-supported patients, I mean for all patients who were operated with that lesion. That's really the question, isn't it?

Del Nido: I think we should expand our concept of VAD or ECMO as purely a rescue. I think there are clearly groups, and you have to define the groups, but there are clearly groups that benefit from a period of time when you can support them mechanically. I think we can all agree that anomalous left coronary artery is one such sub-group. There may be others. Certainly the cardiomyopathy and myocarditis patients are another group that can be successfully weaned. There is experience in the adult world already; there is experience in the pediatric patients who were placed on ECMO support and then weaned.

Castaneda: Would you say that the anomalous left coronary issue is one also not only of a surgical problem, but also one of diagnostics and timing of the referral. If you get the kid with a big dilation, major infarct, and so on at age 3, 4, or 5 months, it's a different issue than when you make the diagnosis very early and you operate on this kid within the first 1 to 2 months of life. So, it's a matter of diagnosis.

Däbritz: But politics may change if you have this assist device as a backup. As I explained, we wouldn't have operated on this 10-week-old transposition child without this backup.

Castenda: That's another worry, because you wouldn't have banded him. That's another issue. The Melbourne group has shown a good number of patients who they managed that way. Rather than banding, they go in if needed, which is a perfectly acceptable way of doing it. Any other hopefully provocative questions?

Watson: I agree with your earlier comment that there has been significant progress over the last 5 years certainly. I wondered if the panelists would discuss longer term support, perhaps even permanent support. I wonder if they could give a better definition to what they meant by that in terms of performance characteristics.

Del Nido: I think our goals should be no different than the goals for the adults, in other words, you want to have a child who is fully supported, who is ideally disconnected from any external machine, who has a totally implantable device, and who can return home having a normal life. I think that should be our goal. That is the goal in the adult world, and certainly that has been reached. I don't see why that cannot be reached for the pediatric world as well.

Watson: In regard to such a system, what are you talking about in terms of performance characteristics and would you see one device for a lifetime, or what would you see?

Del Nido: I think that inherent in the device has to be adaptability to size. As we've learned, it doesn't have to be tremendously adaptable, but it has to have some adaptability, at least two, maybe three size ranges. As far as permanency, I think that's something we don't know. Certainly with cardiomyopathy or viral myocarditis experience adequate time may only be as long as a couple of weeks before they fully recover. They may be very analogous to the anomalous left coronary artery patients that within a year's time have normal cardiac function. Those are certainly the ones who don't require long-term ECMO support, that's the experience. So, I don't believe we need to think in terms of very long term implantation. That's certainly weeks to a few months.

Karl: I think the major issue in supporting small patients is can you get the patient off the ventilator and mobilized. Even with the pneumatic and electrical devices and so on, that goal hasn't been reached in very many patients worldwide. You know, our major drawback with the simpler circuits, VAD and ECMO using a centrifugal pump, is that the patient is ICU bound, often on muscle relaxants and ventilated and so on. We'd be much better off if we had a device which would consistently allow us to normalize things for the patient with the view toward myocardial recovery, transplantation, permanent support, whatever.

Hetzer: Coming back to the question of myocarditis or cardiomyopathy, we had this one case of a child. As Alexi showed it took us 4 weeks. We were surprised that the heart recovered. But as I understand you have some more cases. How long did you support them, how old were those children?

Del Nido: In the Pittsburgh experience, there were two children with myocarditis; one who came off after 10 days and is a long-term survivor with normal heart function. In the Boston experience, there was one child who was treated with LVAD who was supported for 6 days, I believe, discontinued from LVAD and is a long-term survivor.

Castaneda: What does that mean, does that mean the carditis disappeared?

Del Nido: It's reversible. I mean, all we have to do is look at the cardiology literature at the viral myocarditis experience, and if they can keep them out of the surgeons reach who want to transplant them, those kids long-term will recover fully. I don't see why the kids who are sick enough to require mechanical support may not behave the same way. I think the difference is that we don't have a pump that will keep us out of complications for a month, which is what we may need. Although I think some of the problems we bring on ourselves, keeping children, for example, paralyzed, I think that's a bad idea. I think trying to get them weaned, maybe extubated. Let them move around. I think all of those things that we know from the adult experience have certainly helped us. The use of broad spectrum prophylaxis of antibiotics, I think, has been a bad idea. So, there are a lot of things that I think we need to change our own thinking about, how we administer these devices.

Hetzer: I'm extremely interested in this specific topic. You mentioned cardiomyopathy. Are you aware of any case of, let's say, endocardiofibrosis or cardiomyopathy that was weaned or improved by mechanical assistance?

Del Nido: Let me hedge my answer by saying most of the ones, in fact, the ones that I know of were called viral myocarditis. Without a diagnosis, we had biopsies, but the biopsies were inconclusive, but we believed in viral myocarditis, because of the acuteness of the onset, only because of the history. Whether they were bad for a long time and suddenly decompensated, we have no idea. But certainly, there's no question that they can recover if you improve their hemodynamics.

Castaneda: Any other questions?

[Audience]: No one mentioned anything about inotropic drug infusion during ECMO or ventricular assist device. Do you infuse any drugs, such as dopamine or peripheral dilators, or things like that, just to optimize the blood flow, or suppose you have, for instance, some acidosis during full flow, would you try to do some peripheral dilatation in order to increase your flow?

Karl: We use phenoxybenzamine during support for cardiac indications. What full flow means is debatable for patients following surgery, I mean it's not the baseline flow for a child, especially if there is a question of sepsis and so on. We might fall behind by two or three cardiac outputs using the flow that we calculate for a normal cardiopulmonary bypass and you can't always increase your flow to that level with the device that the patient is connected to at the time, so you do often need to give drugs to control contractility and peripheral circulation. With VAD patients, of course, you need to support the right heart and with ECMO patients you need to support the left heart. So in practice I think most patients will be on inotropes, usually in doses that are greatly reduced from what they were receiving before you started the support.

Alexi: We usually do not use inotropes in patients on ECMO before we start to wean the patients from support. Usually, we monitor cardiac contraction and function with transesophageal echocardiography in all patients every day and usually we start to use cathecholamines for improving myocardial contraction only when we start to wean the patient. Another question, many patients have peripheral problems, that is, they have problems with peripheral resistance. Sometimes resistance is very low; sometimes it is very high. In most of the cases you have to use some kind of vasodilatation or vasoconstriction, especially within the first 6 to 7 h after starting ECMO, because usually the patients have vasoconstriction after bypass. This is the problem. Sometimes when you start to use ECMO in the intensive care unit in a patient, and during long-term catecholamine support, they develop peripheral vascular paralysis. So the arterial pressure is absent and you can't do anything. So that's why it's our policy to use catecholamines. The assist patients are another issue.

Castaneda: I suppose the issue of the Medos pump is pulsatility, obviously you people must feel that pulsatile flow is of significant advantage. Do you have evidence that for short-term assist, i.e. not implanting the device permanently, but for short-term assist, do you have objective laboratory evidence that that's truly an advantage.

Däbritz: We haven't inserted a centrifugal pump in children. We use only this pulsatile device in children, so we can't compare both.

Castaneda: No, but you started out by saying surgeons didn't know much about experimental aspects, so I was a little bit surprised, because the whole history of cardiopulmonary bypass and assist devices has been very strongly led by surgical experiments. But, unrelated to that, do you have experimental work to show that pulsatile flow is a very important issue? Do you now have an experimental model that allows you to show that pulsatile flow is superior?

Däbritz: Well, there have been lots of investigations about it, but the final decision has not been made yet. Of course, there are different advantages also corresponding to the costs, for example. The centrifugal pump is much cheaper than an assist device.

Castenada: So, in other words you don't have experimental evidence?

Däbritz: No.

Reul: May I help Dr. Däbritz? We conducted a series of 60 dog experiments in Leuven, Belgium with Professor Flameng and Dr. Waldenberger. He generated a stunning heart model and compared a pulsatile system with the hemopump and showed, and this has been published, that the recovery with pulsatile flow was better than with non-pulsatile flow.

Del Nido: I'd like to interject. This has been a subject of study for many years and I really would defy anyone to show any advantage of a pulsatile pump in children. Certainly there has been some in adult animals to show some advantage here and there, but as far as actual recovery, I think the longest experience in children has been with non-pulsatile pumps and they can certainly be placed and kept on for very long periods of time. For respiratory failure, our longest experience with the non-pulsatile roller pump was 6 weeks in a neonate who recovered fully. So, I don't think that there is hard evidence, either experimental or clinical, that in children, in pediatric patients, that there is a difference.

What is dilated cardiomyopathy?

U. Kühl, H.-P. Schultheiss

Free University Berlin, Universitätsklinikum Benjamin Franklin, Department of Cardiology, Berlin, Germany

Cardiomyopathies are diseases of the myocardium with cardiac dysfunction not due to specific causes such as hypertension, congenital, valvular, coronary, arterial, or pericardial abnormalities. According to the definition of the WHO, primary cardiomyopathies are classified as dilated cardiomyopathy, hypertrophic cardiomyopathy, restrictive cardiomyopathy, and arrhythmogenic right ventricular cardiomyopathy (18). Dilated cardiomyopathy is the most common cause of chronic heart failure. The involved pathogenetic mechanisms, the incidence and exact time course of the disease are yet unknown. It may be idiopathic or familial/genetic although specific causes such as a viral and/or (auto)immune involvement of the heart have been recognized as a possible cause of the disease.

Progress has only recently been made in our understanding of the relationship between the inciting event or agent and the development if dilated cardiomyopathy. Clinical and experimental features suggest that, at least in a patient subset, myocarditis and DCM might represent the acute and chronic stages of a progressive autoimmune disease of the myocardium. This paper, therefore, focusses on the diagnostic and therapeutic possibilities in a subgroup of patients with chronic heart failure in which development and progression of the disease is suggested to be caused by a viral induced active inflammatory process of the heart.

Pathophysiology

Dilated cardiomyopathy is characterized by a variable disturbance of systolic and diastolic cardiac function associated with a normal sized or dilated left and/or right ventricle. With respect to the severity of cardiac dysfunction, the disease may present with normal hemodynamic indices or an elevation of left ventricular filling pressure resulting in an abnormal high pulmonary-arterial pressure, an increase of enddiastolic and endsystolic ventricular volumes, an increase in the arterio-venous difference of oxygen saturation, and the development of insufficiency of the atrioventricular valves due to the ventricular enlargement.

Depressed systolic ventricular function is characterized by a reduction of ejection fraction, stroke volume and cardiac index resulting in clinical symptoms of congestive heart failure. Elevated catecholamine levels produce tachycardia, increase myocardial contractility and elevate left-ventricular enddiastolic pressure. This will result in limited diastolic coronary blood flow and, consequently, in myocardial ischemia. Impaired diastolic relaxation may prolong the compression of the intramyocardial vessels dnad consequently reduce the blood flow to the subendocardial layers. Thereby only reduced amounts of oxygen are delivered to the muscular tissue which further enhance ventricular stiffness influencing ventricular contractility. The resulting subendocardial ischemia could lead to myocardial necrosis, to fiber replacement and, ultimately, to a decompensation of the left ventricle. This will further induce an activation of the neuroendocrine systems resulting in an increasing oxygen demand of the myocardium and a decreasing coronary perfusion. Thus progression of heart failure will continue.

As evident, heart failure is the result of several factors on cellular level. A main question is the energetic state of the myocardium. It has recently been discussed whether a depression of mitochondrial function is present in cardiomyopathic heart failure (20, 21). Changes in the creatine kinase system showing a lower creatine kinase activity, a higher MB creatine kinase isoenzyme content and activity and a lower creatine content in pressure-overloaded hypertrophy may represent an adaptation towards anaerobic metabolism. In addition, alterations in the isoenzyme pattern of the mitochondrial ADP-translocator point to an involvement of disturbed myocyte energy metabolism in failing hearts.

Viral heart disease

The identification of persisting viral mRNA in animal models and humans with myocarditis and dilated cardiomyopathy and the immunohistochemical detection of an active inflammatory process in the myocardium of many of these patients has supported the idea of a postmyocarditic autoimmune process being responsible for development and progression of the disease (1, 2, 4, 7). The term "myocarditis" is commonly used in conjunction with acute infectious or hypersensitive inflammation of the heart, although the existence of a chronic form of cardiac inflammation has been shown by clinical and experimental data. Myocarditis can be caused by a multitude of viruses, but enteroviral infections – especially Coxsackie B_{1-6} serotypes – are the most frequent viral pathogens attacking the heart. Nevertheless, in an isolated case, the diagnosis of viral myocarditis turns out to be difficult. A history of viral infection in relation with onset of symptoms or a systemic viral infection does not necessarily mean that a special organ, e.g. the heart, is affected. Ultimately, after exclusion of blood contamination, the viral origin of myocarditis can only be proven if the virus is detectible within an altered myocardium. One has to keep in mind that myocardial failure can be caused by at least two different mechanisms: (18) the infected myocardium can be injured by the direct cytotoxic effect of the virus or (21 secondary immune responses – triggered by a multitude of agents including viruses – may be responsible for myocardial impairment. In the first case, a viral infection of the heart or its persistence respectively, is required for the development of myocarditis, while in the second a direct attack of the heart by a virus (and its detection later at time of diagnosis) is not necessary.

Although viral infections have been suggested to be one possible precursor of myocarditis and dilated cardiomyopathy they have been discussed controversialy for a long time mostly because virological methods failed to detect the virus in the myocardium. This situation changed completely since molecular biological methods have been developed as diagnostic tools for heart diseases. With the application of in-situ hybridization or polymerase chain reaction (PCR), persisting viral RNA could be demonstrated in the myocardium of some patients with clinically suspected myocarditis and chronic heart failure (dilated cardiomyopathy) (1, 2, 4, 7), (Table 1). In biopsy proven chronic myocarditis enteroviral mRNA is detected in nearly 60% of biopsy specimens. In immunohistologically negative tissues of patients with clinically suspected acute or chronic viral heart disease, mRNA was found in less then 30% of the cases. Viral persistence was not seen in any of analyzed control tissues. These data, demonstrating enteroviral mRNA in the myocardium over months or even years corroborate the concept of viral persistence and suggest that the infection may cause the development of myocarditis further progressing towards chronic heart failure in an unknown percentage of patients with clinically suspected dilated cardiomyopathy.

Inflammatory heart disease

Data obtained from murine models imply that myocardial damage occurs in two phases. In the acute phase of viral invasion and replication, tissue destruction is caused by a direct cytotoxic effect of the responsible virus. The extent of tissue damage and depression of cardiac function at that time depends on the pathogenicity of the infectious agent. This initial phase is followed by a humoral and cellular immune process which might limit further expansion of the destructive process or, by itself, cause an ongoing injury to the myocardium. The developing immune process is characterized by the appearance of organ-specific autoantibodies, immunoglobulin deposits at the cardiac myocyte cell surface, a humoral and/or cellular cytotoxic reactivity directed against cardiac myocytes, and the biopsy proven cellular infiltrations with an enhanced expression of histocompatibility antigens and adhesion molecules (13, 19, 21). At the moment, it is still open whether viral persistence, the viral induced secondary immune process or both are responsible for development and progression of the disease (Fig. 1). This is mainly due to diagnostic reasons.

Diagnosis

Specific clinical parameters to differentiate specific heart diseases from other forms of cardiomyopathies do not exist. This restriction is also true for left heart cath-

Table 1. Persisting viral mRNA in endomyocardial biopsies of patients with histologically and immunohistologically proven myocarditis and dilated cardiomyopathy

	Slot blot Archard et al.	In situ Kandolff et al.	PCR Koide et al.	PCR Pauschinger et al.
Myocarditis	clin. suspected 23/96 (24%)	histology 28/69 (41%)	histology 5/9 (56%)	immunhistology 23/42 (55%)
Dilatated Cardiomyopathy	8/47 (17%)	46/130 (35%)	6/24 (25%)	13/21 (62%)
Controls	0/53 (0%)	2/45 (4%)		0/42 (0%)

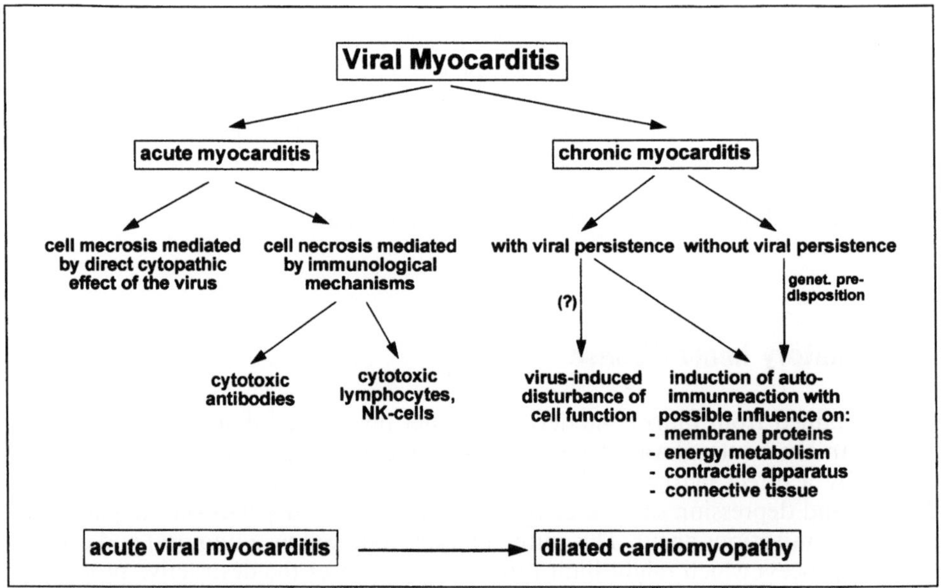

Figure 1. Pathogenesis of inflammatory cardiomyopathy

eterization by which only secondary causes of myocardial dysfunction can be shown or excluded. An indubitable diagnosis for some specific heart muscle diseases can only be obtained from histological analysis of cardiac tissue. The histological analysis of endomyocardial biopsies has been considered as the "golden standard" for diagnosing cardiomyopathies and especially myocarditis. While this is true for some specific (secondary) cardiomyopathies, histologic examination of most cardiomyopathic tissues reveals no specific abnormalities at the cellular level, which allow a definitive diagnosis or determination of the etiology of the disease.

Especially the interpretation of chronic myocarditis can be exceedingly difficult by light microscopy as shown by the great variation of the diagnosis of myocarditis when only based on histological analysis (3, 16). The reason for this is that, at the morphological level, lymphocytes may mimic other cellular elements of the interstitium, and electron-microscopic examination might be necessary in order to evaluate the cell type accurately. The lymphocytic infiltrates are often focally distributed and therefore are easily missed by sampling error (5, 22). Furthermore, it is well established that some lymphocytes can occur in absolutely normal cardiac tissue and therefore the mere presence of lymphocytes in the myocardium, especially if not activated, does not necessarily constitute myocarditis. Other possible causes for the great variation includes patient selection and time point of the biopsy after onset of clinical symptoms, because histological interpretation of endomyocardial biopsies is markedly influenced by the time, the biopsy is taken.

Meanwhile, immunohistological methods have been succesfully introduced into the diagnosis of an inflammatory myocardial process (11, 23, 25). Due to the sensitivity of monoclonal antibodies used against specific epitopes of inflammatory cells, this method allows the identification, characterization and quantification of different cell types infiltrating the myocardial tissue. Thus, in contrast to routine histology with the above explained difficulties in the detection of lymphocytes, cardiac inflammation is immunohistochemically easily identified. This allows a reproducible diagnosis of cardiac inflammation especially in those cases where the involvement of a chronic immune process with focal type of cell infiltration is assumed (8, 9, 11). An active immunologic process is immunohistologically characterized by a lymphocytic infiltration with more than 2.0 cells per high power field (= 7.0 cells/mm^2) (Fig. 2).

Recently, we compared the results of the histological and immunohistological analysis of endomyocardial biopsies from 299 patients with clinically suspected

Cells/antigens	CD	immunohistologically positive if
1. Infiltrating cells	CD3	> 2,0 cells/HPF(7,0 cells/mm^2)
		> 1.5 cells/HPF if focal
and/or		
macrophages	27E10	> 1,5 cells/HPF
2. Markers of cell activation		
HLA-antigens	HLA-I/II	enhanced expression
and/or		
adhesion molecules	CD18, VCAM, CD54	

Figure 2. Immunohistological diagnosis of inflammatory heart disease
((1) High power field (magnification: × 400), equivalent to 0,28 mm^2)

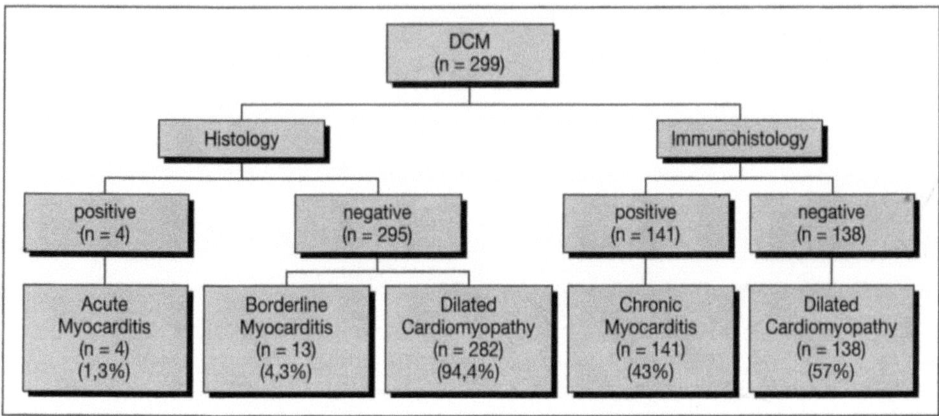

Figure 3. Histological and Immunohistological analysis of endomyocardial biopsies from patients with dilated cardiomyopathy.

dilated cardiomyopathy. Histologically, cardiac inflammation was seen in 1.3% biopsies (4 patients). 4,3% of biopsies were consistent with the diagnosis of borderline myocarditis (13 patients) and 94,4% (282 patients) were classified as dilated cardiomyopathy (Fig. 3). Immunohistochemical analysis revealed an active immune process with pathologically increased lymphocytic infiltrates and enhanced expression of adhesion molecules in 129 biopsies (43%) of patients with dilated cardiomyopathy (Fig. 3). Mean cell counts (per HPF) of lymphocytes and percentages of enhanced expression of histocompatibility antigens or adhesion molecules in immunohistologically positive and negative biopsies are given in Table 2. In immunohistologically negative tissues as well as control tissues only few lymphocytes are detected. Mean lymphocyte numbers of these biopsies were 0.6 (0.4 cells/HPF (11)).

The observed time-course of infiltration depends on the pathogenicity of the infectious agent and on the time the biopsy is taken. Immunohistological analysis of moderate cardiac inflammation revealed that activated macrophages might be the very first and only indication of the beginning immune process. After a short but variable time lymphocytic infiltrates arise, which, in most cases, consist of CD4-positive helper-inducer cells (Fig. 4a). A focal infiltration is more commonly seen than a diffuse distribution. The cellular infiltrates of the persisting immune process in chronic myocarditis contain an infiltrate of activated CD4- and CD8-positive lymphocytes and activated macrophages. The interactions between these immunocompetent cells and with the activated vascular endothelium is mandatory for a further immune cell activation and an ongoing infiltration of blood borne inflammatory cells into inflamed tissues which might be responsible for the progression of the disease. Activation of interstitial cells and of the vascular endothelium is characterized by an enhanced expression of activation markers, the histocompatibility antigen classes I and II, and numerous other adhesion molecules (Figure 4b, c, Table 2).

Table 2. Immunohistological cell markers

Reactive cell compartment	Antigen
T-lymphocytes	CD3
helper/inducer lymphocytes	CD4
cytotoxic/suppressor lympho-cytes	CD8
B-lymphocytes	CD19–22
NK-cells	CD57
macrophages	CD14
activated lymphocytes	HLA-I/II, ILR2, CD25, CD18, CD 54, CD45RO, CD71
activated macrophages	27E10, 25F9, RM 3/1, HLA-DR
activated endothelial cells	HLA-DR, HLA-I, CD54, CD62E, VCAM-1

Table 3. Activated vascular endothelium: Percentage of enhanced expression of adhesion molecules in lymphocyte positive and negative biopsies

Antigen	Positive (> 2.0 T-lymphocytes/ HPF)	Negative (< 2.0 T-lymphocytes/ HPF)
HLA-I/II	93%	31%
HLA-I	58%	10%
HLA-DR	67%	20%
CD54	88%	23%
VCAM-1	85%	20%
LFA-3	60%	13%

Table 4 Expression of immune markers on interstitial cells in patients with DCM

	n	CD3	CD4	CD8	CD45ROmac	CD54	CD18	CD11a	CD11b
DCM	299								
positive (> 2,0 cells/HPF)	129	2.8	1.4	1.4	1.2	1.6	17.8	3.5	3.7	3.0
negative (< 2,0 cells/HPF)	170	0.6	0.3	0.3	0.4	0.8	10.4	2.1	1.9	2.0

Analyzing the data in more detail, it becomes evident that even low numbers of infiltrating lymphocytes characterize an activated immune process with interstitial and endothelial cell activation. Endomyocardial biopsies with more than 2.0 lymphocytes per HPF showed a pathologically enhanced expression of different immune markers, for example histocompatibility antigens (Tables 3 and 4). While a slightly enhanced expression of HLA classes I and II is seen in less then 30% of normal cardiac tissues, expression of these molecules is clearly up-regulated in over 90% of lymphocyte positive biopsies. Similar results are obtained for other adhesion molecules. An enhanced expression of integrins (CD11a/LFA-1, CD11b/ Mac-1, CD11c/p150.95 CD49d/VLA-4, and CD29/VLA-(-chain) can be demonstrated in 55–89% on interstitial cells while members of the immunoglobulin (CD54/ICAM-1, VCAM-1 and LFA-3) and selectin families (CD62E/ELAM-1, CD62P/GMP140) are pathologically enhanced in 36–88%.

Endothelial cell activation, when analyzed by an enhanced adhesion molecule expression, is seen in the majority of lymphocyte-positive biopsies (ICAM-1: 88%, VCAM-1: 85%, LFA-3: 60%). In lymphocyte negative tissues, expression of these molecules is only slightly up-regulated (ICAM-1: 23%, VCAM-1: 20%, LFA-3: 13%). The reason for the up-regulation of HLA- and adhesion molecules in tissues without cellular infiltration is not known. It might be possible that focal lymphocytic infiltrates have been missed in these biopsies due to sampling.

These data confirm impressively that the diagnosis myocarditis can be markedly improved by the use of immunohistologic methods allowing a better characterization of the inflammatory process. A detailed analysis of the different stages of acute and chronic myocarditis will allow a better understanding of the pathomechanisms involved and will improve the therapeutical management of these patients. Light microscopic analysis of the chronic immune process is hampered by the low sensitivity of histological staining procedures due to missing specific histologic changes and therefore should not be the only basis of analysis of inflammatory heart disease.

Differential diagnosis

A combined use of histological, immunohistological and molecular biological analytical methods allows a more detailed differential diagnosis in suspected viral heart disease. As far as acute viral myocarditis is concerned, the Dallas classification has enabled a more standardized assessment of the histologic changes in the myocardium. The clinical benefit, however, is limited by the fact that histological recording of myocytolysis is only possible for a short period of time (10-14 days). These specific histological features are therefore not seen in patients with dilated cardiomyopathy.

Dilated cardiomyopathy has been regarded as the end point of different mechanisms injuring the myocardium in which the harmful agents by definition are unknown. Meanwhile, the use of a combined set of histological, immunohistological and molecular biological analytical methods allows the identification of viral persistence and chronic-immunologic processes as one possible cause for heart muscle injury in a considerable number of these patients. Four different entities of viral induced dilated cardiomyopathy can be identified (3).

1) Postmyocarditic viral heart disease: These patients present clinically as having dilated cardiomyopathy. Immunohistologically, they are characterized by an endomyocardial biopsy without chronic inflammation. Molecular biological methods do not reveal viral persistence.

2) Chronic viral heart disease: Histologically and immunohistologically, these patients cannot be differentiated from postmyocarditic viral heart disease. Viral persistance, however, is diagnosed using in-situ hybridization or polymerase chain reaction.

3) Chronic persistent viral myocarditis: Although histological findings correspond with dilated cardiomyopathy, chronic cardiac inflammation and viral persistance are found by immunohistochemical and molecular biological analysis.

4) Chronic (auto)immune-mediated myocarditis: Immunohistochemical analysis of endomyocardial biopsy reveal an active inflammatory process within the myocardium in the absence of viral persistence.

The rationale for such an etiological separation of "dilated cardiomyopathy" into different phases of the disease is a better understanding of the pathomechanism which might give rise to a more specific treatment strategy. If the developmental process of postmyocarditic heart failure is accelerated by chronic inflammation and/or viral persistence, prognosis of patients might depend on whether virus and inflammation still persist in the myocardium or not (Figure 1).

Immunosuppressive therapy

In the majority of patients, viral induced immune reactivity leads to a reparative process (fibrosis) in the injured myocardial tissue with disappearence of the described immunologic activity (spontaneous resolution of the inflammatory process). In a limited number of patients a persisting (auto)immune process develops, which might cause progression of the disease. This assumption has led to the suggestion that the use of anti-inflammatory agents could be beneficial to prevent development and progression of dilatation and of ventricular dysfunction in this subgroup of patients with a pathologically inflammatory process of the myocardium. The analysis of reported data on treatment of myocarditis, coming from non-controlled treatment studies, in most cases did not provide valid information about the efficacy and safety of immunosuppressive treatment in man. The interpretation of obtained data is limited by the different therapeutic regimen used and the missing homogenicity of studied patient groups, which is mostly due to different diagnostic criteria (6, 12, 14, 15, 17). In most of these studies, myocarditis was histologically characterized according to the Dallas Classification which is not an appropriated approach for the diagnosis of a chronic inflammatory process of the heart as shown above. An inaccurate diagnosis therefore selects a wrong subgroup of patients for therapy. Additionally, in most published studies, natural course of the disease has not been taken into consideration. At present there is no possibility to estimate whether the immunologically active process will resolve or progress with time, and resolving myocarditis therefore might interfere with therapeutic effects. These circumstances might explain the poor response to immunosuppressive therapy reported in most of published treatment trials.

On the basis of the above immunohistological diagnostical criteria, we have selected a group of patients with immunohistologically proven cardiac inflammation for immunosuppressive treatment. Patients underwent biopsy and determination of right and left ventricular function during the initial examination. Baseline data are given in Tables 5 and 6. In order to differentiate clinical and hemodynamic effects caused by a variation in medication from hemodynamic changes caused by therapy or spontaneous remission of the infiltrating process, patients were treated according to general guidelines with digitalis, diuretics, and ACE-inhibitors for an initial 6-month period. Dosage of drugs was individual for every patient but kept constant during the study periode.

After 6 months, patients had a follow-up biopsy and determination of ventricular function. Clinical and hemodynamic data of 49 patients (33 men, 16 women) with globally impaired ventricular function (ejection fraction < 50%) were available for this study. They were required to have no significant improvement of ventricular function or of clinical symptoms and, for enrollment in the treatment group, to have again an immunohistologically positive follow-up biopsy according to the above immunohistologic criteria. A significant change in hemodynamic indices was determined if changes exceeded 5% for EF and 3 mmHg for LVEDP.

Acute myocarditis according to the Dallas Criteria were not seen in any of the initial or follow-up biopsies of these patients. Twenty patients with spontaneous remission of the inflammatory process (but persisting ventricular impairment) were kept on conventional therapy (see above) and taken as control group. Twenty-nine patients with persisting cellular infiltrates but a lack of significant improvement in

Table 5 Resolution of cardiac inflammation caused by therapy and spontaneous remission

	Resolved inflammation		Persisting inflammation		Treatment
n	20		29		29
Biopsy	1.	2.	1.	2.	3.
inflammation	positive	negative	positive	positive	
CD3	2.3 ± 1.3	0.7 ± 0.4*	3.1 ± 3.9	3.5 ± 3.2	1.3 ± 1.1*
CD4	1.3 ± 1.4	0.3 ± 0.3*	0.8 ± 0.5	1.3 ± 1.1	0.6 ± 0.7**
CD8	1.4 ± 0.7	0.4 ± 0.3*	1.1 ± 0.9	2.2 ± 0.7	0.7 ± 0.6*
Mac	1.5 ± 1.7	0.3 ± 0.3*	1.2 ± 1.0	1.1 ± 0.7	1.2 ± 1.1
HLA-DR	1.3 ± 0.5	1.0 ± 0.3	1.6 ± 0.6	1.7 ± 0.7	1.3 ± 0.4

Table 6. Hemodynamic changes during immunosuppressive therapy and spontanous remission of cardiac inflammation

	Resolved inflammation		Persisting inflammation		Treatment
n	20		29		29
Biopsy ₐ	1.	2.	1.	2.	3.
LVEDP	18.2 ± 8.1	11.8 ± 6.8**	18.1 ± 8.9	18.8 ± 9.7	15.2 ± 8.8
PA (mmHg)	22.0 ± 7.5	16.0 ± 8.2	19.3 ± 9.5	18.6 ± 9.6	18.3 ± 6.9
EF (%)	33.0 ± 10.2	35.5 ± 17.1	35.0 ± 12.7	34.0 ± 12.7	43.9 ± 18.3*
EDVI (ml/m^{-2})	183 ± 81	178 ± 79	154 ± 48	155 ± 54	150 ± 20.1
ESVI (ml/m^{-2})	126 ± 66	126 ± 80	102 ± 46	99 ± 41	94 ± 69
SVI (ml/m^{-2})	57 ± 22	52 ± 10	51 ± 18	50 ± 18	54.9 ± 18

*: $p < 0,001$; **: $p < 0,05$
LVEDP: left ventricular enddiastolic pressure
PA: mean pulmonary artery pressure
EF: ejection fraction
EDVI: enddiastolic volume index
ESVI: endsystolic volume index
SVI: stroke volume index

ventricular function or clinical symptoms were enrolled in the study group for immunosuppressive treatment. Daily immunosuppressive treatment with 6-methyl-prednisolone was started with 1 mg/kg body weight. After 3 weeks corticoid dose was reduced in a stepwise fashion by 20 mg and then further reduced every second week until a maintainance level of 12 mg per day was reached. This low dose was maintained until week 24 when a repeated biopsy was taken and measurements of ventricular hemodynamic indices were reassessed.

Follow-up biopsies

After 6 months of conventional treatment with digitalis, diuretics and ACE-inhibitors myocardial inflammation was found to have resolved in 20 patients. These patients reported a significant clinical improvement in training capacity and reduction of cardiac symptoms according to the NYHA-classification from 2.3 ± 1.0 to 1.7 ± 0.8. The LVEDP decreased from 18.6 ± 8.1 mmHg to 11.8 ± 6.8 mmHg ($p < 0.05$). Other hemodynamic indices of the group as a whole did not change significantly. In 29 patients with an ongoing inflammatory process, NYHA-classification of 2.0 ± 0.9 as well as hemodynamic indices remained unchanged (Table 6).

Immunohistologically, myocardial inflammation resolved in 20/29 (69%) (Table 5). CD3-positive inflammatory cells and the enhanced HLA expression normalized during 6 months therapy with 5-methylprednisolon. Macrophages did not change significantly, but it is known that 27E10-positive activated macrophages might be induced by cortisone treatment. Sixteen of these 20 patients (80%) with resolved cardiac inflammation reported an improvement of cardiac symptoms according to the NYHA-classification, while none of the 9 patients immunohistologically not responding to the therapy, improved clinically. NYHA classification improved significantly ($p < 0.05$) from 2.9 (2.5–3,3) to 2.3 (2.0–2.6). A significant improvement was also seen for systolic cardiac function (EF, SVI, LVEDP) and the inflammatory infiltrates while changes of other hemodynamic data (EDVI, ESVI, PA) did not reach a level of significance.

Our findings differ significantly from other reported data which could not demonstrate a clear improvement of ventricular function after corticoid treatment. In our oppinion, this disparity results from differences in the selection of patients studied, due to an inappropriate histologic diagnosis of the inflammatory process. The data in this study show that immunosuppressive treatment of patients with clinically suspected dilated cardiomyopathy results in clinical, hemodynamic and immunohistologic improvement only, if patients with an active, immunohistologically proven, inflammatory process are selected for therapy.

While dilated cardiomyopathy clinically presents as a homogeneous disease which cannot be differentiated according to its responsible pathogenetic causes, new diagnostic methods reveal that, in addition to genetic/familial and toxic origins, viral induced inflammatory mechanisms contribute to the development and progression of the disease. This suggestion is also corroborated by the clinical improvement a subgroup of patients with immune mediated cadiomyopathy attains from immunosuppressive treatment. Above data demonstrate that immunohistological techniques can successfully be used to identify, characterize and quantify mononuclear cell infiltrates in myocardial biopsies, of patients with dilated cardiomyopathy. The combination with molecular biological methods, in addition to the diagnostic advantages, allows a further differentiation of these patients into different entities which might have therapeutical implications. According to this classification (Fig. 5), patients with postmyocarditic viral heart disease should be treated according to general guidelines with diuretics, digitalis, ACE-inhibitors, and possibly β-blockers. As shown above, immunosuppressive treatment has beneficial effects on a subgroup of patients with chronic (auto)immune-mediated myocarditis. Whether patients with chronic viral heart disease and chronic persisting viral myocarditis will derive benefit from a virostatic therapy is still a matter of discussion. These therapies cannot be recommended until safety of these drugs has been shown by randomized studies.

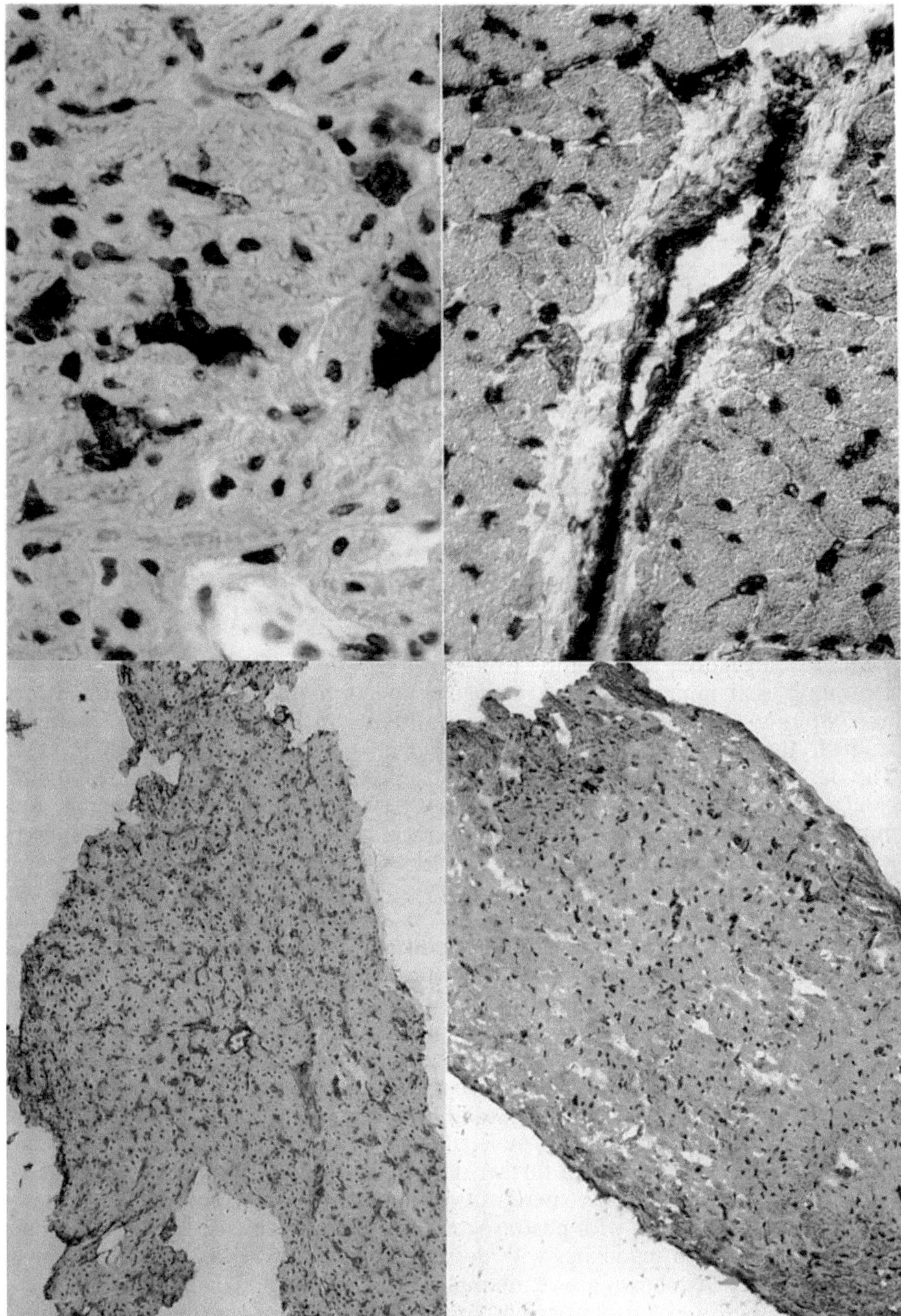

Figure 4. Immunohistological staining of chronic myocarditis. (a) focal infiltration of CD3-positive lymphocytes, (b) activated vascular endothelium (CD54), HLA-DR antigen expression in an immunohistologically positive (c) and negative (d) biopsy. Magnification: a,b x400, c,d x40

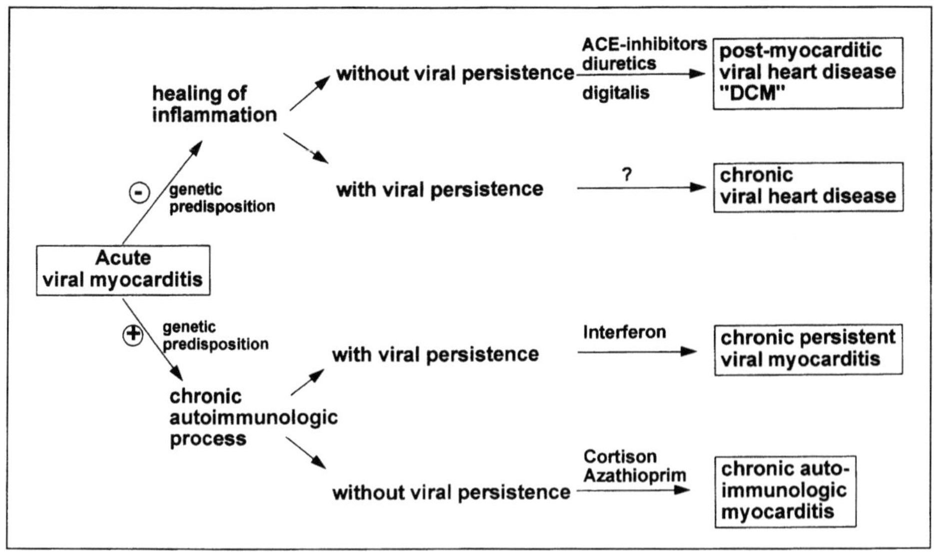

Figure 5. Clinical course of inflammatory heart disease

References

1. Archard LC, Bowles NE, Cunningham L, Freeke CA, Olsen EG, Rose ML, Meany B, Why HJF, Richardson FJ (1991) Molecular probes for detection of persisting enterovirus infection of human heart and their prognostic value. Eur Heart J; 12(Suppl D): 56–59
2. Bowles NE, Ohlsen EGJ, Richardson PJ, Archard LC (1986) Detection of Cocksackie B-virus-specific RNA sequences in myocardial biopsy samples from patients with myocarditis and dilated cardiomyopathy. Lancet; 1:1120–1122
3. Billingham MB (1987) Acute myocarditis: a diagnostic dilemma. B3 Heart J; 58:6–8.
4. Grasso M, Arbusti E, Silini E, Diegoli M, Percivalle E, Ratti G, Bramerio M, Gavazzi A, Vigano M, Milanesi G (1992) Search for coxsackie B3 RNA in idiopathic dilated cardiomyopathy using gene amplification by polymerase chain reaction. Am J Cardiol; 69:658–664
5. Hauck AJ, Kearney DL, Edwards WD (1989) Evaluation of postmortem endomyocardial biopsy specimen from 38 patients with lymphocytic myocarditis: Implication for role of sampling error. Mayo Clin Proc; 64:1235–1245
6. Hosenpud JD, McAnulty JH, Niles NR (1985) Lack of objective improvement in ventricular systolic function in patients with myocarditis treated with azathioprine and prednisone. J.Am. Coll. Cardiol. 6, 217–222
7. Kandolf R, Ameis D, Kirschner P, Canu A, Hofschneider P1H (1985) In situ detection of enteroviral genomes in myocardial cells by nucleic acid hybridization: An approach to the diagnosis of viral heart disease. Proc Natl Acad Sci; 82:4818–4822
8. Kühl U, Noutsias M, Seeberg B, Schannwell M, Welp LB Schultheiss H-P (1994) Chronic inflammation in the myocardium of patients with clinically suspected dilated cardiomyopathy. J Card Failure; 1:13–27
9. Kühl U, Noutsias M, Seeberg B, Schannwell M, Welp LB, Schultheiß H-P Strauer BE Chronic inflammation in the myocardium of patients with clinically suspected dilated cardiomyopathy. J Heart Failure (January 1994), 231–245
10. Kühl U, Schultheiß H-P, Strauer BE (1994) Methylprednisolone in chronic myocarditis. Postgrad. Med. J. 70; S35–S42
11. Kühl U, Seeberg B, Noutsias M, Schultheiß H-P (1995) Immunohistochemical analysis of the chronic inflammatory process in dilated cardiomyopathy: Brit Heart J; 75:295-300

12. Latham RD, Mulrow JP, Virmani R, Robinowitz M, Moody JM (1989) Recently diagnosed idiopathic dilated cardiomyopathy: incidence of myocarditis and efficacy of prednisone therapy. Am. Heart J. 117, 876–882
13. Limas CJ, Goldenberg JF, Limas C (1989) Autoantibodies against β-adrenoceptors in human idiopathic dilated cardiomyopathy. Circ Res; 64:97–103
14. Mason JW, Billingham ME, Ricci DR (1980) Treatment of acute inflammatory myocarditis assisted by endomyocardial biopsy. Am. J. Cardiol. 45, 1037–1044
15. Mason JW, O'Connel JB, Herskowitz A (1994) and the Myocarditis Treatment Trial Investigators. A clinical trial of immunosuppressive therapy for myocarditis. N Engl J Med; 321: 1061–1068
16. Ohlsen EGJ (1985) The problem of viral heart disease: How often do we miss it? Postgrad Med J; 61:479–480
17. Parillo JE, Cunnion RE, Epstein SE, und Mitarb A (1989) prospective, randomized, controlled trial of prednisone for dilated cardiomyopathy. N. Engl. J. Med. 321, 1061–1068
18. Report of the 1995 World Health Organization/International Society and Federation of Cardiology Task Force on The Definition and Classification of Cardiomyopathies. Circulation 1996; 93: 841–842
19. Schultheiss HP, Ulrich G, Janda I, Kühl U, Morad M (1988) Antibody-mediated enhancement of calcium permeability in cardiac myocytes. J Exp Med; 168:2105–2119
20. Schulze K, Becker BF, Schultheiß HP (1989) Antibodies to the ADP/ATP carrier, an autoantigen in myocarditis and dilated cardiomyopathy, penetrate into myocardial cells and disturb energy metabolism in vivo. Circ Res; 64:179–192
21. Schulze K, Becker BF, Schauer R, Schultheiss HP (1990) Antibodies to the ADP/ATP carrier – an autoantigen in myocarditis and dilated cardiomyopathy – impair cardiac function. Circulation 81, 959-969
22. Shanes JG, Ghali J, Billingham ME, Ferrans VJ, Fenoglio JJ, Edwards WD, Tsai CC, Saffitz JE, Isner J, Furner S, Subramanian R (1987) Interobserver variability in the pathologic interpretation of endomyocardial biopsy results. Circulation; 75:401–405
23. Steenbergen C, Kolbeck PC, Wolfe JA, Anthony RM, Sanfilippo FP, Jennings RB (1986) Detection of lymphocytes in endomyocardium using immunohistochemical techniques. Relevance to evaluation of endomyocardial biopsies in suspected cases of lymphocytic myocarditis. J Appl Cardiol; 1:63–73
24. Wolff P, Kühl U, Schultheiss HP (1989) Laminin distribution and autoantibodies to laminin in dilated cardiomyopathy and myocarditis. Am Heart J; 117:1303–1309
25. Zee-Cheng CS, Tsai CC, Palmer DC, Codd JE, Pennington DG, Williams GA (1984) High incidence of myocarditis by endomyocardial biopsy in patients with idiopathic congestive cardiomyopathy. J Am Coll Cardiol 3, 63–70

Corresponding address:
U. Kühl, PhD
Med. Clinic of Internal Medicine
Benjamin Franklin Hospital
Dept. of Cardiology
Freie Universität Berlin
Hindenburgdamm 30
12200 Berlin Steglitz, Germany

Agonistic anti-β_1-adrenoceptor autoantibodies in the serum of patients with dilated cardiomyopathy

G. Wallukat and A. Wollenberger

Max Delbrück Centre for Molecular Medicine, Berlin-Buch, Germany

Introduction

Idiopathic dilated cardiomyopathy (DCM) is per definition a disease of unknown cause (31). However, one of the pathogenic factors observed in patients with this disease is in all probability a chronic adrenergic overdrive (22, 9, 2). Cellular and humoral autoimmune processes may also play a role in the development and maintenance of the DCM. In the blood serum of DCM patients autoantibodies were found that recognize sarcolemmal, myofibrillar, and mitochondrial structures in the cardiac myocytes (15, 16). Moreover, autoantibodies to some of these structures were able to influence the function of the myocytes (19, 25). For example, Schultheiss and coworker (20) described an autoantibody directed against the mitochondrial ADP/ATP carrier which cross-react with the sarcolemmal L-type Ca^{++} channel (17). This autoantibody was able to reduce the cytosolic ATP concentration and to increase the sarcolemmal Ca^{++} current into the myocytes.
Another autoantibody that was found in the serum of patients with DCM and also with myocarditis recognizes the β_1-adrenoceptor (25, 10, 12, 26). This antibody, which was able to influence the function of the cardiomyocytes and which recognized epitopes on either the first or second extracellular loop of the β_1-adrenergic receptor, was detected in approximately 80% of the sera of patients with DCM, using the bioassay system "cultured neonatal rat cardiomyocytes" (26). This presentation characterizes this IgG autoantibody more in detail and suggests that the anti-β_1-adrenoceptor antibody could possibly play a role in the development and maintenance of the DCM.

Pharmacological characterization of the anti-β_1-adrenoceptor autoantibodies

As shown in our first publication on this subject, the immunoglobulin fraction of the serum of DCM patients was able to exert in cultured neonatal rat heart myocytes an increase in beating frequency (25). This positive chronotropic effect was blocked by β-adrenoceptor subtype nonselective and β_1-selective adrenoceptor antagonists. The β_2-selective adrenergic blocking agent ICI 118.551 did not antagonize the observed positive chronotropic effect (27). These findings were the first indications that the autoantibodies which exert in cultured neonatal rat heart myocytes a positive chronotropic effect realize their agonist-like activity via the β_1-adrenoceptor. Furthermore, it was shown that the β_1-selective adrenoceptor antagonists did not only block the agonistic effect of the autoantibodies, but in contrast to the β_1/β_2-adrenergic agonist isoprenaline, which was unable to remove the antibodies from their binding site, they displaced the antibodies from the β_1-adrenoceptor (26,14).

Classic β-adrenergic agonists can realize their effect via the β-adrenoceptor – adenylate cyclase – protein kinase A cascade and can phosphorylate different proteins via this pathway (Fig.1). Phosphorylation of the L-type Ca^{++} channel of the sarcolemmal membrane has been shown to lead to an increase in the Ca^{++} current into cardiomyocytes. On the other hand, a phosphorylation of phospholamban, the regulator protein of the sarcoplasmic reticulum Ca^{++}-ATPase, is connected with a higher activity of this enzyme and an increased uptake of the ion by the reticulum. In an attempt to see whether the anti-β_1-adrenoceptor autoantibodies acted by influencing steps in the above cascade, we looked at first at the initial reaction of this cascade, namely the binding of the agonist or antibody to the β-adrenergic receptor. It was shown in binding studies with radiolabeled ligands that the anti-β_1-adrenoceptor autoantibodies were able to displace the radioligand from the β-adrenergic receptor, supposedly not by competition at the catecholamine binding site (10, 12, 29), but by an otherwise effected change of the conformation of the receptor. The next step in the above cascade is the G-protein-mediated activation of adenylate cyclase. As shown in Table 1, using homogenized cultured neonatal rat cardiomyocytes, the antibodies acted on this enzyme like a β-adrenergic agonist in leading to a significant elevation of the second messenger cyclic AMP (29, 14). Furthermore, the antibodies appeared to induce via this cascade an activation of protein kinase A, as measured indirectly using the specific inhibitor

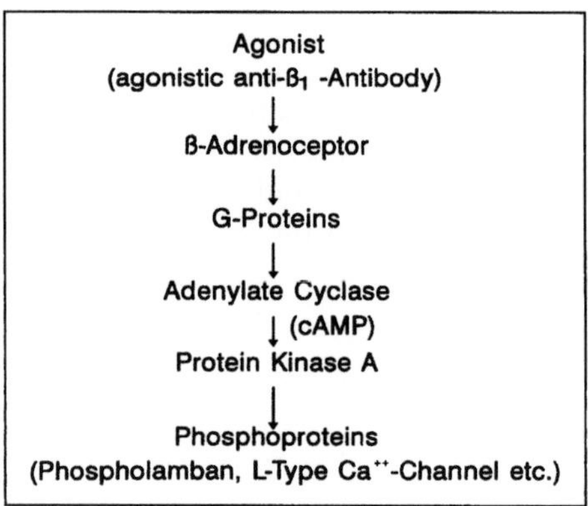

Fig. 1. Reaction cascade of the β-adrenergic stimulation

Table 1. Adenylate cyclase activity of cultured neonatal rat heart myocytes

	Concentration	Activity %
BA		100
NaF	8 mM	443
Iso	10 µM	562
AB (DCM)	1:20	232

BA = basal activity, Iso = isoprenaline; AB = antibody

of this enzyme Rp-cAMPS (29) or directly by measurement of the activation ratio of this enzyme (8). From these data it may be concluded that the anti-β₁-adrenoceptor autoantibodies realize their stimulating effect on the pulsation rate of the spontaneously beating neonatal rat cardiomyocytes like conventional β-adrenergic agonists, probably mainly via the β-adrenoceptor – adenylate cyclase – protein kinase A cascade.

Characterization of the epitopes on the β₁-adrenoceptor recognized by anti-β₁-adrenoceptor autoantibodies

In an antigenic analysis of the β₁-adrenoceptor it was shown that the second extracellular loop of this receptor is one of the main targets of the autoimmune response (11,13). In our functional assay system it was later shown that the serum of some of the cardiomyopathic patients contained anti-β₁-adrenoceptor autoantibodies that recognized the first extracellular loop of the β₁-adrenoceptor as the site of an epitope (Fig. 2) (28). Autoantibodies directed against the third extracellular loop of this receptor were not found in the serum of the DCM patients investigated. In contrast to an earlier study in which 27% of the investigated antibody positive DCM patient contained circulating antibodies against the first extracellular loop

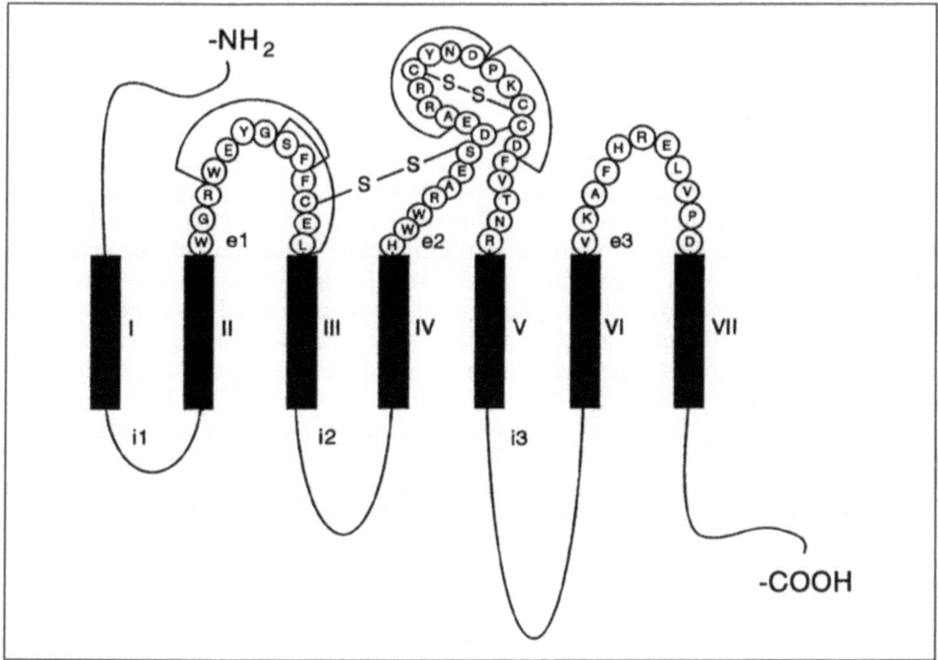

Fig. 2. Schematic representation of the human β₁-adrenoceptor (in analogy to the representation of the β₂-adrenoceptor according to Noda et al. J Biol Chem 1994, 269: 6743–52). The marks represent the main epitopes identified on the first and second extracellular loops.

of the β_1-adrenoceptor (patients from the Berlin area) (30), a second study, involving DCM patients from the southwestern part of Germany, showed that in 58% of the cases the serum samples contained antibodies against the first extracellular and in only 42% against the second extracellular loop (28).

To map the epitopes in the first and second extracellular loops of the β_1-adrenoceptor short overlapping peptides consisting of 6-7 amino acids were used to neutralize the anti-β_1-adrenoceptor autoantibodies. The used sequences derived from the first extracellular loop were, starting from the N-terminal part (in the one letter symbols of amino acids), W-G-R-W-E-Y, E-Y-G-S-F-F, and S-F-F-C-E-L; those corresponding to the second extracellular loop were H-W-W-R-A-E, R-A-E-S-D-E, D-E-A-R-R-C-Y, A-R-R-C-Y-N-D, P-K-C-C-D-F, and D-F-V-T-N-R. Using these peptides the main epitopes on the first and second extracellular loops could be identified by neutralization of the functional antibody action. On the first extracellular loop the sequences E-Y-G-S-F-F and S-F-F-C-E-L were able to oppose the chronotropic effect of the antibodies, recognizing this extracellular part of the β_1-adrenoceptor.

Epitopes recognized on the second extracellular loop of the β_1-adrenoceptor were the amino acid sequences A-R-R-C-Y-N-D and P-K-C-C-D-F. They nearly completely inhibited the action of the antibodies directed against this extracellular loop (28). The sequence H-W-W-R-A-E could partly neutralize the agonistic activity of the antibodies.

Possible pathogenic role of the anti-β_1-adrenoceptor autoantibodies

As mentioned above, the anti-β_1-adrenoceptor autoantibodies realize their effect, at least to a major extent, via the β-adrenoceptor – adenylate cyclase – protein kinase A cascade. But unlike the stimulatory action of a classic β-adrenergic agonist, which causes desensitization and downregulation of the β-adrenergic receptor within 60 min, the autoantibody-induced agonist-like activity remained unchanged for more than 24 h (26). In cultured cardiomyocytes treatment of the cells with the β-adrenergic agonist isoprenaline for 2 hours led to a diminished β-adrenergic responsiveness accompanied by a reduction of the number β-adrenoceptors. Treatment of the cultured cardiomyocytes for the same time with the agonist-like anti-β_1-adrenoceptor autoantibody led neither to a reduction of the antibody-induced positive chronotropic response nor to significant loss of the number of β-adrenergic binding sites. Similar data were obtained by the addition of the β-adrenergic agonist isoprenaline to cardiomyocytes prestimulated by anti-β_1-adrenoceptor antibodies (Fig. 3). In this case the addition of 10 mM isoprenaline did not significantly change the stimulatory effect over a period of 2 h, whereas the effect was reversed after treatment with the β_1-subtype selective adrenergic blocking agent bisoprolol (1 mM). After this treatment and a washing procedure the myocytes reacted to a restimulation by 10 mM isoprenaline with a maximal chronotropic response. These findings demonstrate that an isoprenaline-mediated desensitization did not occur in the joined presence of autoantibodies and isoprenaline. In contrast, myocytes treated for 2 h with 10 mM isoprenaline alone underwent a pronounced desensitization of the β-adrenergic reaction cascade. These isoprenaline-pretreated myocytes responded only moderately to a second stimulation by isoprenaline in the same concentration. The presence of autoantibodies capable of producing an adrenoceptor stimulation without desensitization and of preventing the desensitization of the isoprenaline response could play, in some patients, a role in the pathogenesis of the DCM.

It is widely accepted that a chronic adrenergic overdrive, existing in many patients with dilated cardiomyopathy, could play a harmful role in this disease (5). Activation of the myocardium by elevated levels of circulating catecholamines in combination with the agonistic anti-β₁-adrenoceptor autoantibodies can be expected to lead to a situation in which, independent of the circadian rhythm, a permanently exaggerated β-adrenergic overactivity could be the consequence. Such prolonged adrenergic stimulation could induce metabolic and electrophysiologic disturbances in the myocardium (6, 4) responsible for tachyarrhythmias and sudden death that often is the cause of mortality in DCM patients.

As shown above, β-adrenergic blocking agents were able to break the strong binding of the anti-β₁-adrenoceptor autoantibodies to the β₁-adrenoceptors. Because the β-adrenergic antagonists were able to block the effect exerted by the anti-β₁-adrenoceptor autoantibodies, displacing them from the receptor (Fig. 3), this action could conceivably contribute to the beneficial effect repeatedly reported to be exerted by treatment of DCM patients with β-adrenergic antagonists (23, 21, 24, 7, 3).

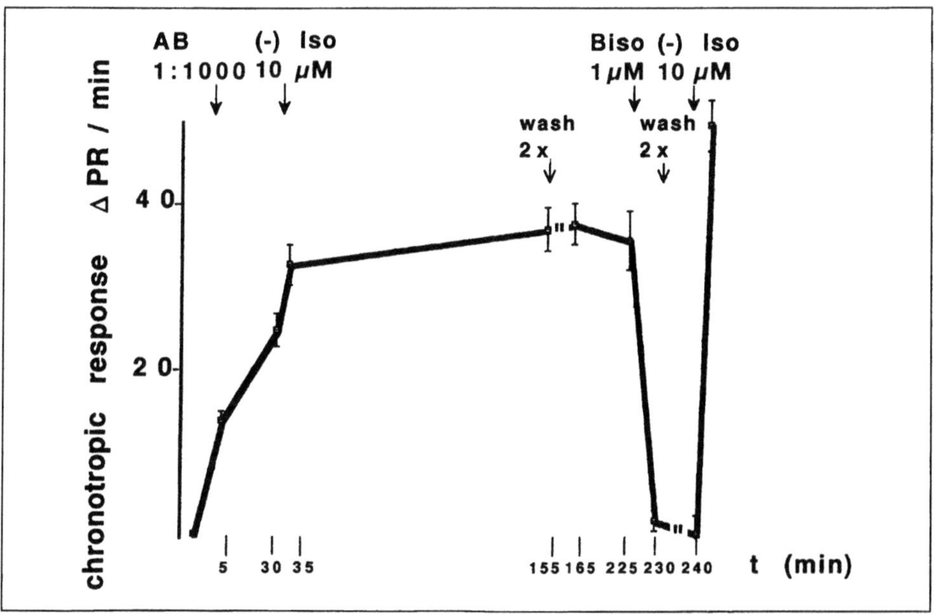

Fig. 3. Chronotropic effect of the anti-β₁-adrenoceptor autoantibodies in the presence of isoprenaline (Iso, 10 μM) and bisoprolol (Biso, 1 μM). Affinity purified antibodies were added to spontaneously beating cultured cardiomyocytes prepared from the neonatal rat heart ventricle. The addition of isoprenaline to the antibody-prestimulated cardiomyocytes did not change the stimulatory effect over a period of 2 h. The stimulation was completely blocked by bisoprolol. A restimulation by the same isoprenaline concentration after the bisoprolol treatment and a washing procedure resulted in a maximal chronotropic effect, confirming that no desensitization occurred in the combined presence of autoantibodies and isoprenaline.

Table 2. Behavior of the anti-β-adrenoceptor autoantibodies, the heart rate, and the ejection fraction in a patient during the process of healing of an acute myocarditis. (EF = ejection fraction, HR = heart rate, AB = antibody)

	EF %	HR (beats/min)	AB-level (relative unit)
acute myocarditis	36	120	30 ± 3.6
7 weeks later	41	65	12 ± 2.4
36 weeks later	59	62	0.4 ± 1.2

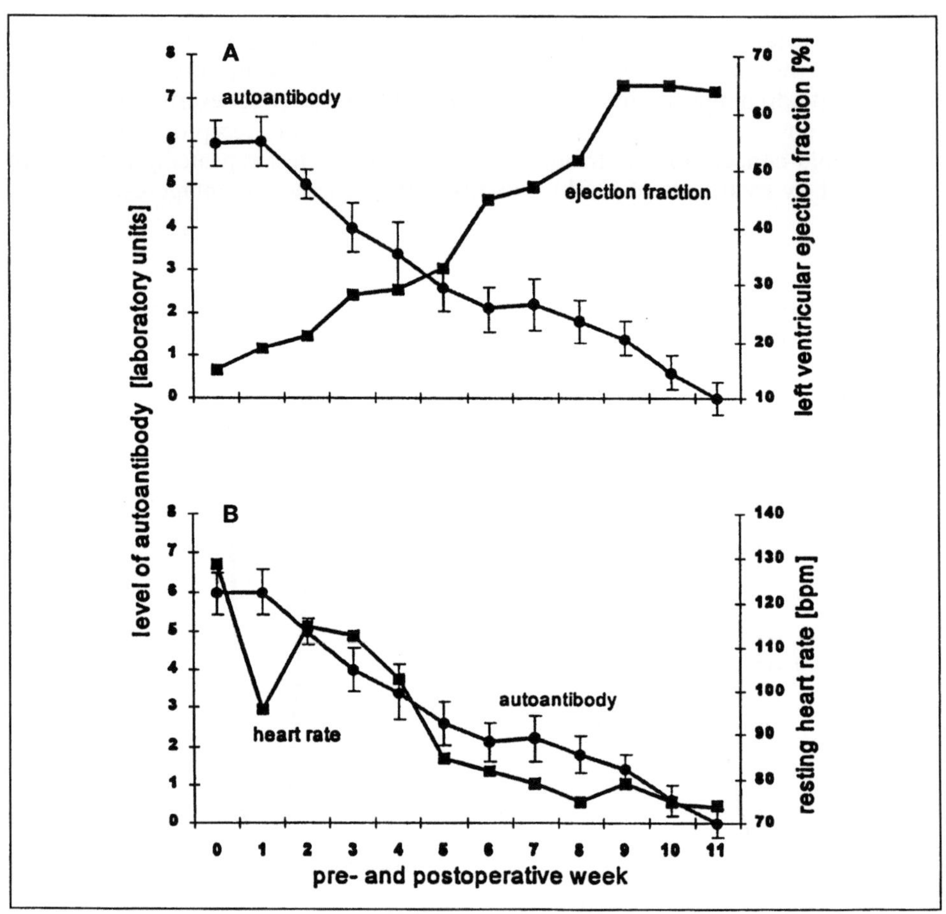

Fig. 4. The antibodies, the heart rate (4B), and the ejection fraction (4A) of a DCM patient supported by a cardiac assist device. After the implantation of the support system there was a reduction in the amount of anti-β₁-adrenoceptor autoantibodies and an improvement of cardiac function.
● antibody, ■ heart rate (4B) and ejection fraction (4A).

That the anti-β_1-adrenoceptor autoantibodies could play a role in the pathogenesis of DCM was indicated by findings in patients with myocarditis, a disease widely held to be a precursor of DCM (1). Patients with this disease do not differ from those with DCM with respect to the presence and the level of circulating autoantibodies that recognize the β_1-adrenoceptor (26). It is therefore also of interest in the present context that in a patient with acute myocarditis the healing process, as reflected by a normalization of the ejection fraction and the heart rate, was correlated with a disappearance of the anti-β_1-adrenoceptor autoantibodies from the blood (Table 2).

A similar correlation between the reduction of these autoantibodies and an improvement of cardiac function was observed in patients with endstage dilated cardiomyopathy treated with a cardiac support system (18). After the implantation of the cardiac assist device in patients containing autoantibodies directed against the β_1-adrenoceptor in their serum a reduction in the amount of these autoantibodies was observed. Their disappearance was accompanied by an improvement of the function of the heart. In parallel with the decrease in the amount of the anti-β_1-adrenoceptor autoantibodies an increase in the ejection fraction and a normalization of the heart frequency and size was observed (Fig. 4).

The remarkable correlation observed between the reduction in the amount of circulating autoantibodies against the β_1-adrenoceptor and the improvement of the function of the heart just described can be interpreted as a hint that the anti-β_1-adrenoceptor antibodies may play a part in the pathophysiology of myocarditis and DCM. At present it is too early to definitely assign a pathogenic role to these antibodies in DCM and myocarditis. At any rate, these antibodies represent a sensitive marker for monitoring the autoimmunological activity in cardiomyopathic and myocarditic patients. The correlation between the decrease in the serum level of these antibodies and the improvement of cardiac function could help to delineate the rehabilation process in these patients.

References

1. Abelman WH (1988) Myocarditis as a cause of dilated cardiomyopathy. In: Engelmeier BS, O'Connel JB (eds) Drug therapy in dilated cardiomyopathy and myocarditis. Marcel Dekker, New York, pp 221-231
2. Charlap S, Lichstein E, Frishman WH (1989) β-Adrenergic blocking drugs in the treatment of congestive heart failure. Med Clin North Am 73: 373-385
3. Engelmeier RS, O'Connel JB, Walsh R, Rad N, Scanlon PJ, Gunnar RM (1985) Improvement in symptoms and exercise tolerance by metoprolol in patients with dilated cardiomyopathy: a double-blind, randomized, placebo-controlled trial. Circulation 72: 536-546
4 Eschenhagen T, Mende U, Diederich M, Nose M, Schmitz W, Scholz H, Schulte Am Esch J, Warnholtz A, Schäfer H (1992) Long term β-adrenoceptor-mediated up-regulation of Giα and Goα mRNA levels and pertussis toxin-sensitive guanine nucleotide-binding proteins in rat heart. Mol Pharmacol 42: 773-783
5. Francis GS, Goldsmith SR, Olivari MT, Levin TB, Cohn JN (1984) The neuronal humoral axis in congestive heart failure. Ann Intern Med 101: 370-377
6. Haft J (1974) Cardiovascular injury induced by sympathetic catecholamines. Prog Cardiovasc Dis 17: 73-86
7. Heilbrunn SM, Shah P, Bristow MR, Valentine HA Ginsburg R, Fowler MB (1989) Increased beta-receptor density and improved hemodynamic response to catecholamines stimulation during long-term metoprolol therapy in heart failure from dilated cardiomyopathy. Circulation 79: 483-490

8. Krause EG, Bartel S, Beyerdörfer I, Wallukat G. (1995) Activation of cyclic AMP-dependent protein kinase in cardiomyocytes by anti-β_1-adrenoceptor autoantibodies from patients with idiopathic dilated cardiomyopathy. Blood Pressure in press

9. Leimbach WN, Wallin BG, Victor RG, Aylward PE, Sundhoef G, Mark AL (1986) Direct evidence from intraneural recordings for increased central sympathetic outflow in patients with heart failure. Circulation 73: 913-919

10. Limas CJ, Goldenberg IF, Limas C (1989) Autoantibodies against β-adrenoceptors in human idiopathic dilated cardiomyopathy. Circ Res 64: 97-103

11. Magnusson Y, Höyer S, Lengagne R, Chapot MP, Guillet JG, Hjalmarson µ, Strosberg AD, Hoebeke J (1989) Antigenic analysis of the second extracellular loop of the human β-adrenergic receptor. Clin Exp Immunol 78: 42-48

12. Magnusson Y, Marullo S, Höyer S, Waagstein F, Andersson B, Vahlne A, Guillet JG, Hjalmarson Å, Hoebeke J (1990) Mapping of a functional autoimmune epitope on the β_1-adrenergic receptor in patients with idiopathic dilated cardiomyopathy. J Clin Invest 86: 1658-1666

13. Magnusson Y, Wallukat G, Guillet JG, Hjalmarson Å, Hoebeke J (1991) Functional analysis of rabbit antipeptide antibodies which mimic autoantibodies against the β_1-adrenergic receptor in patients with idiopathic dilated cardiomyopathy. J Autoimmun 4: 893-905

14. Magnusson Y, Wallukat G, Waagstein F, Hjalmarson Å, Hoebeke J (1994) Autoimmunity in idiopathic dilated cardiomyopathy. Characterization of antibodies against the β_1-adrenoceptor with positive chronotropic effect. Circulation 89: 2760-2767

15. Maisch B, Trostel-Soeder R, Stechemesser E, Berg PA, Kochsiek K (1982) Diagnostic relevance of humoral and cell-mediated immune reactions in patients with acute viral myocarditis. Clin Exp Immunol 48: 533-545

16. Maisch B, Deeg P, Liebau G, Kochsiek K (1983) Diagnostic relevance of humoral and cytotoxic immune reactions in primary and secondary dilated cardiomyopathy. Am J Cardiol 52: 1072-1078

17. Morad M, Davies NW, Ulrich G, Schultheiss HP (1988) Antibodies against ADP-ATP carrier enhance Ca^{2+}-current in isolated cardiac myocytes. Am J Physiol 255: H960-H964

18. Müller J, Wallukat G, Weng Y, Siniawski H, Hummel M, Hetzer R (1995) Abfall der β-Rezeptoren-Autoantikörper in Patienten mit idiopathischer dilatativer Kardiomyopathie (DKMP) während mechanischer Linksherzunterstützung (abstract). Z Kardiol 84 (Suppl): 132

19. Schultheiss HP (1993) Disturbances of the myocardial energy metabolism in dilated cardiomyopathy due to autoimmunological mechanisms. Circulation 87 (Suppl.IV): IV43-IV48

20. Schultheiss HP, Schulze K, Schauer R, Witzenbichler B, Strauer BE (1995) Antibody- mediated inbalance of myocardial energy metabolism. A causal factor of cardiac failure? Circ Res 76: 64-72

21. Swedberg K, Hjalmarson Å, Waagstein F, Wallentin I (1979) Prolonged survival in congestive cardiomyopathy by β-receptor blockade. Lancet i: 1374-1376

22. Thomas JA, Marks BH (1978) Plasma norepinephrine in congestive heart failure. Am J Cardiol 41: 233-243

23. Waagstein F, Hjalmarson Å, Varnauskas E, Wallentin I (1975) Effect of chronic beta-adrenergic receptor blockade in congestive cardiomyopathy. Br Heart J 37: 1022-1036

24. Waagstein F, Bristow MR, Swedberg K, Camerini F, Fowler MB, Silver MA, Gilbert EM, Johnson MR, Goss FG, Hjalmarson Å (1993) Beneficial effect of metoprolol in idiopathic dilated cardiomyopathy. Lancet 342: 1441-1446

25. Wallukat G, Wollenberger A (1987) Effects of the gamma globulin fraction of patients with allergic asthma and dilated cardiomyopathy on chronotropic β-adrenoceptor function in cultured neonatal rat heart myocytes. Biomed Biochim Acta 78: S634-S639

26. Wallukat G, Morwinski R, Kowal K, Förster A, Boewer V, Wollenberger A (1991) Autoantibodies against the β-adrenergic receptor in human myocarditis and dilated cardiomyopathy: β-adrenergic agonism without desensitization. Europ Heart J 12 (Supll. D): 178-181

27. Wallukat G, Boewer V, Förster A, Wollenberger A (1991) Anti-β-adrenoceptor autoantibodies with β-adrenergic agonistic activity from patients with myocarditis and dilated cardiomyopathy. In: Lewis BS, Kimchi A (eds) Heart Failure Mechanisms and Management. Springer-Verlag Berlin, Heidelberg, pp 21-29

28. Wallukat G, Wollenberger A, Morwinski R, Pitschner HF (1995) Anti-β_1-adrenoceptor autoantibodies with chronotropic activity from the serum of patients with dilated cardiomyopathy: Mapping of epitopes in the first and second extracellular loops. J Mol Cell Cardiol 27: 397-406

29. Wallukat G, Kayser A, Wollenberger A (1995) The β_1-adrenoceptor as antigen: functional aspects. Europ Heart J Suppl X: in press
30. Wallukat G, Morwinski R, Magnusson Y, Hoebeke J, Wollenberger A (1992) Autoantikörper gegen den β_1-adrenergen Rezeptor bei Myokarditis und dilatativer Kardiomyopathie: Lokalisation von zwei Epitopen. Z Kardiol 81 (Suppl. 4): 79-83
31. WHO/ISFC Task Force (1980) Report on the definition and classification of cardiomyopathies. Br Heart J 44: 672–673

Author's address:
Dr. G. Wallukat
Max Delbrück Centre for Molecular Medicine
Cardiology
Robert Rössle Str. 10
13125 Berlin, Germany

Weaning from mechanical support after complete recovery in patients with idiopathic dilated cardiomyopathy

J. Müller, G. Wallukat, Yu-Guo Weng, M. Dandel, S. Spiegelsberger, M. Loebe, R. Hetzer

German Heart Institute Berlin, Berlin, Germany

Abstract

Implanting a mechanical cardiac assist system as a bridge to transplantation or for long-term support is ultimately the only immediately available therapy for treating endstage cardiac diseases after conservative drug therapy has failed. The primary indications for implanting a cardiac support system are ischemic heart disease and idiopathic dilated cardiomyopathy (IDC). IDC is frequently associated with the presence of anti-β_1-adrenoceptor (A-β_1-AAB) and other autoantibodies in the sera of patients directed against cardiac structures. This present study assessed whether changes in A-β_1-AAB levels during mechanical cardiac support might be used as an indicator for cardiac recovery with the ultimate goal of weaning patients from the device instead of performing transplantation on them.

Between April 1994 and May 1995, 17 patients with endstage non-ischemic IDC were implanted with univentricular cardiac assist systems (the wearable Novacor N100 system or TCI HeartMate) as a bridge to transplantation. All of the patients were male, in New York Heart Association (NYHA) class IV-D, had a cardiac index below 1.6 liters per minute per square meter of body-surface area (l min^{-1} m^{-2}), a left ventricular ejection fraction (LVEF) below 16%, and a left ventricular internal diameter in diastole (LVIDd) of more than 68 mm. Echocardiographic examinations were performed preoperatively and weekly after implantation. Likewise, the sera of these patients were examined for A-β_1-AAB with a bioassay immediately before device implantation and once a week thereafter.

The mean age of the patients was 49 ± 11 years (range: 32 to 67 years). Six patients died of various causes (3 due to bleeding, 1 due to multiorgan failure, and 2 because of technical reasons). The average duration of support was 160 ± 109 days (range: 37 to 475 days). Presently 4 patients continue to receive support. Three patients were transplanted after 75, 95 and 225 days of assisted circulation, respectively. The sera of all patients were considered positive for A-β_1-AAB preoperatively with a value of 6.5 ± 0.8 laboratory units (LU) (range, 5.2 to 7.5 LU) and within the first 2 weeks postoperatively. During the course of circulatory support, the A-β_1-AAB levels decreased in all of the patients and had completely disappeared 12 ± 5 weeks (range, 8 to 25 weeks) postoperatively. Parallel to this development echocardiographic examinations indicated an improvement in cardiac LVEF to an average of 31 ± 14% (range: 15 to 50%) and a decrease in LVIDd to mean values of 64 ± 10 mm (range: 25 to 81 mm). Four patients who exhibited improvement in cardiac function to near normal values were weaned from the device after

160, 243, 348 and 200 days of support, respectively. To reduce the risk of this new untested procedure, the devices were programmed to operate in an asynchronous drive mode for 3 weeks, which led to a significant increase in afterload of the left ventricle. Under these conditions neither a deterioration in cardiac function was observed through echocardiography nor an increase in A-β_1-AAB through blood samples. Nevertheless, in 1 case it was decided to wean a patient due to thrombo-embolic complications and another due to a severe infection in the assist device pocket. Both decisions were additionally influenced by the unavailability of donor hearts. The device was explanted from a third patient as a planned procedure. As of March 31, 1996, these patients have been off the device for 389, 307, 299 and 185 days, respectively, with no increase in A-β_1-AAB levels while exhibiting stable adequate cardiac function with a tendency towards further improvement

Mechanical cardiac support in patients with IDC and A-β_1-AAB simultaneously leads to a significant improvement in cardiac function and the disappearance of A-β_1-AAB. Assuming that A-β_1-AAB may cause cardiac dilatation and functional impairment, weaning from the device is possible as long as A-β_1-AAB has disappeared and cardiac function improved. However, as the duration of cardiac stability is not predictable, it remains to be seen whether cardiac function has made a long-term recovery. Nevertheless, the results of this study indicate that this procedure may open a new concept in the treatment of endstage IDC. Implanting a mechanical cardiac assist device is often the only means available for supporting the hemodynamic condition in patients with endstage heart failure if a donor heart is not available. As of 1994 this method had been performed approximately 584 times worldwide for bridging to transplantation with an exponentially increasing trend (12, 20, 24, 30).

The possibility of using temporary cardiac assist device support to give the heart an opportunity to recover has been considered for some time. Isolated cases involving patients with acute myocarditis or postcardiotomy have been reported (13, 26, 28, 30, 32).

This idea was conceived after it was clinically observed that cardiac ejection fraction and diameter improved significantly in some patients supported with a cardiac assist device.

It was therefore hypothesized that the macroscopically visible improvement in cardiac function must have a "microscopical" correlate which might show changes during mechanical cardiac support. The investigation was limited to patients who clinically exhibited (non-ischemic) IDC, since significant cardiac improvements were only observed in this cohort.

There is evidence from both clinical and experimental studies that in a subset of patients an autoimmunological mechanism might be primarily or secondarily involved in the pathogenesis of IDC, by definition a disease of unknown origin nevertheless believed to be a sequela of viral myocarditis in many cases. Thus, cardioactive immunoglobulins circulating in patients with these diseases have been found to attach themselves to various structures of the myocardial cells, as indicated by immunofluorescence staining. Cardiac autoantigens identified in myocarditis and IDC include the mitochondrial ADP/ATP carrier, the branched chain keto acid dehydrogenase, the cardiac myosin heavy chain, laminin, and the β_1-adrenoceptor (3, 35, 43, 46). Autoantibodies directed against this receptor have been previously observed in the serum of patients with Chagas' heart disease, whose clinical manifestations resemble those of IDC (1, 3, 4, 8, 10, 18, 19, 21, 22, 34, 35, 36, 39, 41, 43, 46).

Using neonatal rat heart myocytes beating spontaneously in culture as a sensitive adrenergic effector system, as indicated by their chronotropic response to adrenoceptor stimulation, it was possible to show that the serum of patients with myocarditis and IDC contained autoantibodies of the IgG isotype capable of eliciting increases in the beating rate which could be maintained unabated for days.

As a rule such antibodies were not observed in healthy control subjects or in patients with chronic ischemic heart disease and normal cardiac function and size or acute myocardial infarction (44, 45) (Wallukat et al., 1991a, 1991b). The possibility was considered that autoantibodies with chronotropic activity in the anti-β_1-receptor may play a role in the harmful chronic adrenergic drive to which the hearts of patients with IDC are believed to be exposed (5, 9, 17, 40).

In this present study the course of A-β_1-AABs and functional cardiac parameters in patients with IDC who were implanted with mechanical left ventricular assist devices with the primary intention of bridging to transplantation were analyzed. The original goal of this present study was to develop a new therapeutic concept for weaning such patients from mechanically assisted circulation once they exhibited an improvement in cardiac function. This concept is comparable to that of the ESETCID Trial (European Study on Epidemiology and Therapy of Cardiomyopathy and Inflammatory Disease) initiated with the intention of treating patients with dilated cardiomyopathy or myocarditis according to the etiology of their diseases. The aforementioned goal of this study, however, was abandoned after it was observed that the implantation of an assist device alone led to changes in the immunological status of these patients. The following text reports success achieved in weaning patients from assist devices and describes the decision process for explanting the pumps. In 2 cases the decision for device explantation was precipitated due to special clinical conditions (infection and thromboembolism) which represented a significant threat to the patients.

Methods

Patients

Of the 31 patients with endstage cardiac insufficiency implanted with cardiac assist devices at the German Heart Institute Berlin (GHIB) between January 1994 and May 1995, serially 17 with clinically diagnosed IDC were selected for this study. All of the patients exhibited cardiogenic shock at the time of device implantation (27). Before mechanical circulatory support was initiated the patients were in New York Heart Association class IV-D, had a cardiac index below 1.6 l min^{-1} m^{-2}, an ejection fraction below 16%, a left ventricular internal diameter in diastole of more than 68 mm, and had required increasing positive inotropic support over a week's duration. Echocardiographic examinations were performed before implantation and once a week thereafter, whereby the pump was switched off for 2–4 min. Sufficient anticoagulation was ensured at that moment. The following parameters were measured to characterize cardiac function: left ventricular global ejection fraction (LVEF) by planimetry and left ventricular internal diameter in diastole (LVIDd). Regurgitation from the inlet cannula was checked before the parameters were measured. All of the examinations were conducted by the same examiner to ensure a minimum of variability in the echocardiographic parameters.

Table 1. Weaned – patients data at the time of left ventricular assist device implantation (pre) and three days after implantation of left ventricular assist devices (post)

weaned patient	age, sex	body surface area	days on device	positive inotropic medication		arterial blood pressure [systolic/ diastolic] [mm Hg]		Heart rate [beats per minute) ryhthm		mitral valve incompetence; cardiothoracic ratio		left ventricular internal diameter in diastole; left ventricular ejection fraction		cardiac index; mean pulmonary artery pressure; mean pulmonary capilarry wedge pressure; central venous pressure		level of anti-β_1-adrenoceptor autoantibodies (laboratory units [LU])	
				pre	post	pre	post	pre	post	pre	post	pre	post	pre	post	pre	post
1	39 years male	2.00 m^2	160	dobutamine; dopamine	0	95/50	115/65	128 sinus ryhthm	76 sinus rhythm	grade II 0.67	0 0.48	72 mm; < 15 %	53 mm; 50 %	1.5 l m^{-2} min^{-1}; 36 mm Hg; 28 mm Hg; 21 mm Hg	3.1 l m^{-2} min^{-1}; 18 mm Hg; 6 mm Hg; 9 mm Hg	7.2	not detectable
2	43 years, male	2.10 m^2	243	dobutamine; dopamine; phosphodiesterase inhibitors	0	90/55	120/75	125 sinus rhythm	69 sinus rhythm	grade II 0.62	0 0.43	70 mm; 15 %	54 mm; 48 %	1.4 l m^{-2} min^{-1}; 38 mm Hg; 31 mm Hg; 24 mm Hg	3.0 l m^{-2} min^{-1}; 15 mm Hg; 8 mm Hg; 10 mm Hg	6.8	not detecable
3	58 years, male	2.13 m^2	347	dobutamine; dopamine; phosphodiesterase inhibitors	0	100/55	125/80	134 sinus rhythm	75 sinus rhyhtm	grade II 0.64	0 0.45	70 mm; < 15 %	55 mm; 47 %	1.4 l m^{-2} min^{-1}; 19 mm Hg; 29 mm Hg; 27 mm Hg	2.9 l m^{-2} min^{-1}; 19 mm Hg; 11 mm Hg; 11 mm Hg	7.1	not detectable
4	53 years, male	2.08 m^2	200	dobutamine; dopamine; phosphodiesterase inhibitors	0	105/60	110/75	122 sinus rhythm	80 sinus ryhthm	grade I 0.64	0 0.44	69 mm; < 15 %	52 mm; 50 %	1.5 l m^{-2} min^{-1}; 33 mm Hg; 27 mm Hg; 19 mm Hg	3.2 l m^{-2} min^{-1}; 14 mm Hg; 8 mm Hg; 8 mm Hg	6.2	not detecable

Histories of Weaned Patients

Patient number one (Table 1): a 39-year-old man with a 4-year history of dilated cardiomyopathy, presented with cardiac decompensation. He first suffered decompensation during his vacation 4 years ago, yet could regain compensation through conservative therapy. He became clinically conspicuous a second time 3 months before admission. At that time he required high doses of positive inotropic substances and 4 liters oxygen per minute via nasal tube. Phosphodiesterase inhibitors were discontinued due to severe hemodynamically relevant arrhythmias. Creatinine, urea, and liver enzymes had been rising since the day before admission. An electrocardiographic examination upon admission showed a sinus tachycardia with a heart rate of 128 beats per minute and revealed the following data: LVIDd 72 mm, LVIDs 65 mm, LVEF below 15%, and grade II mitral valve incompetence. Important parameters for assessing cardiac function included a cardiac index of $1.5 \, l \, m^{-2} \, min^{-1}$, mean pulmonary artery pressure of 36 mm Hg, mean pulmonary capillary wedge pressure of 28 mm Hg, and central venous pressure of 21 mm Hg. The coronary angiogram was negative. A Novacor N100 wearable mechanical cardiac support system was implanted the day after admission. At 7.2 LU, the level of A-β_1-AABs was pathologic.

Patient number two (Table 1): a 43-year-old man, had a history very similar to that described above. He first suffered cardiac decompensation 3 years before admission to the GHIB, yet regained compensation twice within this time frame through medicamentous therapy. Upon admission the patient presented with severe cardiac insufficiency, tachypnea, and sinus tachycardia (heart rate 125 beats per minute) despite receiving high doses of positive inotropic substances, including phosphodiesterase inhibitors, and 5 liters oxygen via nasal tube. Echocardiographic examination revealed a LVIDd of 70 mm, LVIDs of 64 mm, LVEF of 15%, and grade II mitral valve incompetence. Further clinically important parameters included a cardiac index of $1.4 \, l \, m^{-2} \, min^{-1}$, mean pulmonary artery pressure of 38 mm Hg, mean pulmonary capillary wedge pressure of 31 mm Hg, central venous pressure of 24 mm Hg, and slightly elevated levels of liver enzymes, creatinine, and urea. A Novacor N100 wearable cardiac assist device was implanted on the day of admission. Endomyocardial biopsy was performed during implantation of the outlet conduit and 2 weeks before explantation of the device. The pre-implantation A-β_1-AAB level was 6.8 LU (Table 1).

Patient number three (Table 1): a 58-year-old man with an 8-year history of dilated cardiomyopathy, regained compensation 4 times through medicamentous therapy during this time period. The patient presented with cardiac cachexia, orthopnea, and tachycardia during atrial fibrillation. He was implanted with a Novacor N100 wearable univentricular cardiac support device 2 days afterwards. Echocardiographic examination revealed a LVIDd of 70 mm and a LVIDs of 63 mm. The ejection fraction was below 15%. Doppler sonography indicated grade II mitral valve incompetence. Further parameters included a cardiac index of $1.4 \, l \, m^{-2} \, min^{-1}$, mean pulmonary artery pressure of 40 mm Hg, mean pulmonary capillary wedge pressure of 29 mm Hg, central venous pressure of 27 mm Hg, and chronically elevated values for liver enzymes, creatinine, and urea. Additionally, the patient suffered from non-insulin dependent diabetes mellitus (NIDDM). His serum showed a pathological level of A-β_1-AABs (7.1 LU).

Patient number four (Table 1): a 53-year-old man with a 6 year history of dilated cardiomyopathy. He first suffered cardiac decompensation 5 years before admission to the GHIB. The patient presented with cardiac cachexia, orthopnea, an arterial systolic blood pressure below 85 mm Hg despite of maximal positive inotropic support. He was implanted with a TCI device 2 days after admission. Echocardiographic examination revealed a LVIDd of 69 mm, a LVIDs of 63 mm, an EF of below 15 %, and grade 1 mitral valve incompetence. Further parameters were: cardiac index was $1.5 \, 1 \, m^{-2} \, min^{-1}$, mean pulmonary artery pressure was 33 mm Hg, mean pulmonary capillary wedge pressure was 27 mm Hg, and central venous pressure was 19 mm Hg. The serum exhibited an A-β_1-AAB level of 6.2 LU.

Bioassay

Single cells were dissociated from the minced ventricles of 1 to 2-day-old Wistar rats with a 0.2% solution of crude trypsin, cultured as monolayers on the bottom of Müller flasks as described elsewhere [47], and equilibrated with humidified air in Halle SM20-I medium containing 10% heat-inactivated calf serum and 2 µM fluorodeoxyuridine, the latter to prevent the proliferation of non-muscle cells. The culture flasks were fastened to a metal tray in an incubator and continuously gently rocked back and forth twice a minute at an angle of ± 30° at 37 °C to ensure adequate equilibration of the cell layer with the culture fluid and gas phase. On the third or 4th day the cells were incubated 2 h in 2 ml of fresh serum-containing medium. Afterwards the flasks were transferred to the heated stage of an inverted microscope where 10 small circular fields of the cell layer were observed at 37 °C through the perforations of a metal template. The beats of 7 to 10 selected cells or synchronously contracting cell clusters per flask were counted for 15 s. This procedure was repeated twice in different cultures to yield results representing a total of up to 30 cells or cell clusters for each sample of a given immunoglobulin fraction, affinity-purified antibodies, or drug. Control beating rates on the third and 4th day averaged 162 ± 16 beats/min. The neonatal rats were killed in accordance with the guidelines of the Community Health Service of the city of Berlin.

Ammonium sulfate precipitation at a saturation of 40% was used to isolate immunoglobulin fraction from serum samples of approximately 2 ml. The precipitates were washed, dissolved in a dialysis buffer (154 mM NaCl, 10 mM sodium phosphate, pH 7.2), and dialyzed at 4 °C for 30 h against 1 l of this buffer. The buffer solution was changed 5 times. The immunoglobulins were taken up in phosphate-buffered saline (pH 7.2) and kept frozen at –25d °C until use. The parameter used to quantify the amount of functional effective autoantibodies is expressed as the increase of beats per 15 s (LU) (41, 42).

Cardiac Assist Devices

The wearable Novacor N100 left ventricular assist device (Baxter Healthcare Corporation, Novacor Division; Oakland, CA, USA), which operates with electromagnets, was used in 11 patients and the console-based pneumatically-driven TCI HeartMate assist device (Thermo Cardiosystems Inc., Woburn, MA, USA) in 5. Novacor N100 normally operates synchronously, whereas the TCI HeartMate works asynchronously to the heart rate.

The devices were implanted anteriorly to the fascia musculi recti abdominis posterioris in the left upper abdominal quadrant. The inlet conduit was anastomosed to the apex of the left ventricle and the outlet conduit to the ascending aorta in an end-to-side position. All implantations were performed under extracorporeal circulation.

To avoid postoperative thrombus formation, patients with the Novacor N100 device were administered warfarin (Coumadin) to maintain a prothrombin time at an international normalized ratio (INR) of approximately 2.5, while patients with the TCI HeartMate were orally administered 100 mg of acetylsalicylic acid (ASS) and 225 mg dipyridamole per day.

Weaning procedure

In patients who consented to the weaning procedure, the drive unit was programmed to an asynchronous mode (fixed rate mode) for 3 consecutive weeks to test the stability of the recovered cardiac function. The fixed rate mode led to a separation between the occurrence of cardiac ejection and the filling of the pump, thus increasing afterload of the left ventricle. This explains why the heart and pump were only randomly synchronized. The device was explanted by opening the device-containing pocket along the implantation scar. Inlet and outlet conduits were ligated subdiaphragmatically and the device removed after the conduits were cut through.

Post-implantation management

The early postoperative management of cardiac assist patients is similar to that for any critically ill patient after cardiac surgery. Invasive postoperative monitoring is accomplished through a thermodilution pulmonary artery catheter and left atrial line. Pump output and stroke volume, pulmonary arterial pressure, radial artery pressure, and central venous pressure are monitored continuously during the initial postoperative phase. In addition to the standard postoperative care provided for cardiac patients, the postoperative management of cardiac assist device patients included percutaneous exit-site care and a device-specific anticoagulant regimen. All patient problems and decisions regarding mechanical assist management were assessed by a specially-trained mechanical support team.

Blood samples

During routine clinical visits immediately before implantation and once a week thereafter, 10 ml specimens of peripheral blood were drawn in serum syringes without any additives and handled according to established clinical guidelines. The blood was centrifuged at 3600 RPM to collect sera for tracing A-β_1-AABs by bioassay.

Results

The follow-up courses of 17 patients with IDC who had undergone mechanical left ventricular assist support due to endstage cardiac insufficiency were investigated. All of the patients were male, between the ages of 32 and 67 years (49 ± 11 years), and had a mean body surface area of 2.1 ± 0.2 m^2 (range: 1.7 to 2.4 m^2). Upon admission they all exhibited cardiac decompensation necessitating positive inotropic support with dobutamine and dopamine. Eleven patients had benefited from phosphodiesterase inhibitors. The cardiac index was found to be below 1.6 l min^{-1} m^{-2} in all patients. The patients exhibited elevated levels of creatinine (2.54 ± 0.88 milligram deciliter^{-1}) and liver enzymes, indicative of increasing congestive heart failure.

Since conservative medicamentous treatment was unsuccessful, the decision was made to implant left ventricular assist devices in these patients. Eleven patients received a Novacor device; six patients a TCI. Three patients died between the 59th and 120th postoperative days due to bleeding complications. One patient died due to uncontrollable multiorgan failure on the 93rd postoperative day and 2 because of technical pump-related problems leading to massive bleeding on the 37th and 142nd postoperative day, respectively.

Presently, four patients continue to receive support. Three patients were transplanted after 75, 95, and 225 days and 4 others were weaned from the device 160, 243, 348, and 200 days after implantation, respectively. These latter patients are now (as of March 31, 1996) off the device for 389, 307, 299, and 185 days. The mean duration of support for all patients was 160 ± 109 days (range: 37 to 475 days).

All examined sera were positive for A-β_1-AAB with a mean value of 6.5 ± 0.8 LU (range, 5.2 to 7.5 LU) before implantation. Following assist implantation, A-β_1-AABs decreased in all patients and ultimately disappeared after 12 ± 5 weeks (range, 8 to 25 weeks) in all those 14 patients surviving long enough after implant, and could not be detected at any later time.

During the follow-up course, echocardiographic examinations of these 14 patients who survived at least until A-β_1-AABs had disappeared showed improvement of LVIDd and LVEF from a mean 77 ± 7 mm (range, 69 to 95 mm) to 64 ± 10 mm (range, 52 to 81 mm), and from below 16% to a mean of 31 ± 14% (range, 15 to 50%), respectively.

Cardiothoracic ratio showed improvement from mean 0.69 ± 0.03 (range, 0.62 to 0.74) to mean 0.59 ± 0.11 (range, 0.43 to 0.70).

When these 14 patients are devided into a group (A) of 10 with a LVIDd above 72 mm and a group (B) of 4 with a LVIDd below 73 mm before implantation, certain differences became apparent: in group A, LVIDd decreased from a mean of 80 ± 7 mm (range, 75 to 95 mm) before implantation to 69 ± 8 mm (range, 60 to 81 mm), and LVEF rose to a mean of 23 ± 8% (range, 15 to 35%) at the time after implantation (when the A-β_1-AABs had disappeared), whereas patients in group B showed a better recovery of LVIDd from a mean of 70 ± 1.3 mm (range, 69 to 72 mm) to 54 ± 1.3 mm (range, 52 to 55 mm), and of LVEF to a mean of 49 ± 1.5% (range, 47 to 50%). Group B was comprised of patients weaned from the assist device.

Mean LVIDs had changed from 70 ± 9 mm (range: 61 to 90 mm) to 52 ± 11 mm (range: 39 to 76 mm). Resting heart rate was 127 ± 9 beats per minute (range:

115 to 135 beats per minute) before implantation and 73 ± 7 beats per minute (range: 65 to 82 beats per minute) 14 weeks later.

Weaned patients

Patient number one (Table 1, Fig. 1): With the exception of the necessity for rethoracotomy on the first postoperative day because of bleeding problems, assist device implantation and the postoperative course were uneventful. After all of the central lines had been removed, anticoagulation was changed from heparin to coumarin. Ninety-eight days later the patient was discharged to a family house. Echocardiography was performed once weekly and the serum checked for A-β_1-AABs. After cardiac function had improved, the A-β_1-AABs had disappeared, and the patient had given his consent for weaning, the device was switched to the fixed rate mode to increase loading of the left ventricle as described above to verify the stability of the cardiac improvement and the disappearance of A-β_1-AABs. After the patient suffered abducens paresis induced by thromboembolism, the latter probably caused by the support system, it was decided to avoid further complications by explanting the device. This was accomplished 160 days after implantation.

The following parameters were examined 4 days after explantation: LVIDd 53 mm, LVIDs 39 mm, LVEF 50%, cardiac index 3.1 l m^{-2} min^{-1}, mean pulmonary capillary wedge pressure 6 mm Hg, mean pulmonary artery pressure 18 mmHg, left ventricular enddiastolic pressure 10 mm Hg, and no indications of mitral valve incompetence. Resting heart rate was 76 beats per minute. Examination of the myocardial tissue by immunohistology, immunocytochemistry, and polymerase chain reaction for virus scanning were all negative.

Twelve months after explantation, the patient is in NYHA class 1-A with unchanged cardiac parameters. Angiotensin converting enzyme inhibitors (ACE-inhibitors) were given in a sufficient dosage to maintain a maximal arterial systolic pressure of 110 mm Hg and low dose beta-blockers (2.5 mg bisoprolol per day) are administered to provide further continuous unloading. To prevent embolic complications, long-term anticoagulation was adjusted to prolong the prothrombin time to an international normalized ratio (INR) of approximately 2.5 since the conduits for the assist device were left in place.

Patient number two (Table 1, Fig. 1): The postoperative course was completely uneventful. Anticoagulation was maintained as in the first patient, initially with heparin and later with coumarin. Ninety-six days after implantation the patient was discharged to a family house where he stayed until explantation. As in the first patient, echocardiographic examinations and A-β_1-AAB monitoring was performed once a week. Since his cardiac function had improved (LVIDd 54 mm; LVIDs 40 mm; LVEF 48%) after 13 weeks of support and the A-β_1-AABs had disappeared, the patient agreed to explantation of the pump 243 days after implantation. While immunohistological examination of myocardial tissue taken during implantation exhibited slightly increased numbers of lymphocytes (CD2, CD3, CD4, and CD8 positive cells), these were no longer detected in biopsy specimens taken 2 weeks before explantation. Likewise, virus proof by polymerase chain reaction was also negative. Two days after explantation the following hemodynamic parameters were measured: cardiac index 3.0 l m^{-2} min^{-1}, mean pulmonary capillary wedge pressure 8 mm Hg, mean pulmonary artery pressure 15 mm Hg, left ventricular enddiastolic pressure 8 mm Hg, resting heart rate 69 beats per minute, and

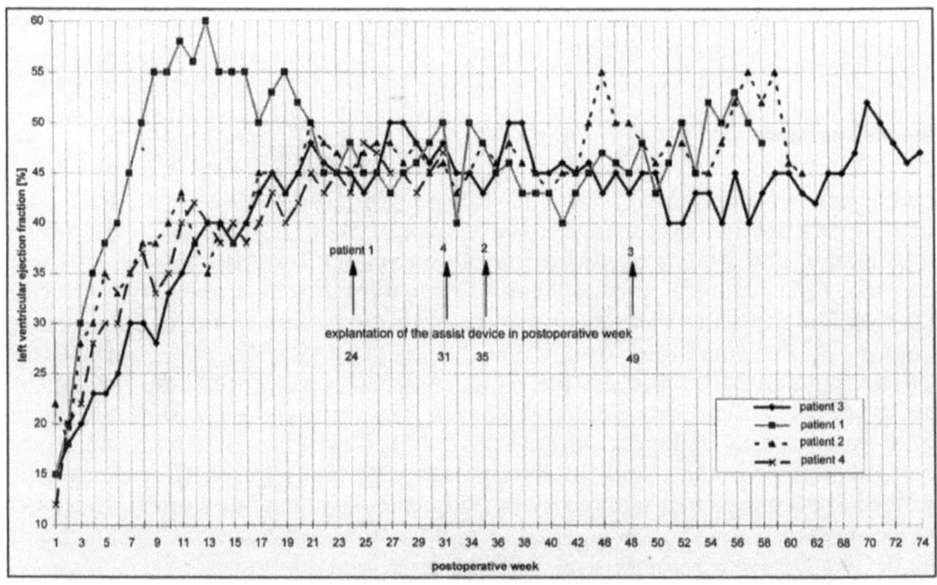

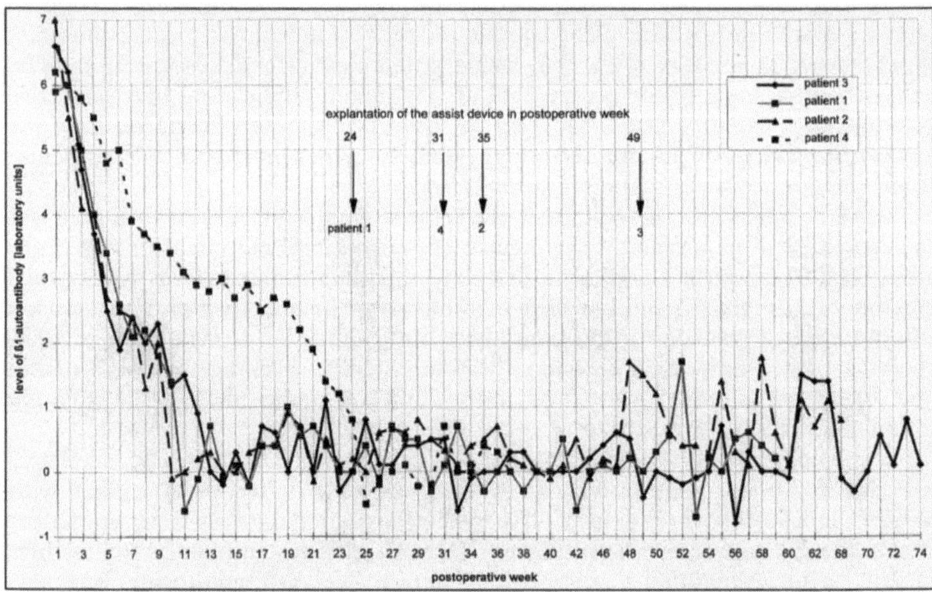

Fig. 1. The weekly course of the left ventricular ejection fraction (upper diagram) and the level of humoral anti-β_1-adrenoceptor auto-antibodies (lower diagram) after implantation of the mechanical left ventricular support system until explantation and the time thereafter in the 4 weaned patients. The arrows indicate the time of explantation of the device.

no indications of mitral valve incompetence. The patient's post-explantation treatment does not differ from that of the patient above. Three months after explantation the patient was also in NYHA class 1-A and exhibited stable cardiac function parameters. Today, nearly 12 months after explantation, he has returned to his former job as an insurance agent.

Patient number three (Table 1, Fig. 1): Due to a distinct transitory postoperative symptomatic psychotic syndrome, this patient had to remain on the respirator for 18 days. On the 22nd postoperative day, he developed clinical signs of infection with an elevated temperature, 17 000 leukocytes in the white blood count, and pus secretion from the pump-containing pocket. Since the patient began to exhibit cachexia, the pocket was lanced along the suture for 6 cm so that the pus could be emptied. Infection remained a constant complication in this patient over the course of mechanical cardiac support. Nevertheless, the A-β_1-AABs disappeared and cardiac function improved significantly after 12 weeks of support, during which time the patient regained normal sinus rhythm. Despite these improvements, the patient became increasingly marasmic. Transplantation therefore represented a significant risk for this patient due to his persistent infection and marasmic condition. Since the patient's cardiac function remained stable during the previously-described loading phase in which the device was switched to a fixed rate mode and the level of A-β_1-AABs did not increase again, the patient gave his consent and was weaned from the device 348 days after implantation. Echocardiography performed at the time of explantation showed an LVEF of 47%, an LVIDd of 55 mm, an LVIDs of 42 mm, and no indications of mitral valve incompetence. Invasive measurement by catheter revealed a cardiac index of 2.9 1 m^{-2} min^{-1}, mean pulmonary capillary wedge pressure of 11 mm Hg, mean pulmonary artery pressure of 19 mm Hg, and a left ventricular end-diastolic pressure of 10 mm Hg. Resting heart rate was 75 beats per minute. 185 days after explantation, the improvement in cardiac function was found to be stable. The patient has since gained weight and recovered significantly. He is now in NYHA class I-A. However, his pocket infection has yet to heal completely. Presently his post-explantation treatment is identical to that in the other 2 patients.

Patient number four (Table 1, Fig. 1): The postoperative course was completely uneventful, too. Anticoagulation was maintained as in the first and second patient, initially with heparin and later with coumarin. As in the first patient, echocardiographic examinations and A-β_1-AAB monitoring was performed once a week. Since his cardiac function had improved (LVIDd 52 mm; LVIDs 38 mm; LVEF 50%) after 25 weeks of support and the A-β_1-AABs had disappeared, the patient agreed to explantation of the pump 200 days after implantation. It is obvious that the time until disappearance of the A-β_1-AABs took much longer in this patient compared to the 3 others which might have been caused by the different type of assist device (25). Three days after explantation the following hemodynamic parameters were measured: cardiac index 3.2 1 m^{-2} min^{-1}, mean pulmonary capillary wedge pressure 8 mm Hg, mean pulmonary artery pressure 14 mm Hg, left ventricular enddiastolic pressure 9 mm Hg, resting heart rate 80 beats per minute, and no indications of mitral valve incompetence. The patient's post-explantation treatment does not differ from that of the patients above. Nine months after explantation the patient is also in NYHA class 1-A and exhibits stable cardiac functional parameters.

Discussion

Weaning patients with IDC from a mechanical cardiac assist system after more than 160 days of left ventricular unloading is a new and untried procedure whose success could not be guaranteed in advance. Confidence in the success of the weaning procedure was based upon the improvement in cardiac function as observed through echocardiography, the unexpected continuous decrease in humoral A-β_1-AABs in the sera of all the positive patients noted within the first 2 weeks after device implantation, and the conclusions derived from the following clinical observation.

A 34-year-old patient with clinically diagnosed IDC required mechanical circulatory support because of endstage cardiac insufficiency. Prior to implantation he had a cardiac index of 1.5 l m^{-2} min^{-1}, a left ventricular ejection fraction below 15%, a LVIDd of 71 mm, and a LVIDs of 67 mm. The patient developed severe cerebral bleeding after 55 days of support. As neurosurgery was indicated, anticoagulation therapy had to be interrupted. Therefore, the decision was made to discontinue mechanical circulatory support to avoid the risk of thromboembolism, whereby it was assumed that explantation and reimplantation of a new device might be necessary. Echocardiographic examinations performed after the pump was switched off indicated an improvement in cardiac function to a LVEF of 50%, LVIDd of 52 mm, and LVIDs of 39 mm. These parameters continued to improve over the next 4 days until the patient died due to neurological complications. The patient's A-β_1-AABs had decreased from 7.8 LU before surgery to 1.1 LU when circulatory support was discontinued.

This experience encouraged the proposal of weaning procedures, however, the scheduled weaning of 2 patients was compelled by the development of pump-related complications. A third patient was weaned as planned.

Following the hypothesis that an autoimmunological process might play a primary or secondary role in the pathogenesis of the development or maintenance of IDC, the disappearance of A-β_1-AABs was considered an immunological marker indicating a process which led to a reduction in cardiac antigenicity. Other anti-heart antibodies which also might have disappeared during the process of chronic left ventricular unloading were not measured. Therefore, the significance of A-β_1-AABs for the cardiac recovery process is difficult to assess. Nevertheless, A-β_1-AABs were noted in all of the 14 patients with IDC. Recent results have suggested that A-β_1-AABs are detectable in 80% of patients with IDC. Other autoantigens, such as the mitochondrial ADP/ATP carrier (35), the branched chain keto acid dehydrogenase (3), the cardiac myosin heavy chain (34), and laminin (23, 46) are observed less frequently in patients with IDC. Moreover, A-β_1-AABs were not found in patients with ischemic dilated cardiomyopathy whose cardiac function improved.

Using bioassay to indicate the presence of A-β_1-AABs is based on the stimulating effect they have and that this effect can be inhibited by beta-blockers. This leads to the hypothesis that A-β_1-AABs may also chronically produce a higher heart rate in patients, which may promote the development of IDC. Furthermore, this hypothesis is supported by the experience of the authors that reducing A-β_1-AABs through the selective immunoadsorption of immunoglobulin G in patients with IDC and a pathologic level of A-β_1-AABs leads to an immediate reduction in heart rate (unpublished data). In animal models chronic cardiac stimulation producing unphysiologically high heart rates (up to 240 beats per minute) leads to the development of dilated cardiomyopathy within 3 weeks (37, 38). Over a span of years the heart rate in affected patients is frequently in the range of more than 100 beats per minute as a result of continuous stimulation by A-β_1-AABs and severe cardiac insufficiency. The patients in this study all presented with heart rates above 115 beats per minute. It should be noted, however, that they all were on catecholamines.

Although β_1-adrenoceptors are not only limited to the heart, the probability that cardiac β_1-adrenoceptors were responsible for the observation of antigen presentation and the development of corresponding autoantibodies was rather high since the intervention achieved led to the disappearance of the antibodies, thus affecting the heart. However, why long-term left ventricular unloading leads to the disappearance of A-β_1-AABs remains unexplained. Nevertheless, a similar, yet inverse process has been observed: exercise in experimental autoimmune myocarditis resulted in associated augmentation of autoimmunity with cardiac dilatation (14). A prolonged delay in the disappearance of A-β_1-AABs has also been noted in patients supported with a cardiac assist device, which led to only temporary left ventricular unloading due to the mode of the device (25).

Within the group of patients whose A-β_1-AABs disappeared, differences were observed in cardiac function improvement compared to the other parameters measured. Although the cause for less improvement was not investigated, hearts with extensive dilatation (LVIDd greater than 76 mm) exhibited the least amount of functional improvement. This may have been due to the fact that these hearts had considerable structural changes and scarred myocardial tissue, and thus would have required much more time before recovering sufficient function. On the other hand, the LVIDd in weaned patients were at the lower range in this study cohort.

Regarding the lymphocytic infiltrate found in the myocardial tissue sample taken from the second weaned patient during device implantation, one has to consider that the clinical diagnosis of IDC was incorrect and actually should have been recognized as chronic myocarditis according to DALLAS classification criteria. Remarkably, this infiltrate could not be detected in 5 biopsy specimens taken after 235 days of mechanical support. However, it is too early to assess this observation. Immunohistology and immunocytology were negative in the first patient; tissue examination was not performed in the third patient.

Although the importance of A-β_1-AABs is still an open question which will require further intensive studies, the fact that today, 185 to 389 days after explantation of the device, all 4 patients exhibit stable cardiac functional parameters and no increase in A-β_1-AABs can be considered as confirmation of the clinical value of weaning. Monitoring A-β_1-AABs and performing echocardiographic examinations in patients with IDC opens the possibility for differentiating in advance between patients who may be weaned from the device and those who may not.

Weaning from the assist device saves donor hearts and costs and improves the quality and perspective of life in these patients compared to those who receive a donor heart. Since choosing the optimal time for assist device implantation has important clinical consequences, this decision should be made carefully after the patient's antibody status is known.

In conclusion, mechanical assisted circulation in patients with IDC and A-β_1-AABs leads to the concurrent disappearance of A-β_1-AABs and improvement in cardiac function. The degree of improvement most likely depends on the extent of cardiac dilatation prior to implantation. To date, four patients could be weaned from left ventricular mechanical support after A-β_1-AABs had disappeared and cardiac function had improved. The duration of support was 160, 243, 348 and 200 days, respectively. Functional parameters measured by echocardiography were found to be stable and no increase in A-β_1-AABs could be detected 389, 307, 299, and 185 days, respectively, after device explantation. This procedure represents a new concept in the treatment of patients with IDC on mechanical support systems which were originally implanted as a bridge to transplantation. At a time when donor hearts are scarce, this method will save donor hearts and health care costs and improve the quality of life and long-term perspective for patients after weaning in comparison to transplantation.

References

1. Abelmann WH. Myocarditis as a cause of dilated cardiomyopathy. In: Engelmeier BS, O'Connel JB (eds.) (1988) Drug therapy in dilated cardiomyopathy and myocarditis. New York: Marcel Dekker, pp 221–31
2. Ansari AA, Wang Y-C, Danner DJ et al. Abnormal expression of histocompatibility and mitochondrial antigens by cardiac tissue from patients with myocarditis and dilated cardiomyopathy. Am J Pathol; 139:337–54
3. Ansari AA, Neckelmann N, Wang Y-C, Gravenis MC, Sell KW, Herskowitz A (1993) Immunologic dialogue between cardiac myocytes, endothelial cells and mononuclear cells. Clin Immunol Immunopathol 68:208–14
4. Borda ES, Pascual J, Cossio PM, Vega M, Arana RM, Sterin-Borda L (1984) Circulating IgG in chagas disease which binds to β-adrenoceptor of myocardium and modulates ist activity. Clin Exp Immunol 57:679–86
5. Bristrow MR (1993) Pathophysiology and pharmacologic rationales for clinical management of chronic heart failure with beta-blocking agents. Am J Cardiol 71:12C–22C
6. Burch GE (1966) On resting the human heart. Am Heart J 71:422
7. Burch GE, McDonald CD, Walsh JJ (1971) The effect of prolonged bed rest on postpartal cardiomyopathy. Am Heart J 81:186–201
8. Caforio AL, Bonifacio E, Stewart JT et al (1990) Novel organ-specific circulating cardiac autoantibodies in dilated cardiomyopathy. J. Am Cell Cardiol 1527–34
9. Charlap S, Lichstein E, Frishman WH (1989) β-Adrenergic blocking drugs in the treatment of congestive heart failure. Med Clin North Am 73:373–85
10. Dec GW, Fuster V (1994) Idiopathic dilated cardiomyopathy. N Engl J Med 331:1564–75
11. Halle W, Wollenberger A (1970) Differentiation and behavior of isolated embryonic and neonatal heart cells in chemically defiend medium. Am J Cardiol 25:292–9
12. Hetzer R, Hennig E, Schiessler A, Friedel N, Warnecke H, Adt M (1992) Mechanical circulatory support and heart transplantation. J Heart Lung Transplant 11:S175–81
13. Holman WL, Bourge RC, Kriklin JK (1991) Case report: circulatory support for seventy days with resolution of acute heart failure. J Thorac Cardiovasc Surg 102(6):932–934
14. Hosenpud JD, Campbell SM, Niles NR, Lee J, Mendelson D, Hart MV (1987) Exercise induced augmentation of cellular and humoral autoimmunity associated with increased cardiac dilatation in experimental autoimmune myocarditis. Cardiovasc Res 21:217–22
15. Koessler A (1972) Myosingehalt und Aktivität der Kreatin-Phosphokinase in Rattenherz-Zellkulturen. Acta Biol Med Germ 29:119–34
16. Krehl L (1891) Beitrag zur Kenntnis der idiopathischen Herzmuskelerkrankung. Dtsch Arch F Klin Med 48:414–31
17. Leimbach WN, Wallin BG, Victor RG, Aylward PE, Sundhoef G, Mark AL (1986) Direct evidence from intraneural recordings for increased central sympathetic outflow in patients with heart failure. Circulation 73:913–9
18. Limar CH, Goldenberg IF, Limar C (1989) Autoantibodies against beta-adrenoceptors in human dilated cardiomyopathy. Circ Res 64:97–103
19. Magnusson Y, Wallukat G, Waagstein F, Hajmarson Å, Hoebeke J (1994) Autoimmunity in idiopathic dilated cardiomyopathy. Characterization of antibodies against the β_1-adrenoceptor with positive chronotropic effect. Circulation 89:2760–7

20. Magovern GL, Golding LA, Oyer PE, Cabrol C (1989) Circulatory support 1988: weaning and bridging. An Thorac Surg 47:102-7
21. Maisch B, Berg PA, Kochsiek K (1980) Immunological parameters in patients with congestive cardiomyopathy. Basic Res Cardiol 75:221-2
22. Maisch B, Deeg P, Liebau G, Kochsiek K (1983) Diagnostic relevance of humoral and cytotoxic immune reactions in primary and secondary dilated cardiomyopathy. Am J Cardiol 52:1072-8
23. Maisch B, Wedekind U, Kochsiek K (1987) Quantitative assessment of antilaminin antiboidies in myocarditis and perimyocarditis. Eur Heart J 8 (suppl. I):233-5
24. Metha SM, Aufiero TX, Pae WE Jr, Miller CA, Pierce WS (1995) Combined registry for the clinical use of mechanical ventricular assist pumps and the total artificial heart in conjunction with heart transplantation: sixth official report – 1994. J Heart Lung Transplant 14:584-93
25. Müller J, Wallukat G, Siniawski H, Weng Y, Hetzer R (1995) Reduction in β_1-receptor autoantibody level in patients with idiopathic dilated cardiomyopathy during mechanical cardiac assist system support. JACC special issue: 23A
26. Nakatani T, Sasako Y, Kumon K, Nagata S, Kosakai Y, Isobe F, Nakano K, Kobayahi J, Eishi K, Takano H, Kito Y, Kawashima Y (1995) Long-term circulatory support to promote recovery from profound heart failure. ASAIO J 41:M526–M530
27. Nomenclature and criteria for diagnosis of diseases of the heart and great vessels (1994) Ninth Edition. American Heart Association. Dolgin M (ed.). Bosotn: Little Brown and Company, p 240
28. Noon GP (1993) Clinical use of cardiac assist devices. In: Akutzu T, Koyanagi H (eds.). Heart replacement. Artificial Heart 4. Tokyo: sprigner-Verlag, pp 195–205
29. Pae WE Jr, Miller CA, Matthews, Y, Pierce WS (1992) Ventricular assist devices for postcardiotomy cardiogenic shock: a combined registry experience. J Thorac Cardiovasc Surg 104:541–53
30. Pae WE Jr (1993) Ventricular assist devices and total artificial hearts: a combined registry experience. Ann Thorac Surg 55:295-8
31. Pennington DG, McBridge LR, Swartz MT (1994) Implantation technique for the Novacor left ventricular assist system. J Thorac Cardiovasc Surg 108:604-8
32. Portner PM (1993) A totally implantable heart assist system: the Novacor program. In: Akutsu T, Koyanagi H (eds). Heart replacement. Artificial Heart 4. Tokyo: Springer-Verlag, pp 71–82
33. Radovancevic B, Frazier OH, Michael JM (1929) Implantation technique for the Heart Mate left ventricular assist device. J Card Surg 7(3):203–7
34. Rose NR, Beisel KW, Herskowitz A (1987) Cardiac myosin and autoimmune myocarditis. Ciba Found Sympos 129:3–24
35. Schultheiss H.P (1989) The significance of autoantibodies against ADP/ATP carrier for the pathogenesis of myocarditis and dilated cardiomyopathy – clinical and experimental data. Springer Semin Immunpahtol 11:15–30
36. Schultheiss H-P (1993) Disturbance of the myocardial energy metabolism in dilated cardiomyopathy due to antoimmunological mechanisms. Circulation 87 (suppl 5):IV43–IV48
37. Spinale FG, Tomita M, Zellner JL, Cook JC, Crawford FA, Zile MR (1991) Collagen remodeling and changes in LV function during development and revocery from supraventricular tachycardia. Am J Physiol 261(2Pt2):H308–18
38. Spinale FG, Zellner JI, Tomita M, Crawford FA, Zile MR (1991) Relation between ventricular and myocyte remodeling with the development and regression of supraventricular tachycardia-induced cardiomyopathy. Criculation Res 69(4):1058–67
39. Taha TH, Mazelka P, Oakley CM, Maisch B (1991) Cardiac-specific antibodies in dilated cardiomyopathy. J Am Coll Cardiol 18:644–5
40. Thomas JA, Marks BH (1978(Plasma norepinephrine in congestive heart failure. Am J Cardiol 41:233–43
41. Wallukat G, Wollenberger A (1987) Effects of serum gamma globulin fractions of patients with allergic asthma and dilated cardiomyopathy on chronotropic β-adrenoceptor function in cultured neonatal rat heart myocytes. Biomed Biochim Acta 46:634–9
42. Wallukat G, Wollenberger A (1988) Die kultivierte Herzmuskelzelle. Ein funktionelles Testsystem zum Nachweis von Autoantikörpern gegen den β-adrenergen Rezeptor. Acta Histochem (suppl XXXV):145–9

43. Wallukat G, Morwinski R, Magnusson Y, Hoebeke J, Wollenberger A (1992) Autoantikörper gegen den β_1-adrenergen Rezeptor bei Myokarditis und dilatativer Kardiomyopathie: Lokalisation von zwei Epitopen. Z Kardiol 81 (Suppl 4):79–83
44. Wallukat G, Boewer V, Förster A, Wollenberger A (1991) Anti-β-adrenoceptor autoantibodies with β-adrenergic agonistic activity from patients with myocarditis and dilated cardiomyopathy. In: Heart Failure Mechanisms and Management. Lewis BS, Kimchi A (eds.), Springer Verlag Berlin, Heidelberg 22:21–29
45. Wallukat G, Morwinski R, Kowal K, Förster A, Boewer V, Wollenberger A (1991) Autoantibodies against the β-adrenergic receptor in human moycarditis and dilated cardiomyopathy: β-adrenergic agonism without desensitization. Eur Heart J 12 (Suppl. D) 178–81
46. Wolff PG, Schulteis H.P (1989) Laminin distribution and autoantibodies to laminin in dilated cardiomyopathy and myocarditis. Am Heart J 117(6):1303–9
47. Wollenberger A, Wallukat G (1993) Adrenergic and antiadrenergic activity of cycloheximide in cultured rat hearts cells. Biomed Biochem Acta 42:917–929

Author's address:
Dr. J. Müller
German Heart Institute Berlin
Augustenburger Platz 1
13353 Berlin, Germany

Discussion Session, Morning of October 22, 1995

Hetzer: I can imagine that there are many questions, and we have many questions to the experts on the panel. I would like to structure the discussion into four main topics. The first one, on the controversies in the pathophysiology and the definition with the aim to maybe guess or delineate those patients who may qualify for such a weaning process. The second, whether we have any criteria on hand which would tell us which patients can be weaned, that is, whether we have any pre-implant or post-implant predictors which might indicate the extent of recovery possible through the use of an assist device. The third one, you have heard the last two presentations focusing on the autoantibodies against the β-1 receptor, as I think it may not be a unique opinion among the panelists as to the significance of those antibodies. And fourthly, to talk briefly about the treatment of a patient after explantation, that is, how to maintain the heart's recovered function and how to prevent the relapse of the underlying disease.

First of all, I understand our friend, Oscar Frazier, would like to show two slides before we go into the discussion.

Frazier: I was very fascinated by the discussion this morning. I have had a long interest in this recoverability of ventricular function, but I just wanted to remind you, the first slide please, in America, when I was a medical student, we had a cardiologist at Tulane University in New Orleans who was a very difficult man. His name was George Birch. He was sort of like the Dr. De Bakey of cardiology. He was a very strong authoritarian; the Germans would like him. But he also devised a plan for bedrest for patients with chronic heart failure. He wrote these patients up in the 1950s and 1960s and he put them to absolute bedrest. If they didn't adhere to absolute bedrest, in his papers he referred to such patients as the deserters, the deserters all promptly died. This is one of the statements he made in 1971 in the American Heart Journal. He was the president of the American College of Cardiology and of the American Heart Association. I think this is something that we have to look at again, that in fact the heart may improve if it's allowed to rest. A lot of the focus this morning was on that. The next slide shows an example of one of these patients. I don't want to belabor it by overextending this privilege, but you see, the patient had chronic heart failure, was put to bedrest for 6 months, his heart improved, he went back to work, his heart worsened, he put him back to bedrest, and the picture on the far right is after 6 years. These next 2 slides show examples of chronic bedrest, you see that the patients received 12 months bedrest. You can't do this today. These are all patients who were treated solely with bedrest. He summarized this from a group with idiopathic cardiomyopathy in 1972. There were 10 patients who obtained normal heart size with such bedrest. Again, it was an impossible situation. Dr. Robicsek reminded me that you had to give many of these patients morphine, I suppose they became morphine addicts, to keep them in bedrest for a year. It's an awful thing, but George Birch could do it. But he couldn't do it with all of them. As you see the ones who left the hospital, those were the deserters, all died. So I would like to say that this is a very important aspect. I appreciate Dr. Hetzer bringing this conference to address this enormous clinical potential of left ventricular assist devices.

Hetzer: Thank you very much. I think this was very important, because bedrest, ACE inhibitors, and left ventricular assist devices may probably all have the same effect on the heart. The difficulty in our patients was just that, at the time of implantation, they were in such bad condition. Regarding the usual criteria for putting a patient on the assist device, we actually would have assumed that they would die within the next 2 days. However, we had no other choice. I think just leaving them in bed would not have solved the problem in such patients. So we are just talking about one step further in the severity of the disease. But let me come back to the first question that I would like to discuss with the panelists. We have heard a more modular system of cardiomyopathy, chronic myocarditis, in contrast to the previous more uniform understanding of this disease. The question is, which type of the disease will probably qualify for recovery, all of them, or only some of them. No one can probably answer this presently, but I would like to ask the panelists for their opinions. In which patients should we attempt such treatment. I would like to start with Prof. Schultheiss.

Schultheiss: Thank you very much. I think that is really a difficult question. I can only surmise, because I think thus far we don't have the data. My personal opinion is that probably, primarily those patients who have chronic myocarditis might be those who have the best chance to improve. I think that unloading the heart probably will decrease cell death. We have a lot of indications that in chronic myocarditis there is a certain amount of cells dying all of the time. So unloading the heart will probably stop this process, and that probably will also stop the immunological process against cell particles of the myocardium. Secondly, the auto-immune reaction goes down and that probably will at least produce a positive result. If you look at the data shown today concerning the β-receptor antibodies, you see that the antibodies go down. We will discuss this later on, but I think, for my opinion, that is only an indication that an immunological process in the beginning was there and that the immunological process slows down. So, it might be cytokines, it might be other antibodies, it might be cellular infiltrates, there are a lot of possibilities, but for me, there is a very strong indication that by unloading the heart you probably bring down the anti-myocardial process, and that probably will be the most important indication for improvement.

Hetzer: Let me extend the question somewhat. How about other types of cardiomyopathy? Toxic? Post-alcoholic? Inherited? And, is there a stage of the disease, as Prof. Maisch has indicated, which probably precludes recovery?

Schultheiss: For alcoholic cardiomyopathy, if it's in the endstage, I have no opinion. What we think is that you get a change in the membrane composition of the proteins and that this change is the main factor making the heart deleterious. For the inherited form, we don't know the percentage yet. What we find in the literature, there are two or three papers now, assumes that it might be about 20%. I think that number is much too high. My personal opinion is that if you have a genetic basis for cardiomyopathy, probably it is the basis to get an immunological process. In my opinion so far, in contrast to hypertrophic cardiomyopathy, we have no indication that there is really a single protein which is the cause for dilated cardiomyopathy. If that is the case, I think this process can't work. If you know, for example, a contractile protein is not processed in the regular way, then I can't understand how an assist device should help. I think it has to be something coming from outside the myocardium which depresses function. If you unload the heart and you stop this process, then the myocardium has the possibility to recover again. I don't suspect a genetic basis for cardiomyopathy.

Maisch: I think it's difficult to really pin down the points. My educated guess today would be that the patient who has an infiltrate, which may be reversible, is probably the one who profits. The patient who has little fibrosis is the one who profits. A patient with increased cytokine levels, observed by monitoring immunological activation, will profit. A patient who may have an antibody to the β-receptor, but also to many other cardiac epitopes, because this is a multi-faceted disease, may profit. A patient in the endstage of fibrosis, and I have shown you slides on this, will have a hard time to profit. Also, we know that unloading the heart and that ACE inhibition will also induce a reparative process that could decrease the content of collagen tissue and perhaps, as observed in animal experiments, reverse hypertrophy. But they will have a harder time. These are the points to which I would fix my opinion about who qualifies for treatment with a mechanical assist device, if this is truly endstage, or who should be ordered bedrest or restrained physical activity and have immunosuppression.

Hetzer: So, you could probably say that at this very point, as to the amount of fibrosis, that two large groups of heart disease, the ischemic and the cardiomyopathic, meet, that is, with ischemia the amount of hibernating myocardium will also predict the extent of recovery. Would you agree with that?

Wallukat: I think the problem with ischemia in all trials that involve unloading the heart or using positive inotropes is that we really cannot define which is truly aneurysm, and that is not cardiomyopathy, and which is the still well perfused part of the heart which has cardiomyopathy of overload. If this is the case, and this is the last proportion, they might profit as well, but their recuperation will be much more difficult the larger the aneurysm. That can't change. It will be there.

Waagstein: I guess that those who will benefit from an assist device will be the same who benefit from β-blockers, because there are two different ways of unloading. That would exclude, to our knowledge, two groups: those with strong heredity which does not react well to β-blockers and those with extreme fibrosis. There is some work from Japan telling us that those with extreme fibrosis might not react as well to β-blockers as those without. To that I would also add those patients with a relatively short history of fast deterioration. If they have had it for 10 or 20 years and are in the endstage, I probably would not expect that they will have such a dramatic improvement from the device. If you have a short history that would of course include the group we suspect to have had myocarditis, which is of course impossible to distinguish between that and dilated cardiomyopathy, as we heard today. So, short history, not too much heredity, and not too much fibrosis, but how can we test that. Well, we try to look at the wall movement by giving an infusion of dobutamine and if they have, let's say, if some of these stunned or hibernating myocardium will start to move a little better, there is the chance that they also will improve on β-blockers. We do that as part of a study, not only with idiopathic dilated, but also ischemic cardiomyopathy.

Regitz: I would agree on most points with Dr. Waagstein. I would focus on his first point that patients where an active disease process occurs might be the first to be treated. We do know there is a group of patients going rapidly down in ejection fraction from 40 to 20% and there is a group of patients that remains stable at 15 to 20% for years and years, where the first group would be the good one. But I would not agree with his point of focusing on fibrosis, because the myocardium really is relatively plastic. As we have seen after treatment of aortic stenosis, there is a relatively large capacity of the myocardium to remodel. I'm not so sure we should just use an acute test to see if there is a contractile reserve. There may be a reserve that only appears with long time testing. To detect acute disease processes, we have so far made relatively bad correlations between auto-immune markers and the disease. I would also like to focus your attention on a group of young patients, perhaps Dr. Wallukat might elucidate further on this, with perfectly normal left ventricular function, just sinus tachycardia, and we had the experience that quite a large number of these patients, where we have sent blood to Dr. Wallukat, have high titers against β-receptor autoantibodies, but observed over a long period, these patients still had normal function. So, there must be something additional which we have not yet discovered. But until we have it, I would take the patients with an active clinical process.

Wallukat: We think that immunological activity is one of the important things for the recovery of the heart function. If the antibodies were removed from the heart by immunoabsorption or by immunosuppression, as shown by Dr. Schultheiss, then I think the recovery of the normal heart function is possible. Dr. Regitz explained that the patients with arrhythmia and tachycardias also have such antibodes. It was very interesting that patients with Chagas disease have the same things. The Chagas patients have all such antibodies against β-adrenoceptors. The first information that the Chagas disease has developed in a patient is arrhythmia. Perhaps some of these patients with arrhythmia would also develop cardiomyopathy later.

Unger: From a surgical point of view, I have a different opinion about these problems. The question is the recoverability. Mostly what we see is that when we unload the heart, partially or wholly, then it's possible to reestablish the normal metabolic situation in the heart. From what we could learn today is that there are different factors, there is myocarditis leading to metabolic disorders, or other diseases, and I see for recoverability three classes. In class 1 are patients who have a metabolic disorder with no scars and no fibrosis in the heart. In class 1 we have a good chance to wean the patient from the device. In class 2, with fibrosis, it's questionable if we can wean the patient and in class 3, with scars to a various extent, and severe fibrosis and, as Dr. Maisch stated, with aneurysm, there is no positive result to be expected. I see the question as being the potential of the recoverability to reestablish the metabolic situation.

Müller: I would like to add something to Dr. Regitz. I think we don't know at which time of cardiomyopathy the autoantibodies develop. We want to find out from the sera we can get from the Robert Koch Institute, the first was taken in 1984, and I think we have to follow up the patient exactly. If you now have a patient with a high level of autoantibodies, it doesn't mean that this patient will remain stable for the next 5 years. It may be you have diagnosed a patient at a very early stage of this process.

Waagstein: We published a paper a couple of years ago and saw no correlation between ejection fraction and the titer of the autoantibody for the β-1 receptor. So, there is no strong correlation there.

Schultheiss: One thing about the fibrosis, I'm not so sure that a high grade of fibrosis is a contra-indication for an assist device. I would just offer the opposite. I think that might be the important difference between medical treatment and a mechanical assist device, because we know, and we are just going on in this study, that it's not only the fibrosis that means more fibrous tissue, but it's a change of the sub-types of collagen, the ratio between collagen 1 and collagen 3 changes. You get a more stiff fibrosis in the myocardium. Over time, if you unload with ACE inhibitors, for example, you change the composition of the collagen. So I just would suspect if you have a heart which has a high grade of fibrosis which is not becoming better under medical treatment, exactly that might be the patient who could improve with a mechanical assist device, because then you give the heart the chance to come back to the normal composition of the collagen content.

Maisch: It is known from physiological experiments that the trigger for hypertrophy is stretch, that the trigger for fibrosis is not load, but neuroendocrine activity. When one unloads the heart mechanically only, then I would not expect very much with respect to regression of fibrosis. If this is combination therapy, unloading the heart mechanically and then giving ACE inhibitors or β-blockers, I would expect that what Dr. Schultheiss has described could work, but it will need much more time than by just mere unloading to improve heart function. It has to be a combined therapy, not mechanical alone.

Hetzer: You know, I think the danger is that we get stuck now with a principle discussion. You understand as a surgeon I have a few pragmatic questions which I would like to discuss with you, since I have you here together today. We have to differentiate. Up to now our indication for implanting of such a device was an emergency situation in a patient whom we could not handle with any other means. When we come to the conclusion that this type of treatment may be something which we should apply electively in patients with severe forms of myocardial diseases, however, not in emergency situations, I think we have to know very well who are the patients who would profit from such treatment. That's my next question. Do we have fairly reliable criteria on hand which would tell us which of those hearts can potentially recover. That means, when you focus on fibrosis, can you tell us what is the amount of fibrosis, when you focus on antibodies, how reliable are those before implantation, or any other criteria or diagnostic tests which can tell us at least with some reliability that this heart may recover. Dr. Müller has shown that the very preliminary data that we have indicates that there may be some relationship to the size of the heart. I'm not so sure whether we can hold this border of 72 mm diameter very closely, but I assume there may be a border somewhere. Could you try to answer this question? Do we have any criteria on hand to tell us beforehand what potential of recovery such a heart may have.

Müller: We have looked at the autoantibodies in a group of 26 patients now. As I showed in my slides, 10 patients had a left ventricular diameter of more than 72 mm and these patients did not recover during left ventricular unloading, well, they did recover, but they didn't recover enough to a level which we consider within the normal range. The patients with an internal diameter of less than 72 mm did recover and achieved a level which we could accept as nearly normal. Patients with a diameter of more than 90 mm didn't recover, even if the autoantibodies decreased to undetectable levels.

Schultheiss: For my opinion, we don't have to give a short answer. You can think about a lot of things, it may be cytokines, it might be fibrosis, it might be a combination, it might be the energetic state of the myocardium, it might be the size. So, I think we just don't know. We have to learn more. I think we really have to sit together and make a program to analyze patients treated with a pump and then look with a second view to see what is at follow-up and what can we then find out afterwards, which might be the good indications.

Hetzer: But you understand, this is a vital question for a surgeon when he goes from the life-saving procedure of implantation of an assist device towards an elective procedure to let the heart recover.

Schultheiss: I agree totally, but for my opinion, we are only speculating. For example, I just talked to my neighbor when you looked at us and he told me we did look for fibrous tissue. But if you only look at histology, you can't quantify fibrous tissue in the myocardium, you have to use molecular biology. So, there are a lot of things to be done to really get an exact answer on what is going on.

Hetzer: How about an advanced type of echocardiography or PET, is there a potential to find out the amount of fibrosis?

Schultheiss: For my opinion not, because it's not only the content of fibrosis, but also the composition of the different collagen types which make the difference in stiffness and so on. That is the main point.

Maisch: I think there is very little to add. This is also my view. We are at the verge of a very interesting fascinating new method and we just don't known to whom it should be applied. As I have said, excessive fibrosis is still a problem, I guess. A very short disease time, I think, is very helpful for making the indication for the pump. An infiltrate in a patient with cardiac decompensation is also a helpful indication, because they don't profit from heart transplantation, you know that from the registry. Those are the three things I would put first and the others are still matters of discussion.

Waagstein: I will say again, I get the question with the β-blockers, who will benefit from it. I still say I don't really know. Since we have a 60% success rate with β-blockers, we can do it with all. I agree with Dr. Schultheiss that we know too little about it and I think we should have some sort of investigation now in a lot of patients. That will again be the short history and maybe not too strong a history of heredity. The fibrosis, I think, as this was pointed out by Dr. Regitz, the heart is plastic and we don't really know that much of the fibrosis could disappear, because they have a short lifetime. So, I think we should not exclude those patients with fibrosis from the beginning. We need to learn more and I think we should include all of the patients with a short history and then we should sit down after the first 100 and discuss what are the results of that. I think we need to do that, otherwise we will be too limited in our patients and we will maybe exclude patients who could benefit.

Hetzer: I will take the liberty to ask Dr. Frazier on the basis of which diagnostic criteria would he place a patient on an assist device, let's say, with advanced cardiomyopathy, but not with untreatable failure.

Frazier: Well, I think this is a very interesting question. This discussion reminds me a little of Shakespeare's comment that a thought which quartered had but one part wisdom and there were three parts cowardice. We might be thinking too much about this to some degree. I think as surgeons we are often cowardly, to quote Shakespeare again, the hue of resolution is sickled over with the pale cast of thought. We're thinking too much, I think. One of the questions I would ask Dr. Schultheiss is if the etiology of this couldn't be a common toxin that results in an abnormal physiology or anatomical state of the heart such that by chronic unloading, we may restore the function of the heart? I think this is a fundamental question. It's not so much why they get bad, as why they get better. It's important that in Birch's studies, the average duration of heart failure on those patients was 4 years. Dr. Maisch I think commented on his patients being acute, but he had recovery in patients with long-term heart failure. So, with a long-winded approach, I would say first of all, it's good to do the studies which Dr. Müller has pointed out, and we reported those also, that the heart does improve with long-term unloading. What we'll discuss in America, I think, is trying to start a chronic trial. The cardiologists are well familiar with these large volume trials, and I think this is like an area that we are going to have to approach the β-blocker studies. We're going to have to get enough volume of patients with a strict protocol of entry for long-term study of recovery in European and American centers to dictate this. For the present, I have been reluctant to remove any of these patients, because I didn't have criteria of recovery. But I think these criteria of recovery might well be delineated in a protocol fashion that we could study properly with controls. That's going to be hard also. As far as right now, we're restricted by the FDA in that we can't use those devices except in the same group of patients that you use them in, the very sick patients. It would be, when we start our study which we're going to assess this afternoon of elective implantation, if you will, to core out a sub-group of these patients to study for recovery. My impression would be to take the ones that are the dilated cardiomyopathies, because in spite of Dr. Schultheiss' ruminations on the nature of fibrosis, I think generally as a surgeon when the heart is fibrotic, it doesn't recover. But I do think that the cardiomyopathic patients, idiopathic cardiomyopathy, would be the best class of patients and certainly to try to intervene before the heart is too deformed. I discussed the 7.2 cm, I think there is going to be a limit. So, I think the anatomic size, the etiology, and the age of the patient would be the three determining criteria in this study.

Schultheiss: I would just like to add one thing, because I think you understood me wrong. Every dilated cardiomyopathy has an enormous amount of fibrous tissue, much more than in a normal heart. I didn't talk about ischemic cardiomyopathy with an aneurysmatic situation, or things like that. I just talked about dilated cardiomyopathy with a certain amount of collagen in it. That's what I mean. The more severe dilated cardiomyopathy is, the higher the collagen content is. Also, it is very broadly around every single cell, you find collagen if you look for it. That is what I mean. In this diffuse collagen content, you get the shift I was talking about. So, that is not contradictory, what you said and what I said. That's exactly what I mean.

Regitz: Well, I don't have any really good criteria. We know there is a change in gene expression in the failing heart and we have to work harder to understand these changes in gene expression. It may be that if these changes are not hereditary, but are induced by any external stimuli, then we should be able to describe these changes and by unloading the heart, we should give the cells a chance to recover their initial gene expression, to come back to the normal program, and then could try to maintain this. So, I think we have to look in more detail what really happens at the level of gene expression in the failing and the recovering heart.

Wallukat: I think that unloading plays a very important role, because we have some data from some patients with the assist device operating synchronously and asynchronously. In the patient in which the assist device operated asynchronously, the antibodies disappeared nearly 5 weeks later and the improvement of the heart function was also later than in the hearts which were supported by an assist device which operated synchronously.

Robicsek: After several of the speakers this morning have said that they don't know what dilative cardiomyopathy is, you very unfairly ask them to divide it into groups. I would stipulate that besides not knowing what the disease is, we don't really know how this mechanical support helps. The mere word "unloading" as the key word for cure reminds me when, while in the operating room, we "send the heart on holiday", that is leaving it on bypass. I think the key word is really to relieve myocardial stretch and decrease the size of the heart. The decrease in the size of the heart is not a symptom of improvement, but it is the cause of improvement. I think both are indications of measuring the success, we may concentrate on heart size. There are some very interesting data pouring out right now from Brazil. It's very interesting that Prof. Wallukat mentioned Chagas disease, which is really a physiological model, and cardiac surgeons are cutting out half of the heart's in Brazil very wildly and are finding an amazing improvement in cardiac function by decreasing the size of the heart and decreasing myocardial stretch. So I think the crux in the whole matter is to decrease heart size with mechanical circulatory support and you get improvement secondary to the decrease, and not vice versa.

Hetzer: Does anyone in the audience have any questions or comments about these two fields, pathophysiology and diagnostic criteria for recovery?
    Let me come briefly to the question of the significance of the β-1 autoantibodies. It's fascinating to see how they inversely correlate with the function of the heart. However, I would like to ask the panelists, is this, as Dr. Wallukat has indicated, a pathophysiological mechanism, or are they a marker for heart failure on the whole, visible in every kind of heart failure on the contrary? I would like to hear your opinions on this.

Müller: For all of our trial the β-1 autoantibodies were used as a marker. This has to be very clear. We use it as a marker and nothing else. I think there is no correlation between the reduction in autoantibodies and the increase in ejection fraction. This relationship may be caused by things we don't know at the moment. We also observed β-1 autoantibodies in the sera of patients with infarction. I think some patients not only have ischemic heart disease, they have a mixture of chronic myocarditis or immunological myocarditis and ischemic heart disease.

Schultheiss: I have two opinions. I also think it's only one indicator that an immunological process is going on. I think before we can say that these antibodies against the β receptor are really the cause or the consequence for failure or recovery, we really have to look for other factors, for example, cytokines, and so on. I think we don't have to discuss that. But there's a second idea which comes up in my mind, and that is myasthenia gravis, where you have antibodies against the acetylcholine receptor. We know very well that the disease is paralleled by these antibodies. Again, that's an epitope on the cell surface, like the β receptor is too. There you can show if you make immunoabsorption and you put out the antibodies, the patients become better. I think the data Dr. Wallukat showed today at least go in the same direction. For my opinion, it might be that the antibodies against the β receptor are important for myocardial function, but so far I don't think we have enough data to draw this conclusion.

Hetzer: I think Dr. Müller should reply to this, because we have the first patients whom we have treated with immunoabsorption only.

Schultheiss: Yes, I saw that and that gave me the idea about myasthenia gravis, where you make exactly the same. I think so far you haven't shown that there are other factors which might be as important or even more important and that these are removed through immunoabsorption, too. I think that is the problem with looking for only one thing and, before we have proven it, that means we exclude other factors, we can't say that is the single factor.

Maisch: I think as with any inflammatory disease, as with myocarditis as well, there is a microheterogeneity of antibodies. If we use one marker and then correlate with that marker, we always get some type of correlation. In 1974 we did that with the anti-myolemal antibody, Hans Peter Schultheiss did this with the ANT antibody, and he does it with the β-adrenoceptor antibody. I think that from that historical experience one would say that most of those antibodies do their job quite well as being disease markers, but if they are really markers of prognosis and markers of pathophysiology, you can always prove in vitro and not in vivo. My personal feeling is that since this is a picture with many facets, it will be an important one. As long as the correlation is positive, we use ours and you use your markers for monitoring the disease process. If we do have pathophysiological data available in vivo or in vitro that they contribute to the deterioration or the improvement of function, this is fine, but always keep in mind, this is a complex disease and not a one protein, one antigen operation.

Waagstein: We have to be honest, we don't know. We have some evidence both pro and contra. We are investigating if you can cause the disease in animals by immunizing with β-1 antigen and it seems like we could at least have early stages of cardiomyopathy, but we don't know if it is the cause of the disease. What we know is that β-blockers work. If it fits with the theory that it could be so that we are antagonizing these antibodies, it should be one way of treating them. We need to do more work, we need to study it, and we need to follow these titers and see whether they are different when we have a β-blocker or when the β-blocker is not there.

Regitz: According to Dr. Waagstein, we need much more work. I think you have found in your setting that the antibody is a wonderful marker, at least of cardiac function, but there are other papers. A paper from Dr. Linas where it is not a marker of decreased function and also in patients with normal function and tachycardia it is not a marker of depressed function. But I think you can be very close with the data with the patient sera which you have now. Perhaps in about half a year you will be at a point where you can answer this question.

Wallukat: I think that the antibodies which induce a functional effect, for example the antibodies against ATP carrier for the cross reaction with the calcium channels of the sarcolemma or the β-1 adrenoceptor or antibodies against the muscarinic M-2 receptor which were also found in some of the DCM patients and in most of the Chagas patients, that such antigens could have an effect. I think that not only one antibody alone makes it. I think that the concept of different autoantibodies which are detectable in the sera of the patients could have an influence on cardiac function and can disturb the function of the cardiomyocytes.

Hetzer: So, there is more uniformity among the cardiologists than I expected. You're probably surprised why I didn't ask more surgical questions, for instance, the amount of unloading that is necessary to let the heart recover, but I don't think that we have enough time to go into this very interesting topic. I would like to briefly still ask the question: is there a need, and a need for what, to treat those patients after their hearts have recovered, after the pump has been explanted. As Dr. Müller has shown you, we administered ACE inhibitors and β-blockers. The question is, should we consequently treat those patients with immunosuppression, for instance, with steroids.

Müller: We treat the patients with ACE inhibitors and β-blockers more or less for safety reasons, because we don't know how their hearts will react after the explantation of the device. I think there is no need to treat the patient with steroids, because we have just shown that our immunological marker, the β-1 autoantibody, had disappeared. Why should we give the patients immunosuppressants?

Hetzer: But isn't this something which should be considered according to the type of disease?

Schultheiss: I agree with what you ask. I think it really depends on what the cause of the disease was. For example, I'll just ask you one question. If you have viral persistence, you won't eliminate the virus by pumping. We think, and there are a lot of data, for example by molecule mimicry, that the viral persistence might be the main factor for reactivating the immunological process. It would be very important to know whether these patients who improve have viral persistence. If they have it, I would suspect that it probably will reactivate this immunological process. So far they had it before. So again that is a question I think we can't answer yet, but we have to look before we put them on the pump, after we have weaned them from the pump, and we have to see what the follow-up is. So I could speculate that if there is a patient with viral persistence where you get a reactivation of the immunological process, these patients will probably profit, if you provide a specific treatment. If that is not the case and you have no virus in the myocardium, you have no cellular infiltrates, you have no other indications of an on-going immunological process, I wouldn't do that. I'm not sure that there are not factors which might reactivate it.

Müller: We didn't find any viruses in our four patients.

Hetzer: Yes, but I think it has to be considered in the future, and I would like to hear your opinion, although it is probably speculative in any case.

Maisch: I think if the pathogenic process still goes on and that you evaluate in this case after pumping, not by hemodynamics, but simply by biopsy, one should consider pathophysiologically or pathogenetically oriented treatment which may involve all the 3 treatment arms I have suggested for the European study on treatment. I read with great interest on the patient who was remodeled positively by pumping, and still has an inflammatory process in the heart, and still has viral persistence, either one of those, and then let that develop. If I may just add another sentence, I think you can really evaluate the value of pumping only and the effect of further therapy if you do it in a double blind controlled manner. It's extremely difficult to convince my cardiological colleagues to do a treatment study in a controlled manner, to have a controlled group and randomize. It would be important to have that also done with the mechanical assist devices that you have, because I think that spontaneous recovery in the DCMs we are talking about is extremely high, it's between 10 and 40%. As long as we don't know what the spontaneous recovery in your patients is, we can really judge only from a double-blind or at least randomized trial.

Hetzer: Yes, but you see, as I pointed out at the beginning, our indication for implanting the pumps was an emergency situation, that means it would be ethically unacceptable to randomize those patients, because that would mean death.

Maisch: But if you do it electively, it would be good.

Hetzer: I cannot take this responsibility upon myself. I know that some surgeons have been speculating on doing this. I guess it has been discussed to conduct such a trial. I think I'll wait for the results before I do this to the patients.

Maisch: If you have elective patients, I think one should consider it, not of course in patients in an emergency situation. I would agree on that.

Waagstein: I think your specific question was what to do with a patient after you have weaned him. I always say that since I am a believer in β-blockers, we should do a controlled study without β-blockers also. That means that we should maybe put them an ACE inhibitor, which is an accepted treatment, and that half of them go on with β-blockers and half of them without β-blockers. Then follow titers, follow their function, let's say up to 3 or 6 months, and then make a re-evaluation and then maybe we can get the answer on that. I would also follow the autoantibodies, not only against β-1 receptors, but also against ATP, ATP carriers, and myosines, or whatever you could find to see if there is a general activation of these autoantibodies and whether they could be suppressed by β-blockers or not. I think that is a very important question I would like to have answered.

Regitz: β-blockers in combination with ACE inhibitors might be the appropriate therapy of these patients after weaning, because the alterations in gene expression that characterize failing myocardia can be induced by the β-adrenergic system as well as the angiotensin system. It might be really better to block both systems than to block only one of them. But this treatment clearly has to be evaluated in a randomized trial after weaning.

Wallukat: I would like to point out that the patients treated with assist devices are not completely healed. The clone which produces the antibodies can be induced again by any infection. I think it's very important to monitor the patients after explantation.

Hetzer: But no immunosuppression?

Wallukat: I think it is also important to do the things that Dr. Schultheiss mentioned, because it is very important to detect if the viral infection is persistent or not, or is it coming back again. I think general treatment with immunosuppression is not needed.

Unger: If I were to be in the lucky situation to have four patients weaned from a cardiac assist device who have good ventricular function, I would stop any medical therapy. I would wait a little bit and make some echo studies and after a time I would re-evaluate them all. Maybe we could wait 2 or 3 months.

Hetzer: I'll tell you honestly, although the patient who has been off the pump longest now, 8 months, is doing well, I am still very concerned whether he will have the same type of disease a year from now. I think nobody knows this. I think it's just fair to really seriously consider prohibiting any kind of degeneration after such a procedure. It would only be logical to put those patients on afterload reduction, and if you are convinced of the concept, also on β-blockers.

Introduction to Afternoon Session, October 22, 1995

Hetzer: This afternoon's session focuses on the topic which I personally find the most exciting at present and for the near future. As you know the dream of all artificial heart developers since 1950 has been to develop a real substitute for the heart for permanent use. As you also all know, this has failed in several epochs and in several attempts. Also here in the city, such a development has a long tradition. Professor Bücherl and his group at the Berlin Free University in Charlottenburg have worked on an artificial heart for about 20 to 25 years. In fact, as of the early mid-80's, this was a fairly good substitute which I also had the pleasure to implant in 1987 in two instances for the purpose of bridge-to-transplantation.

But as you also know, those devices were not compatible with patient quality of life and the complications observed were tremendous. Now with more advanced assist devices which give the patients a high degree of mobility and also a very low complication rate in the long run, the concept of using such devices for permanent use has re-emerged. It has come to us, more or less automatically, because the patients who were put on such devices for the purpose of bridge-to-transplantation had in some instances such long waiting times for a suitable donor organ, that it already was a sort of semi-permanent use. It occurred to us as well, and as Dr. Loebe will show you, we now have eight patients who were on such devices for longer than 200 days. We have a patient who, after 470 days with an assist device, represents the longest ongoing case of such mechanical support worldwide. I have arranged for this patient to come visit us, so that he might answer any questions you may wish to pose.

Of course, this has also brought up the idea to purposely implant such pumps for permanent use, which we have also done in a few patients who we thought did not qualify for transplantation. This has opened a very important question. Of course society, and especially the insurance companies, are very concerned whether in the future no 90-year-old or 100-year-old person may be allowed to die peacefully, but instead will receive an artificial pump to prolong the life for a year or two. So, I think we as surgeons are now asked, at least in our country, to define the criteria and also the excluding criteria for such treatment. I think we have to do this in the immediate future.

I would like to ask the panelists, and the audience also, to try to give us some help and some ideas about how to approach this topic in the future. This is why I have asked for the opinions of Prof. Fox, an ethicist who for many years has dealt with patients with major surgery and artificial organ implants, of Dr. Watson from the FDA, who can explain the viewpoint of a national regulatory institution, and from prominent surgeons from around the world who have patients with permanent or very long-term implants. So I hope and expect that this will be a very interesting session.

The session is chaired by Dr. Noon from Houston who has witnessed one of the major developments in this field since the late 1960s or early 1970s and by my friend Reiner Körfer who heads one of the other large programs involving artificial devices in this country.

Dr. Noon:
There is certainly a need for artificial devices for the heart transplantation population. For instance, in the United States, there are approximately 2500 transplantations per year, and that is the limit of donors we have, with a potential of 40 000 patients who could be heart transplant recipients. Thus, the supply of donors will never meet the need for this population of patients. The other consideration is extending assist device support to patients with chronic heart failure who are not necessarily transplant candidates. I think that if we have a good device for this type of patient that it could very well be economical in that it would reduce the medicine requirements of these patients, it would reduce the hospitalization that these patients have, it also would improve their living and their ability to go back to work. So, it might prove to be very economical when we do have a permanent device which we can put in such patients. The question also is, which type of device are we going to be using, a pulsatile device, which is the only real long-term device we have available at the present time, or whether we should consider using a non-pulsatile device in these patients.

Epidemiology of heart failure

R. Dietz

Franz-Volhard-Klinik, Max-Delbrück-Centrum, Humboldt-Universität zu Berlin, Berlin-Buch, Germany

Introduction

Despite continuous improvement of diagnostic tools and therapeutic possiblities heart failure remains a major public health problem. Even worse, congestive heart failure (CHF) does not only represent a common, but also a growing and fatal disease.

CHF as a common disease

First, congestive heart failure is common. In the United States, more than 3 million adults are affected. Every year 400 000 new cases appear in addition. For Germany, the figures are somewhat less in proportion to the smaller population: about 1 million patients are treated for this disease, with about 100 000 new cases year (6, 9, 10, 15, 19, 20, 22).

CHF as a growing disease

Second, congestive heart failure is a growing condition. It is important to recognize that heart failure is the only major cardiovascular disorder that is increasing in:
– incidence
– prevalence
– and mortality.
   The "growing" of this disease occurs despite considerable advances in diagnosis and treatment.
   Therefore, the question arises, why do we observe this untoward trend?
   There are two possible answers:
– first, doctors and patients are now more aware of the symptoms of congestive heart failure. With improving of the diagnostic tools – especially echocardiography – more cases with impaired left ventricular function are detected.
– second, all our efforts in improving treatment of major cardiovascular diseases: i.e. valvular heart disease and coronary heart disease ultimately lead to an increasing number of patients who still have a cardiac problem. They will finally

either present as sudden cardiac death or – more likely – as patients with the chronic disease of cardiac failure. Thus, the more we are successful in treating the basic cardiac diseases, the more we get a growing population with heart failure.

CHF as a fatal disease

Third, congestive heart failure is a fatal disease. Its survival rates compare to malignancies.

This short summary may require some more exact data on prevalence and incidence of congestive heart failure.

Prevalence of CHF

Data from the Framingham Heart Study of 2 years ago concerning the prevalence of the disease in an unselected population (8, 20).

Prevalence is about 2% at the age of 60 and increases to more than 7% at the age of 80 (6, 11, 12, 15).

Incidence of CHF

The annual incidence of heart failure is less than 1% at the age of 60 and increases further with age (7, 10, 15).

Both in men and women coronary heart disease and hypertension prevail as underlying causes of heart failure.

Discharge rates for CHF

What data do we have to support the assumption that heart failure is a growing condition?

The rates of discharges for heart failure from US hospitals during the years 1973 throughout 1986 progressively increase for ages 55 to 74. The rate of rise is even steeper when we look at discharges for heart failure in individuals over 75 years (5).

This is not only true for the USA, but a similar trend is observed in Europe. In a study from Sweden the progressive increase for heart failure in the past 15 years is also obvious.

Survival after the onset of CHF

What are the data on survival when heart failure occurs?

In comparison to an age-matched population sample, life expectancy is sharply reduced after onset of congestive heart failure. This reduction in life expectancy is more pronounced in men where half of the heart failure patients are dead within 4 years after onset.

In women the comparable figure is 6 years (4, 14, 15).

For survival in terminal heart failure we may use the data of the CONSENSUS I trial (24).

The inclusion criteria fit well with the diagnosis of terminal heart failure; in the group treated conventionally at that time, survival rates amounted to 50% in 12 months.

Addition of ACE-inhibitors to the therapeutic regimen slightly improved the poor prognosis.

Prognosis related to the cause of CHF?

When prognosis in heart failure is related to the underlying disease, we are confronted with different sets of data: In the study of Franciosa, patients with coronary artery disease had a poorer prognosis as compared to patients with primary cardiomyopathy. In contrast, in the study by Wilson from the same year prognosis was equally poor in both subgroups with heart failure (23, 27).

There were no marked differences with respect to the survival rates when four large studies in severe terminal heart failure were compared: life expectancy is in the range of 1 year under these circumstances.

Vicious Cycle in CHF

These findings give reason to believe that once a critical point in the development of heart failure has occurred, then a vicious cycle is begun (Fig. 1).

It starts from a marked impairment in left ventricular function resulting in an increase in wall stress. An augmented wall stress is the biological signal which triggers a cascade of events ultimately leading to a change in phenotype of the left ventricle.

The change in phenotype consists in a change in mass and in composition of the myocardium. The response to the increased wall stress results in the activation of several growth factors. Since adult myocytes cannot enter the cell cycle again, the result is an unnatural growth response of the myocardium. However, these growth factors may not only lead to hypertrophy of the myocardium, but in addition to programmed cell death.

Our knowledge about factors regulating these processes in terminal heart failure is rapidly expanding. Especially the role of cardiac angiotensin II becomes progressively more clear. Its inhibition either by ACE-inhibitors (or more specific

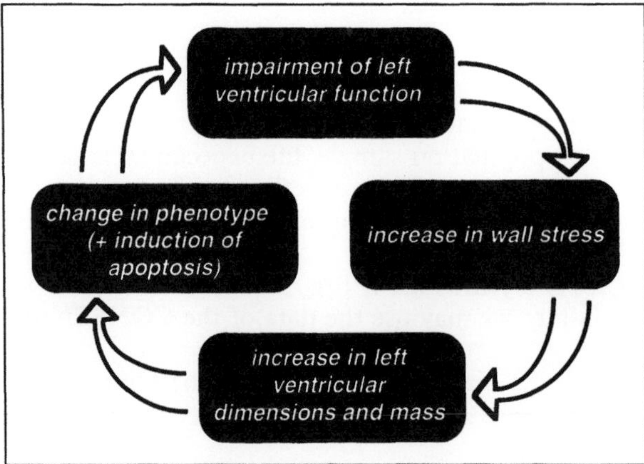

Fig. 1. Vicious cycle in CHF

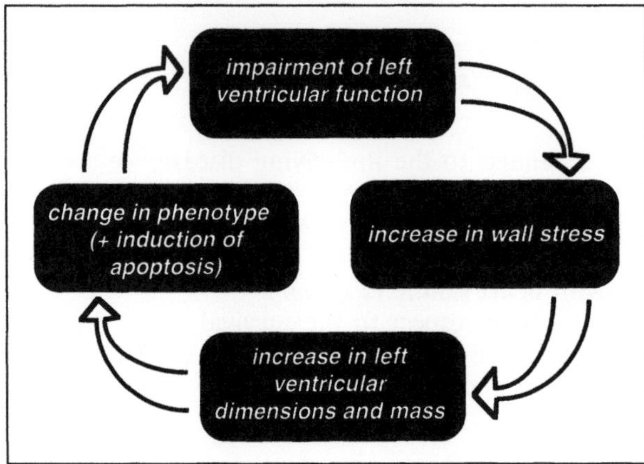

Fig 2. Reverse remodeling

AT-1receptor antagonists) represents the cornerstone of modern treatment of severe heart failure. However, we have to admit that even with the addition of this kind of drug, prolongation of life expectancy is modest. The success of treating heart failure is mainly restricted to symptomatic improvement (1, 17, 21, 26). New strategies require expansion of our present knowledge (3, 13, 16).

Reverse Remodeling

The concept of unloading, however, is still promising. It is expanded in its original conception by adding mechanical unloading to the therapeutic regimen when pharmacologic unloading has reached its end.

The emerging concept of reverse remodeling follows the idea of fully unloading the failing heart not only as an instant therapeutic measure but in addition as a means of interrupting the vicious cycle in heart failure.

First data presented by Dr. Levine's group indeed demonstrated a normalization of enddiastolic pressure volume relationships in hearts supported by left ventricular assist devices.

Reinforcement of such findings would clearly open a new scenario in the modern treatment of "refractory" congestive heart failure.

Impact of new therapeutic strategies

What is the impact of such a concept in treating terminal heart failure?

From an economic point of view, congestive heart failure is already a major health problem. It affects nearly 15 million people worldwide. It is listed in almost 800 000 discharge records in the USA representing a total of 5 million hospital days which equals 8 billion US dollars. In Germany, we spent about 7000 million marks for treating heart failure in 1985 (2).

Offering a new perspective for patients at the end of a common, growing and fatal disease during times of severe financial restrictions requires a thoughtful evaluation of new options for treatment.

References

1. Cohn JN, Archibald DG, Ziesche S, Franciosa JA, Harston WE, Tristani FE et al (1986) Effect of vascodilator therapy on mortality in chronic congestive heart failure; results of a Veterans Administrations Cooperative Study. N Eng J Med 314:1547–1552
2. Dinkel R, Büchner K, Holtz J (1989) Chronic heart failure Socioeconomic relevance in the Federal Republic of Germany. Münch Med Wschr 131:689–9
3. Eichhorn EJ (1992) The paradox of β-adrenergic blockade for the treatment of CHF. Am J med 92:527–538
4. Firth BG, Yancy CD Jr (1990) Survival in congestive heart failure: have we made a difference? Am J Med 88 (1N): 3N–8N
5. Ghali JK, Cooper R, Ford E (1990) Trends in hospitalization ates for heart failure in the US 1973–1986: evidence for increasing prevalence. Arch Intern Med 150:769–773
6. Gibson TC, White KL, Klainer LM (1966) The prevalence of congestive heart failure in two rural communities. J Chron Dis 19:141–52
7. Gillum RF (1987) Heart failure in the United States 1970–1985. Am Heart J 113:1043–5
8. Ho KKL, Anderson KM, Kannel WB, Grossmann W, Levy D (1993) Survival after the onset of congestive heart failure in Framingham Heart Study subjects. Circulation 88:107–115
9. Kannel WB, Belanger AJ (1991) Epidemiology of heart failure. Am Heart J 121, 3 (Pt 1); 951–7
10. Klainer LM, Gibson TC, White KL (1965) The epidemiology of cardiac failure. J Chron Dis 18:797–814
11. Landahl S, Steen B, Svanborg A (1980) Dyspnea in 70-year-old people. Acta Med Scand 207:225–30
12. Littmann D (1971) The natural history of congestive heart failure. N Engl J Med 285:1481–2
13. Litwin SE, Grossmann W (1993) Diastolic dysfunction as a cause of HF. J Am Coll Cardiol 22:49A–55A
14. Massie BM, Conway M (1987) Survival of patients with congestive heart failure: past, present and future prospects. Circulation 75 (suppl IV) 75:IV-II-IV 19

15. McKee PA, Castelli WP, McNamara PM et al (1971) The natural history of congestive heart failure: the Framingham study. N Engl J Med 285:1441–6
16. Packer M (1992) The neurohormonal hypothesis: a theory to explain the mechanism of disease progression in heart failure. J Am Coll Cardiol 20:248–254
17. Packer M (1992) Long-term strategies in the management of heart failure: looking beyond ventricular function and symptoms. Am J Cardiol 69:150G–154G
18. Packer M, Gheorghiade M, Young JB, Constantini PJ, Adams KF, Cody RF et al (1993) Withdrasal of dioixin from patients with chronic heart failure treated with angiotensin-converting-enzyme inhibitors. RANDIANCE Study. N Engl J Med 329:1–7
19. Parameshwar J, Shackell MM, Richardson A, Poole-Wilson PA, Sutton GC (1992) Prevalence of heart failure in three general practices in north west London. Br J Gen Pract 42:287–289
20. Schocken DD, Arrieta MI, Leaverton PE, Ross EA (1992) Prevalence and mortality rate of congestive heart failure in the United States. J Am Coll Cardiol 20:301–306
21. Sumita PD, Kunth KM, Eagle KA, Weinstein MC (1994) Costs and effectiveness of ACE inhibition in patients with CHF. Arch Intern Med 154:1143–1149
22. Sutton GC (1990) Epidemiologic aspects of heart failure. Am Heart J 120; 6 (Pt 2):1538–40
23. Teerlink JR, Goldhaber SZ, Pfeffer MA (1991) An overview of contemporary etiologies of congestive heart failure (editorial). Am Heart J 121:1852–1853
24. The CONSENSUS Trial Study Group (1987). Effects of enalapril on mortality in severe congestive heart failure: results of the Cooperative North Scandinavian Enalapril Survival Study (CONSENSUS). N Eng J Med 316: 1429–35
25. The SOLVD Investigators (1991). Effect of enalapril on survival in patients with reduced left ventricular ejection fraction and congestive heart failure. N Engl J Med 325:293–302
26. Uretsky BF, Young JB, Shahidi FE, Yellen LG, Harrison MD, Jolly MK et al (1993) Randomized study assessing the effect of digoxin withdrawal in patients with mild to moderate chronic congestive heart failure: results of the PROVED trial. PROVED Investigative Group. J Am Coll Cardiol 22:955–962
27. Yusuf S, Thom T, Abbott D (1987) Changes in hypertension treatment and in congestive heart failure mortality in the United States (2):174–9

Author's address:
R. Dietz
Franz-Volhard-Klinik
Max-Delbrück-Centrum
Humboldt-Universität zu Berlin
Wiltbergstraße 50
13125 Berlin-Buch

On the way to permanent support: Battery-powered, vented ventricular assist systems and other innovative new systems

O. H. Frazier

Cardiopulmonary Transplant Service, Texas Heart Institute, Houston, Texas, USA

Introduction

Ever since the beginning of research into cardiac support systems, the ultimate goal has been a mechanical device that can provide permanent circulatory support (defined as $\geq$ 5 years) and an enhanced quality of life, including maximal patient freedom. To fulfill this goal, such a device must be totally implantable, i.e., free of external connections. Ideally, it would also be durable, biocompatible, nonthrombogenic, infection-resistant, readily available in numerous sizes, and reasonably priced.

With respect to type of flow, cardiac assist devices are divided into two categories, pulsatile and continuous flow. Research efforts are being directed toward the development of both types. Continuous flow pumps are well suited to providing short-term (7-day) support, but they have not yet been evaluated for long-term implantation. On the other hand, pulsatile assist devices are able to offer prolonged safe cardiac support, as has been well documented in cases involving bridging to cardiac transplantation (5).

In designing pulsatile systems for permanent use, investigators have been hindered by the need to compensate for the gas volume created by the action of a stroke-type pump. The solution of an implantable volume compensation mechanism or compliance chamber has yet to be developed. However, pulsatile devices now exist that present ingenious solutions to the problem of volume compensation. These include vented left ventricular assist systems (both pneumatically and electrically actuated), which are being used clinically, and a redesigned total artificial heart, which is still at the experimental stage. These systems offer excellent potential for permanent implantation and are major focuses of research at our institution.

Vented ventricular assist systems

In the HeartMate left ventricular assist systems, volume compensation is provided by an externalized vent tube. In the electrically actuated (battery-powered) version, the vent tube exits from the motor chamber. The two most widely investigated battery-powered left ventricular assist systems are the Novacor Ventricular Assist System (VAS) and the HeartMate Vented Electric Left Ventricular Assist System (VE-LVAS). Because the latter device has undergone extensive evaluation at our institution and was the first to be used clinically (1), we will focus on it.

Novacor ventricular assist system

The Novacor VAS (Baxter Healthcare Corporation, Novacor Division, Oakland, California, USA) is an implantable blood pump monitored by an external drive console. The pump's outer housing is a fiberglass-reinforced polyester resin shell. In response to an internal solenoid that serves as an electromechanical energy converter, the pump's two pusher plates undergo compression, causing as much as 70 mL of blood to be ejected from the polyurethane pump sac. The inflow and outflow conduits are valved to maintain unidirectional blood flow. The pump and console are connected by a drive cable, which provides both power and venting. The pump may be operated in synchronous, automatic, or fixed-rate mode. The implantation technique is described elsewhere (7). The Novacor VAS is especially useful for staged cardiac transplantation. While being supported by this device, many patients are able to undergo rehabilitative treatment. Maximal mobility, entailing the option of outpatient treatment, is afforded by a wearable, battery-operated Novacor VAS that is currently undergoing clinical trials.

HeartMate

The HeartMate VE-LVAS (Thermo Cardiosystems, Inc. Woburn, Massachusetts, USA) is an abdominally positioned pump that comprises a flexible polyurethane diaphragm within a rigid titanium outer housing. The diaphragm separates the pump into two chambers, one for the motor and the other for blood. The inflow and outflow conduits consist of woven Dacron grafts, each containing a 25-mm caged porcine xenograft valve. The outflow graft has a 20-mm extension that is tailored to fit during implantation. To promote the creation of a pseudoneointimal lining, all blood-contacting surfaces except the valves are textured.

The pump is actuated by an electric torque motor located within the pump housing, on the nonblood side of the diaphragm. This motor activates the pusher plate and diaphragm by means of ball bearings. Once blood has been ejected, the pump fills passively. An electric lead and a vent tube exit from the motor chamber and are tunneled out the patient's left side. The system can operate in the fixed-rate and automatic modes.

With a total blood volume of 90 mL and a maximum effective stroke volume of 83 mL, the HeartMate VE-LVAS can provide a blood flow of up to 12 L/min. The entire device weighs about 680 g. Implantation necessitates a median sternotomy and an extended midline abdominal incision (6).

After implantation, the initial goals of therapy are appropriate nutrition and ambulation. Once patients can walk short distances, they gradually build up to energetic treadmill exercise. As the need for routine medical therapy becomes increasingly minimal, they are able to assume total self-care. Because the VE-LVAS requires only a small system controller and a pair of batteries, selected patients can leave the hospital and return to their normal physical and social activities. The batteries provide 6 to 8 h of power and are usually worn in an unobtrusive shoulder pack. For home use, patients are given a battery charger with a 51-cm power cable and a display unit. Because pump operation and maintenance require no specialized training, these tasks can easily be performed by the patient or a family member.

The HeartMate VE-LVAS has been implanted in 47 cases worldwide. At the Texas Heart Institute, clinical trials of this device began in 1991. As of July 1995, we had implanted the device in 9 patients. The longest support period undergone by a single individual has been 503 days (1). In that case, the explanted blood pump was remarkably free of wear and structural failure.

The HeartMate VE-LVAS has an implantable pneumatic counterpart (the IP-LVAS) that was approved for commercial use in the United States in 1995 and is now also commercially available in Europe and Japan. Both models have identical blood pumps and similar operating modes. Furthermore, both models permit treatment on an outpatient basis, because the pneumatic device has a portable console. Nevertheless, the VE model is the HeartMate with the most potential for use as an alternative to transplantation.

The Abiomed/Texas Heart Institute (THI) Artificial heart

The Abiomed/THI artificial heart is a pulsatile blood pump that has a centrifugal, electrohydraulic pump as an energy converter. The artificial heart was created jointly by Abiomed Cardiovascular, Inc. (Danbury, Massachusetts, USA) and the Texas Heart Institute (8). In this system, left- and right-sided flows are balanced by an internal volume compensator (an atrial flow balancing chamber).

The Abiomed/THI heart has reciprocating rotary valves, as well as an electromechanical switching mechanism that allows the flow of hydraulic fluid to be reversed with each heartbeat. Two trileaflet valves ensure unidirectional blood flow. Because commercially available valves are so expensive, Abiomed produces its own valves out of polyetherurethane (Angioflex), a material that the company itself developed.

Basically, the pump's stroke volume depends on the motor speed, which can change from beat to beat. The beat rate depends on the filling pressure, which is determined by a hollow center within the pump. As the right atrial pressure rises, flow increases accordingly, yielding an output of up to 10 L/min. Atrial attachment is achieved by means of textured, smooth-surfaced twist-lock connectors. During pump implantation in calves, the aortic cross-clamp time averages about 60 min, which is quite acceptable for this type of device.

The Abiomed/THI heart's unique method of volume compensation has proved highly satisfactory in calf experiments extending up to 162 days. Transcutaneous energy transfer is quite feasible with this system. Blood flow is exceptionally smooth and not at all hemolytic. Moreover, renal and hepatic function are well compensated. Another important benefit is the heart's near-total silence.

Thanks to its innovative design, the Abiomed/THI heart offers excellent potential for permanent implantation, and short-term clinical trials are expected to begin sometime after 2000.

Rotary pumps

Although rotary blood pumps are not yet suitable for long-term implantation, the current experimental versions have many benefits over pulsatile systems: they can be completely implanted without the need for either a vent or a compliance chamber, they can be small (thereby making them suitable for implantation in women and children as well as adult males), they do not require valves or flexing membranes, and they are less complex mechanically (thereby having the potential for greater reliability and durability). Further, they require minimal power, use fairly simple control systems, and tend to be relatively inexpensive.

One such pump, the Jarvik 2000 heart, is showing considerable promise in calf studies at our institution. No larger than the cardiac cannula of a conventional LVAS, this device is implanted via a left thoracotomy and placed in the left ventricle through a sewing ring in the apex. The 16-mm outflow graft is anastomosed to the thoracic aorta. In our laboratories, it has supported the cardiac function of five calves for an average duration of 120 days (range, 70-162 days). Like other axial flow pumps, it operates on the principle of Archimedes' screw. An important key to the potential of the Jarvik 2000 heart is the decision to use blood-immersed bearings in the pump (2). Blood-immersed bearings do not require lubrication and enable the device to be mechanically very simple and very small. Although the Jarvik 2000 heart is still in the experimental stage of its development, if its full potential is realized, it may be the most promising alternative to transplantation as we approach the 21st century.

Comments

Although a permanent cardiac substitute still eludes investigators, ongoing experience with temporary assist devices is paving the way for permanent support. So far, the most extensive experience has been gained with ventricular assist systems in bridge-to-transplant cases. The newest of these devices, battery-powered to provide maximal patient freedom, are offering patients an almost normal quality of life, including the option of outpatient treatment. Such treatment entails innumerable economic, psychological, and social advantages. Further, by augmenting end-organ perfusion, mechanical assistance improves a patient's overall status, thereby increasing the chance of successful transplantation and ensuring that scarce donor hearts are used effectively.

The innovative pumps that are the subject of this article appear to have overcome some of the obstacles that have plagued systems designed for permanent use. Indeed, the HeartMate's ability to support patients for extended periods is primarily due to the system's reliability, as well as the biocompatibility of its blood-contacting surfaces. Moreover, venting in the HeartMate and Novacor systems and the volume-compensation method used in the Abiomed/THI heart prove that a pulsatile pump can be used in ambulatory outpatients.

The next step on the way to permanent support involves defining the group of patients who would be expected to derive the most benefit from implantation of these systems on a permanent basis. The most likely candidates for initial clinical trials are patients with end-stage heart disease who are ineligible for transplantation and have exhausted all other conventional therapeutic options (1). Once permanent implantation has proved safe and effective in this population, it can be offered as an alternative to cardiac transplantation or long-term medical therapy.

In the United States, the need for permanent cardiac support is becoming increasingly urgent as the average age of the population rapidly increases. Experts have predicted that, by the year 2010, when America's "baby-boom" generation reaches retirement age, circulatory support may be needed by 70 000 patients per year in this country alone (2). In the long run, permanent mechanical assistance should prove less expensive than transplantation or the long-term care of patients whose cardiac status is severely compromised. It is to be hoped that such assistance will be available by the end of this century, if not sooner.

Despite the remaining obstacles, researchers are steadily advancing along the road to permanent cardiac support. As major milestones on that road, the above-described systems prove that the destination is well within our reach.

References

1. Frazier OH (1994) First use of an untethered, vented electric left ventricular assist device for long-term support. Circulation 89:2908-2914
2. Jarvik RK (1995) System considerations favoring rotary artificial hearts with blood-immersed bearings. Artif Organs 19:565-570
3. McCarthy PM (1995) HeartMate Implantable Left Ventricular Assist Device: bridge to transplantation and future applications. Ann Thorac Surg 59:S46-51
4. McCarthy PM, James KB, Savage RM, Vargo R, Kendall K, Harasaki H, Hobbs RE, Pashkow FJ, and the Implantable LVAD Study Group (1994) Implantable left ventricular assist device: approaching an alternative for end-stage heart failure. Circulation 90:II-83-II-86
5. Mehta SM, Aufiero TX, Pae WE Jr, Miller CA, Pierce WS (1995) Combined Registry for the Clinical Use of Mechanical Ventricular Assist Pumps and the Total Artificial Heart in Conjunction with Heart Transplantation: sixth official report – 1994. J Heart Lung Transpl 14: 585-593
6. Radovancevic B, Frazier OH, Duncan JM (1992) Implantation technique for the Heartmate® left ventricular assist device. J Cardiac Surg 7:203-207
7. Shinn JA, Oyer PE (1993) Novacor ventricular assist system. In: Quaal SJ (ed) Cardiac mechanical assistance beyond balloon pumping. Mosby, St. Louis, pp 99-115
8. Yu LS, Finnegan M, Vaughan S, Ochs B, Parnis S, Frazier OH, Kung RT (1993) A compact and noise free electrohydraulic total artificial heart. ASAIO J 39:M386-391

Author's address:
O. H. Frazier, M.D.
Texas Heart Institute
M.C. 3-147
P.O. Box 20345
Houston, TX 77225-0345, USA

The wearable Novacor LVAS at Henri Mondor Hospital

D. Loisance, D. Tixier, C. Baufreton, P. Le Besnerais

Service de Chirurgie Thoracique et Cardiovasculaire CNRS URA 1431 et Association Claude Bernard C.H.U. Henri Mondor

Summary

From March 1993 to February 1996, 8 patients have been selected, from a group of 40 patients in cardiogenic shock, referred for urgent cardiac transplantation. Immediate hemodynamical improvement allowed a rapid favorable evolution of organ dysfunction, a weaning off any IV inotropic support. The late evolution was as follows: one patient still on device after 164 days living at home. One patient died at 201 days as a result of the psychological sequellae of an embolic episode. Six patients have been transplanted, with a successful outcome in 5.

The experience allows comments on the problems related to right ventricular function, hemorrhagic and thrombo embolic complication and infection.

In the early 1970s, P. Portner introduced the concept of an implantable left ventricular assist device, connected between the left ventricular apex and the aorta, electrically powered, allowing prolonged survival. The system was designed to offer an alternative to cardiac transplantation. Since that period, continuous technological developments have permitted to evolve from an extracorporeal console based system towards the fully implantable system: in 1993, the wearable configuration was used clinically for the first time at Henri Mondor's hospital and rapidly adopted by many groups throughout Europe. This initial experience allows to evaluate the real problems raised by the survival of patients, suffering a major cardiac dysfunction, and about to die. These problems are of a clinical and technological nature. They also include ethical issues and economical considerations.

Analysis of the first eight cases of our group is the substance of the present report.

Clinical experience

Clinical material

Since March 17, 1993, the date of the first implantation of a wearable Novacor LVAS, to February 1, 1996, eight patients in cardiogenic shock, unresponsive to optimal medical treatment, have received a wearable LVAS Novacor as a bridge to transplantation. The pump was a N100 A in the very first case. The other seven patients received a N100 PC Novacor. These patients have been highly selected (1) among a population referred, in the same time frame, for urgent cardiac transplantation and/or mechanical bridge (n = 40): 13 presented some type of contra-indication for mechanical support and/or transplant (1), patients were treated with an external system including a centrifugal pump (n = 7) or a pneumatically driven extracorporeal pump (n = 11) (Nippon-Zeon system).

The characteristics of the 8 patients selected for wearable LVAS implantation are as follows: 7 male, 1 female, mean age = 34 years (range 17–45). Cause of shock was an acute idiopathic cardiomyopathy in all but two who suffered from a toxic myopathy and from myocarditis. Implantation occurred after 5.7 days (2–14) of intensive pharmacological support, because of the lack of improvement of the cardio-circulatory condition. At time of the decision, the main hemodynamical parameters were as follows: systolic aortic pressure: 88 ± 7 mmHg; cardiac index: 1.7 ± 0.4 l/min/m^2; range: 1.2–2.1; mean pulmonary arterial pressure: 33.7 ± 4 mmHg; capillary wedge pressure : 24.4 ± 5 mmHg ; right atrial pressure 21 ± 5 mmHg. Organ function was rapidly deteriorating, evidenced by anuria in 3.

Every patients was operated according to the protocol previously published (2).

Clinical evolution

Every patient could be weaned off IV drug within a period of 8 days. Free mobilization around the bed, in ICU, was achieved in all but one, before 11 days (range 8-15). In one case, free ambulation was made impossible because of a major right ventricular insufficiency. Discharge from ICU occurred after 14 days.

The patients were transferred to the regular ward, and submitted to an active physical rehabilitation program except for one. In the meantime, confidence in the system was enhanced by a progressive training in a self control of the driver, charger and batteries, and by temporary visits outside the hospital. Seven patients become fully ambulatory inside the hospital. The eighth had to be readmitted to ICU, for IV inotropic support of the right ventricle after 40 days. The seven patients doing well were proposed for being sent home; for reasons related to the living conditions, the first 4 patients were kept hospitalized and were allowed free ambulation, in and out of the hospital, until transplantation. The three other patients were sent home, and lived within a 2-h driving time distance. They lived with their relatives, as before implantation of the Novacor, taking care of the daily wound dressing themselves. They were readmitted once a week for 1 day to allow complete clinical examination, blood coagulation testing, and various tests such as transthoracic echocardiography, transcranial ultrasound echography (weekly), isotopic ventricular ejection fraction measurements, and stress testing on a treadmill (monthly).

Hemodynamical evolution

Rapid improvement during immediate post-operative period is observed in every patient (Table 2). As inotropic support was progressively reduced over a period of 5 to 7 days, cardiac index remained stable, associated to a low left ventricular preload, and there was progressive normalization of right atrial pressure. This profile was similar in every patient except two in whom right ventricular dysfunction remained severe (echocardiographic right ventricular ejection fraction stable, below 20%) or increased (case F.P.) The etiology in this last case was an evolving myocarditis.

Table 1. Clinical characteristics of the 8 patients, selected for Baxter Novacor LVAS bridge to transplantation

Patients	Date	Age (Years)	ABO type	Weight (kg)	Etiology
Re	3.93	44	A	78	Idiopathic
Vi	11.93	45	AB	70	Toxic
Li	1.94	35	A	50	Idiopathic
Ja	10.94	23	AB	54	Idiopathic
Cr	2.95	27	A	70	Idiopathic
Le	3.95	44	A	85	Idiopathic
Mo	9.95	21	O	65	Myocarditis
Pa	11.95	17	O	70	Myocarditis

Table 2. Hemodynamical evolution following LVAS implantation

	Cl $L/min/m^2$	Systolic AoP mmHg	PCWP mmHg	RAP mmHg
Before	1.6 ± 0.4	66 ± 12	25 ± 6	19 ± 7
12 hours	2.7 ± 0.3	98 ± 10	8 ± 1	12 ± 1
p	0.01	0.05	0.001	0.001

During the period of chronic support, hemodynamics were remarkably steady without any pharmacological support, except in the patient with persistent RV failure, who required diuretics.

Complications

Four groups of complications have been observed.

Effusion, both intrapericardial and in the pump pocket. Two episodes of tamponade, significant hemodynamically (decrease in stroke volume) occurred in 2 patients at days 13 and 10. The episode resolved after surgical drainage under local anesthesia.

Seven episodes of pocket effusion occurred in 6 patients, always early in the evolution (from day 8 to 27). They were treated by surgical drainage.

Septic complications: isolated fever without any positive culture was observed in 3 patients, resolving under IV anti-staphylococcic antibiotherapy. In one patient, a positive blood culture (acinotobacter) was observed and successfully treated. Pocket infection was observed in 2 cases after 19 days and 27 days, requiring temporary local irrigation.

Besides these minor episodes, one major complication occurred: inflow valve endocarditis, due to aspergillus infection, leading to inflow valve obstruction. Both valve conduits were changed via two small incisions under sedation. The patient condition immediately improved, both hemodynamically and on the mycotic point of view. Recurrence of aspergillus infection occurred despite prolonged encapsulated Amphotericin B IV therapy 3 months post transplantation.

Thrombo-embolism : two patients presented embolic complications: the first case presented one episode at day 22, (1-min episode of aphasia), followed at day 156 by a major complication (seizure, followed by coma, related to vertebral artery embolism). Each time, the episode occurred as atrial fibrillation spontaneously resolving into sinus rhythm. The last episode was followed by a progressive recovery of the cerebral function, but psychological disorders were observed, leading to death on day 201.

The second patient who presented embolic episodes at 47, 48, 49 days (hemiplegia and aphasia, transient) was the one with an increasing right ventricular dysfunction. The pump flow was reduced to 3.8 liters as right atrial pressure was increasing, tricuspid regurgitation maximal, right ventricular dimensions enlarged. The embolic episodes stopped when inotropic support (Dobutamine IV) permitted a rise in the pump flow in the 5.0 liters range.

In both cases, at time of explantation, the valves and the ventricle were free of any thrombus.

Right ventricular dysfunction

In two cases, the RV function did not improve during the period of assistance. In one, the clinical expression was minimal, limited to leg edema and oliguria, easily treated by lasex. In the second case, every echocardiographic index of right ventricular dysfunction progressively deteriorated after a 2-week stabilization. After 1 month on assistance, free ambulation became impossible. Orthostatic hypotension associated with a drop in pump flow were observed. Clinical condition became more severe, leading to IV inotropic support; During the period of low flow, three embolic episodes occurred over few days. The patient was listed for cardiac transplantation and transplanted on an urgent basis on day 62 post implantation.

Transplantation

Six patients have been transplanted, 5 electively, 1 on an urgent basis (case PA) after 100 days (52-169). One patient is still on the device, after 164 days. In the first 4 cases, the evolution was uneventful. In the last case, the urgent transplantation, death occurred rapidly, because of a disseminated intravascular coagulopathy. The pathological examination of the explanted native heart showed an envolving myocytolysis, extended to both ventricle, associated to a plasmocytic and lymphocytic diffuse infiltration, and subsequently explaining the lack of improvement of the right ventricular function.

Discussion

The experience accumulated since 1993 permits some comments on the actual evolution of prolonged mechanical circulatory support, both as a bridge to transplantation and as an alternative to transplantation.

The first comment deals with the major change induced by the wearability of the controller and energy power : it allows full mobility of the patient, making possible a full physical rehabilitation, a genuine feeling of return to an almost normal life. The real magnitude of the clinical impact of the change from a console based system to a wearable configuration – every other component of the system being identical – is by far more spectacular than we expected. One may even speculate that the additional improvement in quality of life due to the implantation of the controller and the primary energy pack will be minimal when compared to the one recently observed by the miniaturization of the extracorporeal components of the system.

The recent experience clearly illustrates the real issues of prolonged mechanical support. First, the acceptance of the system by the patient himself. The inconvenience related to the noise of the pump, to the necessity of an adequate management of the batteries appears surprisingly minimal. In the meantime, the facility with which the patient can take care of the system himself is also surprising, making obsolete the requirement of a caregiver, fully trained, living permanently with the patient. These observations confirm the feasibility of a long-term or permanent use of the system. Further technological developments such as reduction in the noise level, a more compact and efficient energy pack will increase confidence in the system and acceptance by the patient.

The second comment is related to the concept of monoventricular support itself. It is now clear that adequate circulatory support may be achieved in most cases by left ventricular assistance only as far as pulmonary resistances are not elevated. The adequate function of the left ventricular prosthesis is obviously best observed in case of a recovery of the right ventricular dysfunction. It is also observed (despite not being optimal) in case of persistent right ventricular failure and even in case of further deterioration due to the persistence or recurrence of the pathological process: in one of our patients, temporary periods of diuretics and inotrope therapy were required to maintain a satisfactory circulatory support. In another case, return to IV sympathomimetic therapy was made necessary, after 6 weeks of assistance, because of a continuously increasing further damage in the right ventricular dynamic by the initial pathology (myocarditis). The risks related to a major right ventricular dysfunction appears to be a limitation in the physical performance and, consequently, a reduction in the autonomy of the patient and an increased risk of embolic complication directly related to a low flow condition in the circuit.

The actual risks of the system are now more clearly seen than before. They are related to infection and thrombo-embolism. Infectious complications include minimal problems such as pocket contamination, which can be controlled successfully by local debridement, or irrigation, and major complications such as septicemia and endocarditis. The evaluation of the actual risk deserves more experience in each individual center or a well defined multicenter study. At the present stage of the experience, one may say that active treatment of major complications is possible, including replacement of parts of the system affected by the infectious process such as valve conduits.

Embolism is obviously the second major concern. This specific risk has led to an efficient anticoagulation, eventually associated with an antiaggregant therapy. In the two patients who suffered embolism, a hemodynamical problem was present, suggesting the major responsibility of flow conditions in the para-ventricular circuit and the native cardiac cavities as well: a reduction in the assist flow due to atrial fibrillation in one and major additional deterioration in the right ventricular function in one. It may be of interest to observe that transcranial Doppler studies of the cerebral arteries performed on a systematic basis brought different information: unusual high intensity transient signals the day before a major complication in one, no abnormal signal in the second case. In this domain also, more experience is needed to allow the technique its full potential to predict high risk of clinically significant embolic complications and consequently adjust the therapy : conversion of atrial fibrillation into sinus rhythm, additional inotropic support to the right ventricle or enhanced anticoagulation.

The last observation, made possible by the present experience, is related to the change in the level of investment, both in personnel and economics allowed by the wearable system, when compared to extracorporeal assist systems. A drastic reduction in the time spent by registered nurses and intensivists in the early stage of the post operative period reflects the more rapid return to a stable condition of the patient. The reduction in time requirement for practical nurses reflects the more complete autonomy of the patient and his higher mobility. These observations correlate with the drop in costs allowed by rapid discharge from ICU and hospital. The extent of the reduction in the various costs is such that after a few weeks, the difference in the initial cost of the system itself is reimbursed.

In conclusion, the present experience with the wearable Novacor assist system clearly shows that expectations are becoming reality, that risks related to the prolonged use of the system are minimal, and that a step towards permanent use as alternative to transplantation is being progressively made.

References

1. Loisance D, Dubois-Randé JL, Deleuze PH, Hillion ML, Duval AM, Tavolaro O, Romano P, Castaigne A, Tarral A, Cachera JP (1989) Pharmacological bridge to cardiac transplantation. Eur J Cardiothoracic Surg 3:196–202
2. Loisance D, Cooper GF, Deleuse PH, Castanie JB, Mazucotelli JP (1995) Bridge to Transplantation with the wearable Novacor left ventricular assist system, operative technic Eur J Cardiothoracic Surg 9: 95–98

Author's address:
Professeur D. Loisance
Centre de Recherches Chirurgicales Henri Mondor
Faculté de Médecine,
8, rue du Général Sarrail
94000 Créteil, France

Long-term mechanical circulatory support

R. Körfer, A. El-Banayosy, O. Fey

Department of Thoracic and Cardiovascular Surgery, Heart Center North Rhine-Westphalia,
Ruhr University of Bochum, Bad Oeynhausen, Germany

Introduction

Over the past decades major progress has been made in the field of heart transplantation; with a 5-year survival rate of 65% (3), it remains the only therapy for patients with end-stage heart failure. However, the resulting increase in potential organ recipients has not been met by an equivalent increase in organ donors. As an alternative, several devices for mechanical circulatory assistance have been developed. Since the waiting time for heart transplant candidates has increased, there is the need to provide devices for prolonged support and even for permanent support.

Our mechanical circulatory support program was initiated in September 1987 with the application of a Biomedicus centrifugal pump in a patient with postcardiotomy cardiogenic shock. Since October 1990, we additionally apply the Abiomed BVS system 5000; since March 1992 the Thoratec ventricular assist device, since March 1993 the implantable Novacor left ventricular assist device, and since April 1994 the pneumatic HeartMate (Thermo Cardiosystems, Inc.) (5). In our institution the last three systems are available for bridging to cardiac transplantation and for long-term support (1, 2, 4, 6).

The aim of our study is to compare our mechanical circulatory support collective as a whole with those patients under long-term support (> 60 days).

Material and methods

From September 1987 to August 1995 altogether 220 patients (176 men, 44 women) ranging between 11 and 82 years of age (mean 50.9 ± 13.4) received mechanical circulatory support. In 16 of these patients the assist device had to be replaced by a different system. The application of the systems with regard to different indications is detailed in Table 1. In 145 patients the MCS was applied as left ventricular assistance, in 56 patients as biventricular assistance, in 6 patients as right ventricular assistance, in 5 patients as total artificial heart, and in 20 patients as femoral-femoral cardiopulmonary bypass. In 12 of these patients femoral-femoral cardiopulmonary bypass was replaced by a different kind of assistance. Duration of support was 1 h to 67 days (mean 5.4 ± 9.4 days) in patients with postcardiotomy cardiogenic shock, 2h to 342 days (mean 38.3 ± 46.3 days) in bridging patients, and 2 h to 111 days (mean 13.3 ± 22 days) in patients with miscellaneous indications.

Twenty of these patients (17 men, 3 women) between 15 and 64 years of age (mean 46.58 ± 15.76 years) were supported for more than 60 days (long-term sup-

Table 1. Application of VAD by Indication

	PC n = 86	Bridging n = 102	AMI n = 15	Myocarditis n = 4	HLTx n = 1	Rejection n = 6	PGF n = 2	RHF n = 4
CP (n =53)	36	3	8	1	1	0	0	4
A (n = 54)	37	14	0	1	0	1	1	0
Th (n = 67)	7	52	3	1	0	3	1	0
N (n = 18)	0	18	0	0	0	0	0	0
TCI (n = 12)	0	12	0	0	0	0	0	0
CP + A (n = 5)	3	0	2	0	0	0	0	0
CP + TH (n = 7)	2	0	2	1	0	2	0	0
CP + TCI (n = 2)	0	2	0	0	0	0	0	0
A + TH (n = 1)	1	0	0	0	0	0	0	0
TH + N (n = 1)	0	1	0	0	0	0	0	0

PC = postcardiotomy cardiogenic shock; AMI = acute myocardial infarction; HLTx = Heart-lung transplantation; PGF = primary graft failure; RHF = right heart failure; CP = centrifugal pump; A = Abiomed; TH = Thoratec; N = Novacor; TCI = HeartMate

Table 2. Clinical results

	Postcardiotomy n = 86	Bridging n = 102	Miscellaneous n = 32
Weaned	39 (45.3%)	–	4 (12.5%)
Transplanted	12 (14.0%)	69 (67.6%)	5 (15.6%)
Discharged	38 (44.2%)	66 (64.7%)	8 (25%)
Waiting	–	5	–
Alive	38 (44.2%)	61 (59.8%)	8 (25%)

port). The indications were bridging to heart transplantation in 18 patients, one patient had suffered postcardiotomy cardiogenic shock, and in one patient mechanical circulatory support had become necessary following fulminant myocarditis. Seven patients received the Novacor LVAD, another 7 patients the Thoratec system (biventricular assistance in 6 cases, left ventricular assistance in 1 case), and 5 patients the HeartMate (TCI) as left ventricular assist device. In 1 patient both Novacor and Thoratec assist devices were applied for biventricular support. Duration of support in this patient group was 63 to 342 days (mean 109.7 ± 61 days).

Results

The outcome of the whole collective is summarized in Table 2. Sixteen of those patients with long-term support were transplanted (88.8%), all of them could be discharged (post-transplant survival rate 100%). The patient supported with Thoratec and Novacor was a 17-year-old boy with dilated cardiomyopathy and cardiogenic shock. Prior to implantation of the device he had mycoplasma pneumonia with acute respiratory failure and sepsis. This patient received the Novacor device for left ventricular assistance. Since he developed severe right heart failure, Thoratec right heart support was initiated, from which he could be weaned successfully

Table 3. Complications

	Postcardiotomy n = 86	Bridging n = 102	Miscellaneous n = 32	Long-term n = 20
Bleeding	36 (42%)	31 (30%)	7 (22%)	8 (40%)
Neurological	13 (15%)	9 (9%)	4 (12.5%)	3 (15%)
System-rel. inf.	–	5 (5%)	1	2 (10%)
Pat.-rel. inf.	10 (12%)	12 (12%)	7 (22%)	–
MOF	14 (16%)	9 (9%)	8 (25%)	1
Liver failure	4 (4.6%)	16 (15%)	3 (9%)	3 (15%)
RHF (LVAD)	2	9 (9%)	–	3 (15%)
Hemolysis	4 (4.6%)	5 (5%)	–	1
Renal failure	9 (10%)	5 (5%)	–	–
Gastrointestinal	3	12 (12%)	–	2 (10%)

after 17 days. Three weeks postoperatively, he recovered from acute respiratory failure and pneumonia and could be extubated. On POD 52 the patient had to undergo appendectomy. 140 days following the implantation of the support device he underwent heart transplantation and has meanwhile been discharged from hospital.

The patient supported for myocarditis was a 15-year-old girl with severe cardiogenic shock at a referral hospital. Upon arrival at our Center she had to be resuscitated and was immediately supported with biventricular Thoratec device. She recovered and could be successfully transplanted after 111 days of support. The patient supported for postcardiotomy cardiogenic shock received TCI left ventricular assistance for 67 days, before he could be transplanted and discharged.

Two patients with mechanical circulatory support as a bridge to heart transplantation died under long-term support. One patient under Novacor left ventricular assistance suffered intestinal perforation and had to undergo hemicolectomy. Thereafter, he suffered liver failure (bilirubin 16 mg/dl), from which he recovered as well. As a result of a hypertensive crisis he developed severe cerebral bleeding from which he died after 103 days of support. The other patient was supported with biventricular Thoratec device. Prior to implantation he had suffered klebsiella pneumonia from which he recovered. Under support he unfortunately developed hemiparesis and died of sepsis on the 98th postoperative day. Two patients are still waiting for transplantation, one of them is at home and is working partially.

Table 3 provides a survey of the complications in the whole collective as well as in patients under long-term support. Regarding these 20 patients neurological complications occurred in both patients who died as well as in 1 surviving patient. Three patients with liver insufficiency prior to implantation had reversible liver failure under support. In another 3 patients right heart failure occurred, one of them was the 17-year-old by who required mechanical RV support. In the other 2 patients right heart failure could be treated medically, in one of them right heart failure occurred after 40 days of support with a Novacor LVAS.

Out-of-hospital experience

Seven out of 20 patients under long-term support (> 60 days) were discharged from hospital under mechanical circulatory assistance with the implantable Novacor LVAD. Four of them went home for the weekends, three were at home completely. Two patients were even working partially (at a butcher shop and bakery, respectively).

Criteria for patient selection for home circulatory support:
- no organ failure, fully recovered patients
- no hemodynamical and technical problems
- fully mobilized
- good general and psychological condition
- no anxiety about the technique
- optimal help by the family
- possibility to introduce patient and family members to the system (intellectually)
- adequately furnished patient home with the possibilty of the system installation

Protocol for out-of-hospital management of patients with MCSS
Every 4–6 weeks the patients undergo an ambulatory "in-hospital" examination. This includes clinical, neurological/psychological, and laboratory examination, echocardiography, x-ray if needed, ECG, stress testing, wound inspection, as well as a detailed conversation between the VAD team and the patient. During the first month every 2 weeks, then every month the LVAS operator visits the patient at home. In addition to a short clinical, neurological and psychological examination and a wound inspection, he performs a complete VAD function check (patient and equipment) and discusses any problems with the patient, family members and the family physician.

Protocol for patient/family member
- daily weight control
- blood pressure control twice a day
- daily control of pump output, pump rate, residual volume, fill rate, ejection rate
- daily temperature control
- daily wound inspection and change of wound dressing

We organized a 24h on-call duty for our VAD team for technical and psychological support of the patient and family members.

Technical problems at home
There were 4 cases of device-related technical problems. In 1 patient a massive air filter obstruction occurred 120 days after the implantation leading to a high residual volume and a low pump output. In another patient the pump stopped for 15 min resulting from the rupture of a connector adapter cable after 220 days of support. In addition, there were two cases of controller malfunction.

Discussion

As a result of the shortage in donor organs there has been an increasing demand in long-term mechanical circulatory assistance (7). Long-term support, however, implies a high financial burden for the community as well as psychological stress for the patient. For the first 3–4 months of support the patients generally are in a good psychological condition, because they are aware of their physical improvement. The situation often deteriorates when they begin to suppress their severe condition prior to implantation, realize the waiting time ahead of them and consequently, feelings of anxiety arise. For this reason, we thought about the possiblity of discharging patients under support until heart transplantation could be performed.

So far, only two systems allow out-of-hospital support: the wearable Novacor LVAS, which has been applied in all of our patients discharged under support, and the electrically driven HeartMate. Other investigators have reported on patients being allowed to leave the hospital on a daily basis or on patients discharged to an outpatient facility (1, 4). In July 1994 our first patient, a 62-year-old woman, was discharged home under support, where she partially worked in a butchery shop. After 342 days of support she was successfully transplanted in May 1995 and is at home again. Another patient was at home for 4 months. Life quality of these patients can be described as near normal. The most important limitation results from the weight of the controller and batteries and from the exit site.

Although major progress has been made in the field of mechanical circulatory support systems suitable for long-term support, they can not yet be regarded as a true alternative to heart transplantation. A further development of devices is urgently required.

References

1. Frazier OH (1994) First Use of an Untethered, Vented Electric Left Ventricular Assist Device for Long-term Support. Circulation 89:2908–2914
2. Hill JD, Farrar DJ, Hershon JJ, Compton PG, Avery GJ, Levin BS, Brent BN (1986) Use of a prosthetic ventricle as a bridge to cardiac transplantation for postinfarction cardiogenic shock. N Engl J Med 314:626–8
3. Hosenpud JD, Novick RJ, Breen TJ, Daily OP (1994) The Registry of the International Society for Heart and Lung Transplantation: Eleventh official report – 1994. J Heart Lung Transplant 13: 561–570
4. Kormos RL, Murali S, Dew MA, Armitage JM, Hardesty RL, Borovetz HS, Griffith BP (1994) Chronic Mechanical Circulatory Support: Rehabilitation, Low Morbidity, and Superior Survival. Ann Thorac Surg 57:51–8
5. Körfer R, El-Banayosy A, Posival H, Minami K, Körner, MM, Arusoglu L, Breymann T, Kizner L, Seifert D, Körtke H, Fey O (1995) Mechanical Circulatory Support: The Bad Oeynhausen Experience. Ann Thorac Surg 59:S56–63
6. Loisance DY, Deleuze PH Mazzucotelli JP, Le Besnerais P, Dubois-Randle JL (1994) Clinical implantation of the wearable Baxter Novacor ventricular assist system. Ann Thorac Surg 58: 551–4
7. Mehta SM, Aufiero TX, Pae WE, Miller CA, Pierce WS (1995) Combined Registry for the Clinical Use of Mechanical Ventricular Assist Pumps and the Total Artificial Heart in Conjunction with Heart Transplantation: Sixth Official Report – 1994. J Heart Lung Transplant 14: 585–93

Author's address:
Dr. A. El-Banayosy
Herzzentrum NRW
Klinik für Thorax- und Kardiovaskularchirurgie
Georgstr. 11
D-32545 Bad Oeynhausen, Germany

Left ventricular assistance with Novacor device: the "Pavia Experience"

G. Minzioni, M. Rinaldi, L. Martinelli, F. Pagani, N. Pederzolli, M. Vigano'

Department of Cardiac Surgery, IRCCS Policlinico S. Matteo, Pavia, Italy

Introduction

The shortage of donors is responsible for the majority of patients dying while awaiting transplantation. To rescue these critically ill patients, a wide variety of devices has been proposed for circulatory assistance as bridge to heart transplantation (1, 2). The necessity of long periods of bridging because of donor scarcity and because of the need to allow the recovery of the patient before transplantation, has led to the consolidation of left ventricular assistance with electrically-powered devices (4). The wearable system of the Novacor device is the result of the effort to miniaturize the previous large external console. It can be now worn on a belt, allowing high degree of mobility and good quality of life during the waiting period (5). For this reason its use has spread to a large number of transplantation centers and the duration of the assistance has increased significantly over time. In some centers under assistance have been discharged and followed-up as outpatients, thus decreasing the economical impact of circulatory assistance on health care resources.

Aim of this presentation is to discuss the experience in Novacor implantation at the Cardiac Surgery Department of I.R.C.C.S Policlinico S. Matteo – University of Pavia with particular attention to the new technique of implantation used at our Center and to the response of the right ventricle and the pulmonary circulation to the left ventricular assistance. The issues of the discharge and the outpatient care of the individuals while on assistance are also addressed.

Patients and methods

From November 1992 to December 1995, 11 patients underwent Novacor N100 LVAS (Novacor Division – Baxter Healthcare, Oakland – California) implantation for end-stage cardiac failure as bridge to transplant. In the first two cases the system was console-driven. In subsequent cases the wearable system was used. In the latest seven cases PC valved conduits were implanted.

In Table 1 the anagraphics and hemodynamics of the patients are summarized. Nine patients had dilated cardiomyopathy (DCM) and two had ischemic cardiomyopathy (ICM) and they were all awaiting heart transplantation. They were all in NYHA class IV: 10/11 were under continuous inotropic or vasodilator infusion. Two patients were under intra-aortic balloon pump (IABP). The extremely compromised hemodynamic picture was reflected in an initial deterioration of parenchymal functions. Renal function was compromised and they were all oliguric with a mean

Table 1

Age	Sex	Pathology	BSA m²	Bilirubine mg%	Creatinine mg%
48.7 ± 8.5	10 M, 1 F	DCM 9 ICM 2	1.88 ± 0.16	2.4 ± 1.4	1.4 ± 0.5

Table 2

CVP mmHg	PAm mmHg	PCWP mmHg	C.O. l/min	C.I. l/min/m²	PVR dyne/m²/sec⁻⁵	REF %
12 ± 4	44.3 ± 9.0	28.3 ± 8.8	3.3 ± 0.6	1.7 ± 0.2	351 ± 134	9.4 ± 3.5

creatinine level of 1.4 ± 0.5 mg%. The mean bilirubine level was 2.4 ± 1.4 mg%. As shown in Table 2 pulmonary circulation was extremely compromised in most of the patients with high mean pulmonary pressures and transpulmonary gradients.

Severe right cardiac failure was present in all 11 patients with a PVC of 12 ± 4 mmHg and a RV ejection fraction of 9.4 ± 3.5%. The level of pulmonary vascular resistance was 351 ± 134 $dyne/m^2/s^{-5}$.

Surgical Technique

In all cases we adopted a modified "ortho-dromic" technique using aortic cross-clamping and hypothermic cardioplegic arrest of the heart (7). After sternotomy, the pocket is tailored dividing the insertion of the diaphragm to the lower ribs, for an easier bleeding control. On cardiopulmonary bypass, the aorta is cross-clamped and cardioplegia administered. Apical cannulation is performed first on a dry, still field. The device is then easily deaired, with blood flowing in the physiologic direction. The aorta is declamped and the outflow conduit is anastomosed. Before tying the suture, the final deairing is obtained. This technique allows extreme precision in apical cannulation, easier control of bleeding and accurate deairing of the pump. The ischemic time is short (around 30 min).

Postoperative course

The operative mortality was 0. One patient required surgical re-exploration for bleeding and another one surgical debridement and mediastinal irrigation for mediastinitis which eventually resolved. A prolonged inotropic support with dobutamine (11.5 ± 5.6 days) was needed in all cases to support the right ventricle during the postoperative period. Pulmonary vasodilatation was also obtained in 10 cases with sodium nipride (0.5–2.0 ng/kg/min) and in one case with nitric oxyde (10–20 ppm). A mechanical right ventricular assistance was not necessary in any case. The average stay in ICU of the nine patients with the wearable device was of 5.0 ± 3.6

Table 3

	Pre-implantation	Post-implantation	p
PAM mmHg	44.3 ± 9.0	21.1 ± 2.4	< 0.01
PCWP mmHg	28.3 ± 8.8	8.0 ± 3.6	< 0.01
C.I. l/min/m^2	1.7 ± 0.2	3.0 ± 0.3	< 0.01
PVR dyne/sec/cm^{-5}	351 ± 134	182 ± 71	< 0.02
RVEF %	9.4 ± 3.5	21.1 ± 5.0	< 0.01

days. All the patients but one were successfully extubated after 4.0 ± 5.4 days. One patient died from a multi-organ failure 16 days after the Novacor application. All the hemodynamic parameters improved during assistance as shown in Table 3. The renal and hepatic function improved gradually with a significant creatinine reduction (from 1.4 ± 0.5 to 0.7 ± 0.5; p < 0.01) and bilirubine reduction (from 2.4 ± 1.4 to 0.9 ± 0.7; p < 0.01). A critical issue in mechanical assistance is the prevention of bleeding in the immediate postoperative period and of thromboembolism in the long term. For the first three cases we adopted the Szefner protocol. In the later cases the anticoagulation treatment was greatly simplified introducing calcium heparin (7500 UI subcutaneously) as soon as the surgical bleeding stopped, to maintain PTT at 1.5 times the basal value and subsequently switching to oral acenocumarole aiming at a PT of 20–40%. An anti-platelet agent is also added (aspirin 100 mg/day) to prevent micro-aggregation.

The mean implant duration was 95 days (range: 7–330 days), with a significant extention of the period in the latest cases. Four patients were discharged from our Department to a rehabilitation center and three of them were subsequently discharged home and followed-up weekly as outpatients. Five patients were transplanted. One of them died on day 15 due to multiorgan failure as a consequence of a severe anaphylactic shock after aprotinine administration at the time of transplant. The other four patients are alive and well after transplantation (mean follow-up: 17 months, range 5–26). Five patients are currently under assistance; one of them has performed cytotoxic antibodies and has been waiting for a compatible graft for 11 months. We have observed two strokes; one completely resolved and the other one resulted in minor psychic disturbances. An interesting observation is that both patients were in atrial fibrillation at the time of the event.

Out-of-hospital management

The wearable setting of the Novacor LVAD allows a complete mobilization of the patient. This fact outlines the importance of an adequate protocol of rehabilitation for a long period of support. Continuous hospitalization is no longer necessary, because once the patient has been physically rehabilitated and trained to take care of the controller and the batteries, he can be discharged home. Our protocol is based on the discharge of the patient to a rehabilitation center as soon as the clinical situation is stable, when the patient is fully mobilized and complete healing of surgical wound is obtained. At the rehabilitation center physical training is completed, with serial controls of the hemodynamic profile. A further step towards the normalization of the quality of life consists in the complete autonomization of the patients at home. The first step is to discharge them from the rehabilitation center during the week-end and subsequently these periods can be extended to a permanent discharge. A limiting factor is represented by the excessive distance of a patient home from the transplant or rehabilitation center. This would preclude routine control of the device, monitoring of anticoagulation, and rapid admission in case of transplant.

Four patients (three males and one female, ages 58, 39, 62, 44 years) were discharged from our Center 39, 100, 78 and 36 days after implantation and were admitted to the Rehabilitation Center. The functional status of all patients was dramatically improved at that time. They all moved from NYHA class IV to class I, in respect to their daily life. The rehabilitation program was based on appropriate physical training and psychological support to allow patients to be discharged home. All patients attended an appropriate training in order to either improve their self-sufficiency or to minimize any associated risk related to the device.

As far as the psychological aspects are concerned, all patients soon became optimistic. They really felt themselves to be on a bridge linking heart failure with heart transplant. The improvement in their health status overcame any discomfort. The device was highly accepted and its sound was not annoying, but rather reassuring them. Cardiopulmonary exercise test was performed respectively at day 59, 107, 106 and 42 from implant. This test showed the high degree of physical deconditioning of some of the patients (peak VO2: 18.2, 11.7, 6.7, 17 ml/kg/min).

An individualized physical training program was then scheduled. This program was based on 5 days/week cycle of treadmill sessions, calistenics and stretching exercises. The stretching exercises were mainly oriented for the back muscles and aimed at avoiding or treating possible contractures due to abnormal postures caused by the weight of the device (about 4 kg). No complications occurred during physical sessions. The percentage of attendance at the gymnasium was 90%, 78%, and 29%, of the scheduled sessions respectively for the three discharged patients. In fact, a staged program for discharging at home LVAS recipients was set up concertedly with Baxter Novacor Service support. It was based on several weekend trips home. These excursions started respectively 47, 37, 30 days after admission to the rehabilitation unit. Up to now, three patients are at home, in satisfactory general condition with a restored normal social life. One of them was transplanted 139 days after system implant. Two patients have been discharged from the Rehabilitation Center after three weekend trips home and are closely followed-up by all the team involved. One patient is still in the rehabilitation center.

Discussion

The use of mechanical assist devices as bridge to transplantation has spread in most of the transplant centers in recent times. The great enthusiasm and expectation has recently been attenuated by some skepticism mainly due to social costs and the scant impact of this approach on global mortality of patients listed for transplantation. Clearly, even a wide application of prolonged mechanical assistance does not increase the total number of transplants which is only affected by graft availability. The wider application of mechanical support contributed to the technological development and engineering of biocompatible materials. The miniaturization of the energy sources and the controlling computer has made possible to have totally wearable and portable systems with great advantages in terms of quality of life for the assisted patients. These technical advances now make it possible for prolonged assistance in such a way that their application is not only as a life-saving procedure but also as a strategy to normalize compromised patients and to get them to transplantation with better chances of success. This philosophy is confirmed by the longer period of bridging as experience increases and confidence in the device becomes broader.

With the same attitude, we are accepting more high-risk patients in the Novacor protocol. Particular interest is developing in the study of the acute and chronic behavior of the right ventricle during a left ventricular assistance (3, 6). During the immediate postoperative phase the right ventricle suffers because of the increased pre-load and because of the leftward shifting of the interventricular septum due to total left heart decompression. This geometric alteration causes right ventricular distention with increased tricuspid regurgitation. Usually this situation can be overcome by inotropic support of the right ventricle with dobutamine and pulmonary vasodilatation with sodium nipride and/or nitric oxide. The efficacy of this treatment can be easily monitored by intraoperative trans-esophageal echocardiography. This support must be prolonged for some days after the implant to allow right ventricular adaptation.

During the long-term support we have observed a gradual decrease of the pulmonary vascular resistances and of the transpulmonary gradient, despite that cardiac output increases. This is of paramount interest because of the possible application of such devices to normalize pulmonary vascular resistances allowing a low-risk heart transplantation. A very convincing proof of the good adaptation of the right ventricle in the long-term is given by the execution of serial effort tests with hemodynamic monitoring. These tests showed a progressive increase of the cardiac output and of the maximum oxygen consumption along with the stress. This means a right ventricle which can very efficiently stand the increased work of the artificial device. This behavior can be regarded as extremely positive in view of a permament application of the LVAD systems and can theoretically guarantee a normal life style.

The surgical technique must allow a safe, quick and precise insertion of the device. We adopted a new "orthodromic" technique which in our opinion minimizes the risk of inflow and outflow cannulas malpositioning air embolism and bleeding. The only criticism that can be made is that the aortic cross-clamping and the cardioplegic arrest could damage the right ventricle. This was not the case in our series. The short cardioplegic arrest allows a complete decompression of the right ventricle and the damage can be considered negligible. As a matter of fact, all our patients had a severe right ventricular failure preoperatively as demonstrated by the extremely low right ventricular ejection fraction and the high pulmonary vascular resistances. Despite this, the recovery was rapid in all cases and none required right ventricular assistance.

References

1. De Vries WC, Anderson JL, Joice LD et al. (1984) Clinical use of the total artificial heart. N Engl J Med 310: 273

2. Ferrar DJ (1994) Thoratec Ventricular Assist Device Principal Investigators: Preoperative predictors of survival in patients with Thoratec: Preoperative predictors of survival in patients with Thoratec Ventricular Assist Device as a bridge to heart transplantation. J Heart Lung Transplant 13: 93
3. Kormos RLK, Gasior T, Antaki J et al (1989) Evaluation of right ventricular function during clinical left ventricular assistance. ASAIO Trans 35: 547–550
4. Portner PM, Oyer PE, Pennington G et al (1989) Implantable electrical left ventricular assist system: bridge to transplantation and the future. Ann Thorac Surg 47: 142
5. Vetter HO, Kaulbach HG, Samithz C et al (1995) Experience with Novacor left ventricular assist system as a bridge to cardiac transplantation, including the new wearable system. J Thorac Cardiovasc Surg 109: 74–80
6. Vigano' M, Martinelli L, Rinaldi M et al (1994) Efficacy of LVAD in normalizing pulmonary circulation and allowing complete rehabilitation before transplantation. Circulatory Support, Pittsburgh. Abstract book pp 4–5
7. Vigano' M, Martinelli L, Minzioni G, Rinaldi M, Pagani F (1996) Modified method for Novacor ventricular assist device implantatioin. Ann Thorc surg 61: 247–249

Authors' address:
Dr. Gaetano Minzioni
Department of Cardiac Surgery
IRCCS Policlinico S. Matteo
27100 – Pavia, Italy

Long-term mechanical circulatory support: The Berlin Experience

M. Loebe, Y. Weng, E. Hennig, J. Müller, S. Spiegelsberger, R. Hetzer

German Heart Institute, Berlin

Over the last 10 years more than 1000 intrathoracic transplant procedures have been performed at the German Heart Institute Berlin, 840 of which were orthotopic heart transplantations. From early on, it became apparent that medical treatment alone would not be sufficient for supporting patients through an ever-expanding waiting period before transplantation (1, 2, 3, 5–7).

Since 1989, a total of 221 mechanical circulatory support procedures have been executed, primarily as a bridge to transplantation. Ten patients were supported with the pediatric Berlin Heart device (12 ml); this experience is discussed in greater detail in the chapter by Alexi-Meskishvili. A total of 19 patients were under the age of 16 (5). Figure 1 shows a Berlin Heart patient enjoying the gardens at our Institute. One notes, however, that his ability to walk about freely is somewhat impaired by this biventricular support system. Since prospective transplant recipients increasingly have an extremely long wait before a suitable donor organ is procured, patient mobility has become an important concern. Today, patients im-

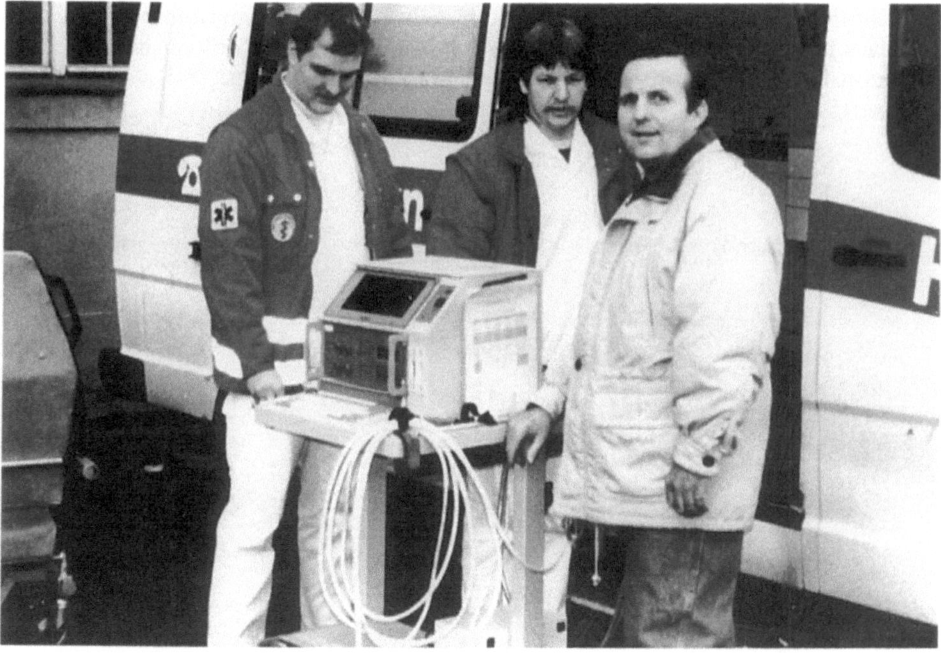

Fig. 1. 47-year-old patient with the biventricular Berlin Heart support system. The battery of the Heimes drive unit provides up to 180 minutes operation.

planted with wearable LVADs are discharged home, thereby regaining a high degree of physical activity and quality of life (3, 4, 7).

Figure 2 shows the development in our use of different support systems. As mentioned above, we have primarily used the Berlin Heart assist device, but in recent years a growing number of left ventricular assist devices (27 Novacors/10 TCIs) have been used in our institution. In the 37 patients with left ventricular assist devices the diagnoses included cardiomyopathy in 23 patients and ischemic heart disease in 14. Figure 3 shows two of our patients strolling along the Kurfürstendamm. The patient on the left has now been on the device for more than 500 days. The patient on the right has been transplanted after 260 days on Novacorsupport. A total of 100 patients underwent heart transplantation after mechanical circulatory support at German Heart Institute Berlin. Transplantation was only performed after the patient's condition had stabilized (2).

Regarding experience with long-term support, which we define as more than 3 months, a total of 6 patients have been supported with a TCI device, 13 with a Novacor, and 10 with a Berlin Heart. Three of the patients in the TCI group subsequently underwent transplantation, 1 was weaned, 1 awaits transplantation, and 1 died after 3 months of support. In the Novacor group, 3 patients have undergone transplantation, 3 were weaned, 3 continue to await transplantation, and 1 remains on support after more than 500 days. Six of the Berlin Heart patients have undergone transplantation after more than 90 days of mechanical support. Due to heparin coating of the Berlin Heart systems, thromboembolic complications have not been observed in our recent long-term biventricular support recipients (5)

Cardiac recovery has been extensively addressed in the chapter by Müller. It should be kept in mind that this is part of our long-term support experience. All four of the patients weaned from Novacor devices remain asymptomatic more than 60 days after the discontinuation of mechanical support. Looking at those who were on the device more than 200 days, presently 12 patients, 8 have been fully

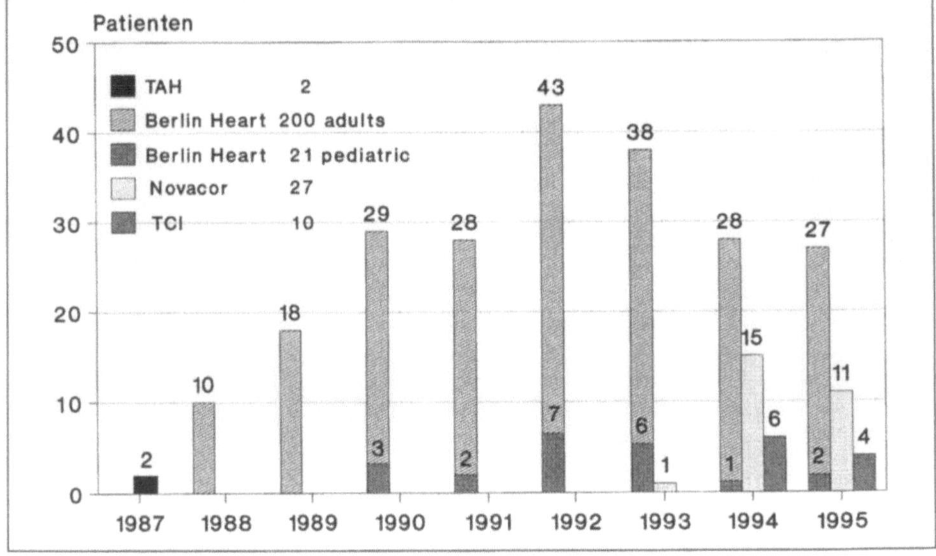

Fig 2. Use of mechanical assist devices by year at the German Heart Institute Berlin

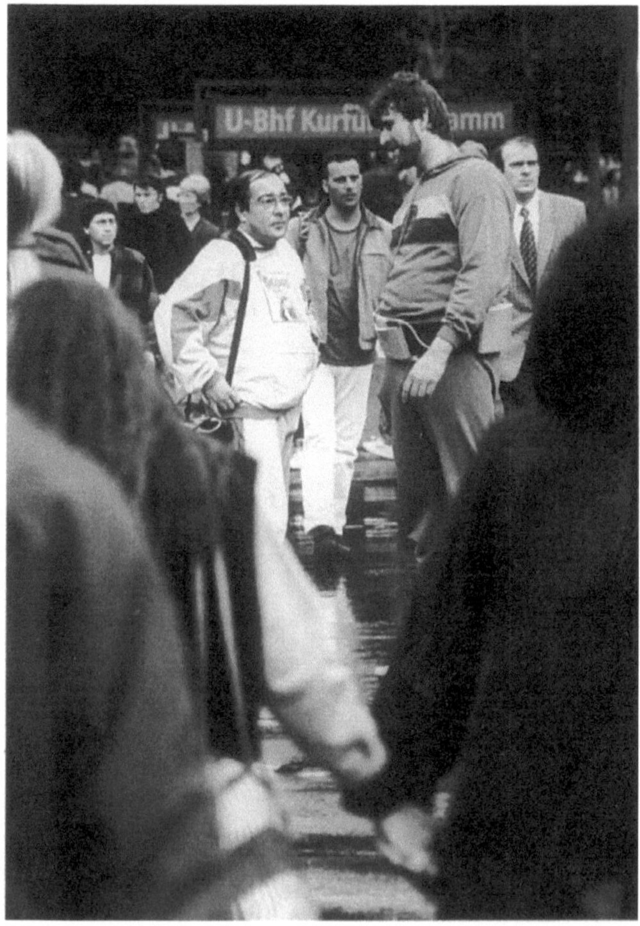

Fig 3. Two patients with wearable Novacor LVADs enjoying a stroll along the Kurfürstendamm.

mobilized and 2 died shortly after crossing the 200-day mark. Both of these latter patients suffered long-term impairment due to cerebrovascular embolisms during the early postoperative course. Three of the other eight patients underwent transplantation, all of whom survived. I have already mentioned the 3 patients who were weaned from the left ventricular assist device. Two patients presently remain on the device for more than 200 days, and as mentioned before, the longest ongoing support totals more than 500 days.

Figure 4 shows the inner surface of the TCI pump at the time of transplantation after 220 days of support. Complications during long-term support included mainly thromboembolism in 3 patients, 2 suffered from sepsis, 1 from bleeding due to technical problems with the left ventricular assist device (TCI). In the BVAD group 2 patients suffered from sepsis, 2 from multi-organ failure, and 2 from cerebral bleeding. Seven of the 13 patients with a wearable Novacor system were discharged from the hospital for 1 or even more than 400 days now.

As far as discharging patients with wearable LVADs from the hospital is concerned, we were initially quite reluctant to send them home. Our early patients

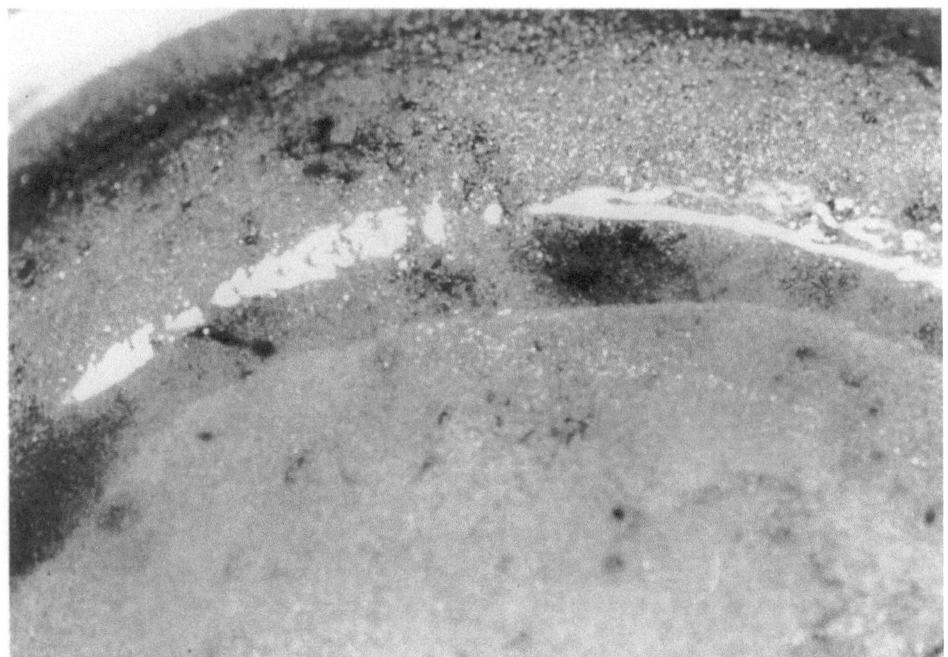

Fig 4. The inner surface of a TCI explanted at the time of heart transplantation after 220 days of trouble-free support. Note the smooth inner lining of the chamber.

stayed for more than 100 days at the German Heart Institute Berlin. As their status improved they began exploring the hospital grounds and soon discovered that day-trips well beyond the hospital grounds were both safe and exciting. Some patients even went by taxi or subway across Berlin without notifying the hospital staff of where they were going and what they intended to do. This clearly demonstrated the great confidence these patients had in the technical reliability of their respective support systems. One patient traveled by taxi to a shopping mall some 50 kilometers away from our hospital. Excited by the new mall, he bought several items, including a pair of roller skates and a TV. On his way back to our facility the taxi got caught in a traffic jam near the Brandenburg Gate during rush hour. Eventually the battery in the Novacor became discharged and, since the patient had forgotten to carry spare batteries with him, he asked the taxi driver to call the police for help. The officers were quite surprised to find a man with roller skates in a cab who claimed that his artificial heart had run out of energy.

Such adventures prompted us to find a family house for patients with LVADs some 15 km from our hospital grounds. Five patients went there and stayed at the Paulinenkrankenhaus for up to 5 months. Once a week they visited our Institute for a general examination including WBC, Hb, x-rays, and ECG.

Now, we discharge the patients home. Prior to this the patient and his caregivers receive extensive training in the use of the device and its driving unit. The local physician, who is responsible for managing anticoagulation treatment and for providing emergency treatment, if required, is also provided information. The electrical circuit at the home of the patient has to be checked by an electrician who ensures that no other major electrical appliances are connected to the fuse the drive unit will be supplied by. One of our perfusionists accompanies the patient home and rechecks the local circumstances. The patient visits our facility once every 2 weeks for a routine examination. Hospital staff members call the patient and his physician twice a week to check on the patient's condition.

Based upon our experience with bridging, long-term support appears to be quite feasible and safe. Patients who were on the device for more than 100 days without complications did not develop any afterwards. The quality of life for these patients was, of course, extremely good. This led us to implant devices in some patients who exhibited many contra-indications to heart transplantation with the intent of providing permanent isolated left ventricular assistance.

At the meeting in Bad Oeynhausen about a month ago, we presented our first four patients, all of whom were substantially above the age of 60, had diabetes, were multi-morbid and impaired for long periods, and bedridden due to their cardiac disease. Three were implanted with a Novacor device; one with a TCI device- all with the goal of permanent support. One patient died early, after 11 days of support, and the other 3 were still alive. As I also pointed out at the Oeynhausen meeting, it is very difficult to rehabilitate these patients after their long history of heart disease. Their care makes substantial demands on the nursing staff.

Looking at the same group of patients today, we must report that three of them have died due to various causes in their multi-morbid history. Only one of the four patients is still alive, rehabilitated, and home with his Novacor system, some 700 kilometers away from Berlin.

I presented these rather sobering details of our experience to raise the following questions: which patients should be selected for permanent support, and if a patient does not fulfill the criteria for heart transplantation, can he still be safely supported with a ventricular assist device?

Nevertheless, one can conclude from our experience gained in the bridge-to-transplantation group that long-term support is not only technically feasible, but also safe. Patients with wearable devices regain a surprisingly high level of physical activity, social reintegration, and quality of life. The systems available are very easy to handle. With adequate training, every patient and his family is able to use the device without requiring in-depth technical knowledge. System related complications are extremely rare during long-term support.

Provided the patient is in the condition to undergo a major surgical procedure, the assist systems presently available can be used for long-term support in patients with endstage heart failure with the expectancy of a high degree of rehabilitation and safety.

References

1. Frazier OH, Macris MP (1994) Current methods for circulatory support. Texas Heart Institute Journal. 1994; 21:288–95.
2. Friedel N, Viazis P, Schiessler A, Warnecke H, Hennig E, Hetzer R (1991) Patient selection for mechanical circulatory support as a bridge to cardiac transplantation. Int J Art Organs 14:276–279.
3. Hetzer R, Hennig E, Schiessler A, Friedel N, Warnecke H, Adt M (1992) Mechanical circulatory support and heart transplantation. J. Heart Lung Transplant; 11:175–181.
4. Loebe M, Hetzer R, Schüler S, Hummel M, Friedel N, Weng Y, Schiessler A (1992) Herztransplantation- Indikation und Ergebnisse. Zentrbl Chir 117:681–688.

5. Loebe M, Weng Y, Alexi-Meskishvili V, Hausdorf G, Hennig E, Schüler S, Warnecke H, Hetzer R (1993) Mechanical circulatory support as a bridge to transplantation in children. J. Heart Lung Transplantation 12:S85
6. Müller J, Wallukat G, Wenig Y, Siniawski H, Hofmeier M, Kupetz W, Hetzer R (1995) Effect of synchronized-non-synchronized pumping mode of (-receptor autoantibodies (RAAB) in patients with cardiac assist devices. ASAIO 41(suppl.):50
7. Schiessler A, Warnecke H, Friedel N, Hennig E, Hetzer R (1990) Clinical use of the Berlin biventricular assist device as a bridge to transplantation. ASAIO Trans 36:M 706–708

Author's address:
Dr. M. Loebe
Deutsches Herzzentrum Berlin
Augustenburger Platz 1
13353 Berlin

Mechanical circulatory support systems 1995 – New devices under investigation

E. Hennig

Humboldt University of Berlin, Germany

Introduction

With the first generation of implantable left ventricular assist devices intended for semi-permanent or permanent use, clinical experiences have been gathered worldwide during the last 8 to 10 years. The development phase of these devices started in the early 1970's, it took 15–20 years until initial clinical applications.

Based on this experience, one can calculate that new devices today under development will reach clinical readiness in the second half of the first decade of the 21st century.

This overview includes 35 groups with more than 40 systems under development, with at least the results of working laboratory types today.

The systems described are characterized according to their pumping principle and kind of energy conversion (Table 1).

Table 1. MCSS-Characterization

Pumping principle	Energy conversion
– displacement pumps	– electromechanically
– hydrodynamic pumps	– electromagnetically
– combinations	– electrohydraulically
	– indirect
	– direct
	– thermomechanically
	– biological – mechanically

Most displacement pumps today under development have a free or supported moving diaphragm separating a blood chamber from a gas-filled chamber. However, some models are equipped with rotary or linear pistons. In hydrodynamic pumps, the fluid is transported by tangential or axial-acting forces induced by rotating impellers or turbines.

Today, in most systems electrical energy is converted into linear, rotating, or oscillating movement of pistons, turbines, or elastic walls. As the first step, electrical energy is converted into electromagnetic fields to drive electromotors or move compact solenoids, magnetic fluids, or magnetic particles embedded in elastic walls.

As a second step, the rotational movement of the electromotors has to be converted into mechanical linear movement by different kinds of gearing, into hydraulic pressure to drive linear pistons or elastic displacement chambers. Direct conversion of the rotational movement of the motor into blood transportation is possible with centrifugal or axial blood pumps. In thermomechanically-driven energy converters, the electric energy produces heat to drive miniaturized steam engines (Stirling principle). In these systems nuclear energy sources could be used as well.

Electromechanically-activated left ventricular assist devices and total artificial hearts

Displacement pumps under development in combination with electromechanical energy conversion are compiled in Table 2. Listed are the developer (principle investigator/location), special features of the system under investigation, the status achieved at the end of 1995 (hardware, results of animal experiments) and a reference for further information.

Table 2. Electromechanically Activated LVAD and TAH

Developer P.I./Location	System description special features	Status 1995	Ref.
G. Noon, Y. Nosé Baylor; Houston	reversing DC-Motor roller screw pusher plate LVAD, TAH	in vivo TAH < 1 w. LVAD < 2 w.	(1–3)
W. Pierce, G. Rosenberg Hershey		in vivo TAH < 23 w. LVAD < 35 w.	(4, 5)
E. Okamoto, Y. Mitamura Sapporo		in vitro LVAD < 24 w.	(6)
B. Mambrito, Rome		in vivo TAH < 2 w.	(7)
H. C. Kim, B. G. Min Seoul	reversing DC-Motor pendulous moving actuator epicyclic gear train	acute in vivo	(8)
V. L. Poirier, O. H. Frazier TCI & THI; Houston	unidirectional low speed torque Motor cam-follower	long term clinically LVAD	(9)
H. Reul, R. Kaufmann Aachen	unidirectional DC-Motor hypocycloidic crank pusher plate	TAH working prototype	(10)
I. M. Sauer, J. Frank Berlin	unidirectional DC-Motor inner oval of cogs	TAH working prototype	(11)
J. Bykowski, C. Christensen Milwaukee	unidirectional DC-Motor cycloidal activator	durab. test < 2,7 y	(12)
J. R. Monties Marseille	unidirectional low speed Motor hypocycloidical pump "Wankel" principle	LVAD, TAH working prototoype	(13)
Y. Abe, K. Imachi K. Atsumi; Tokyo	"Undulation pump" nutating disc	LVAD, TAH working prototype	(14)

Eleven groups have been identified which fulfill the above-mentioned criteria.

The first four systems listed work with the same principle of energy conversion. The total artificial heart is an implantable, electromechanical one-piece pump with left and right blood chambers sandwiching a thin centerpiece with an actuator assembly. The driver is a miniature electromechanical actuator that consists of a direct current (DC) motor and a planetary roller screw. The rotational motion of the motor is converted to a linear motion of the roller screw. During systole, the roller screw mechanically pushes a pusher plate to ejection, whereas the pusher plates are completely decoupled from the roller screw during diastole. Hall effect commutation sensors and the left pusher plate position sensor are used to control the motor speed and run the left and right pumps in a left master alternate variable rate mode. Polyurethane or polyolefin rubbers are used as a diaphragm material. The pumps are miniaturized to fit within the thoracic cavity as orthotopic heart replacement or in the preperitoneal space with the blood drained from the apex of the left ventricle as a ventricular assist device. Figure 1 shows as an example the mockup of the totally implantable total artificial heart and associated components of the Baylor design. The pump and compliance chamber are implanted into the chest cavity, an internal power pack is implanted into the submuscle space, the secondary coil and emergency port are implanted subcutaneously. The primary coil and external power pack are fixed outside the body. The electric power of this pump is transferred from the external battery to the internal battery through transcutaneous energy transmission system (TETS). If some deterioration or accident occurs, power can be supplied using the emergency port. The hybrid controller circuits are miniaturized and divided into a microprocessor and controller hybrid,

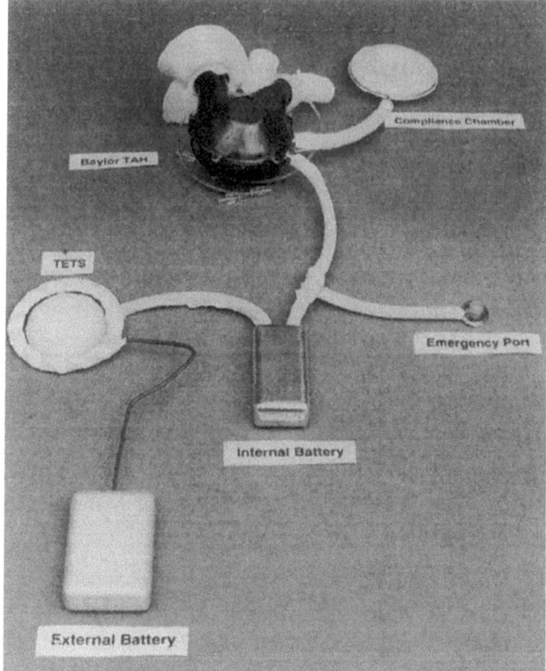

Fig. 1. Mock-up of the totally implantable artificial heart and associated components of the Baylor design (1).

a motor driver hybrid, left and right hall sensors hybrids, and a commutation sensor hybrid. All electronic components fit in the centerpiece motor housing of the Baylor heart (Fig. 2).

Figure 3 shows the assembly drawing of the Baylor total artificial heart. The motor stator is first mounted in the centerpiece, followed by insertion of the rotor-nut assembly; they are fixed to the centerpiece by the motor end bells with a bearing at each end. The rotor-nut assembly freely rotates and is suspended by the radial bearings. Then the rotor screw and the support plate assembly will be screwed into the rotor-nut with linear translation rods guided through the slide bushings mounted in the centerpiece. Both left and right pusher plates with flexing diaphragms will then be inserted inside the roller screw from each side. The pusher plate shafts are guided inside the roller screw, not only to prevent free motion of the pusher plate, but also to allow passive filling during the diastolic phase. The final step is to place the left and right pump housings and fix them to the center-piece so as to compress the diaphragm between the housing and the centerpiece. Figure 4 shows the assembled Baylor total artificial heart in left ejection and right fill phase (left side) and right ejection and left fill phase (right side). The electro-mechanical energy converter is compact and fits in the space available between the left and right shaped pusher plates. With the same energy converter and associated components, a left ventricular assist device has been developed where one side of the motor housing is covered by a back plate (Fig. 5). Mechanically very similar, but different in the type of blood contact surface and prosthetic heart valves used, are the systems under development by W. Pierce, E. Okamoto, N. Shapiro, and B.

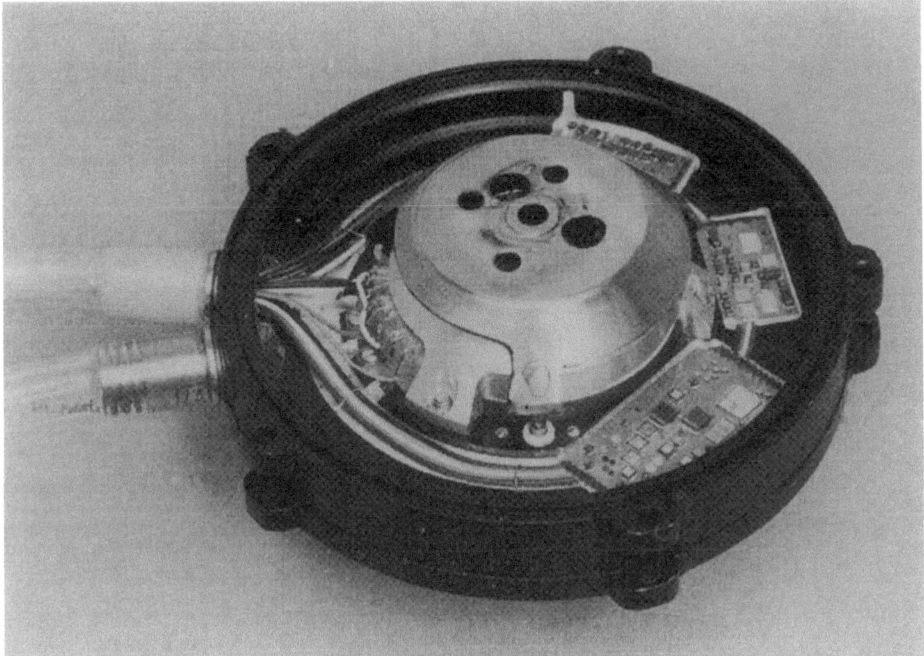

Fig. 2.   Centerpiece motor housing of the Baylor heart (1).

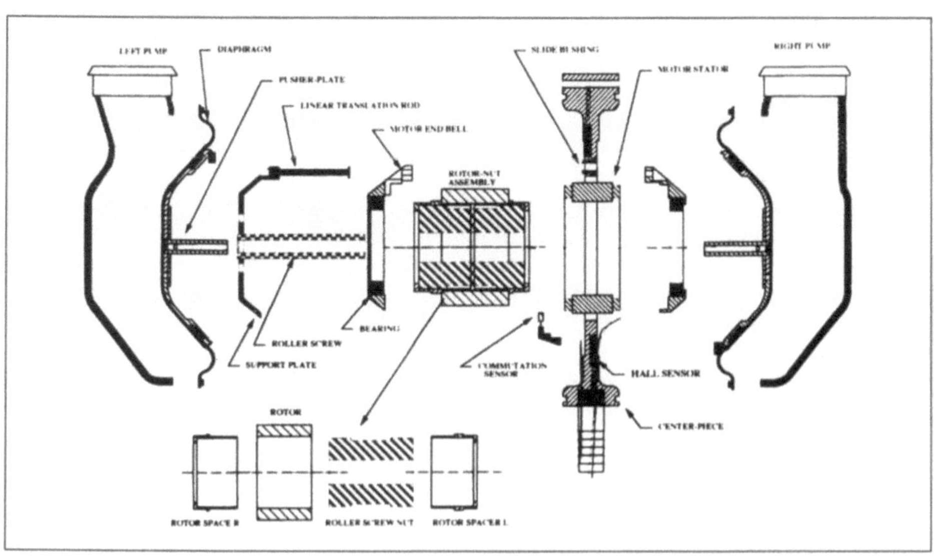

Fig. 3.   Assembly drawing of the Baylor total artificial heart (1).

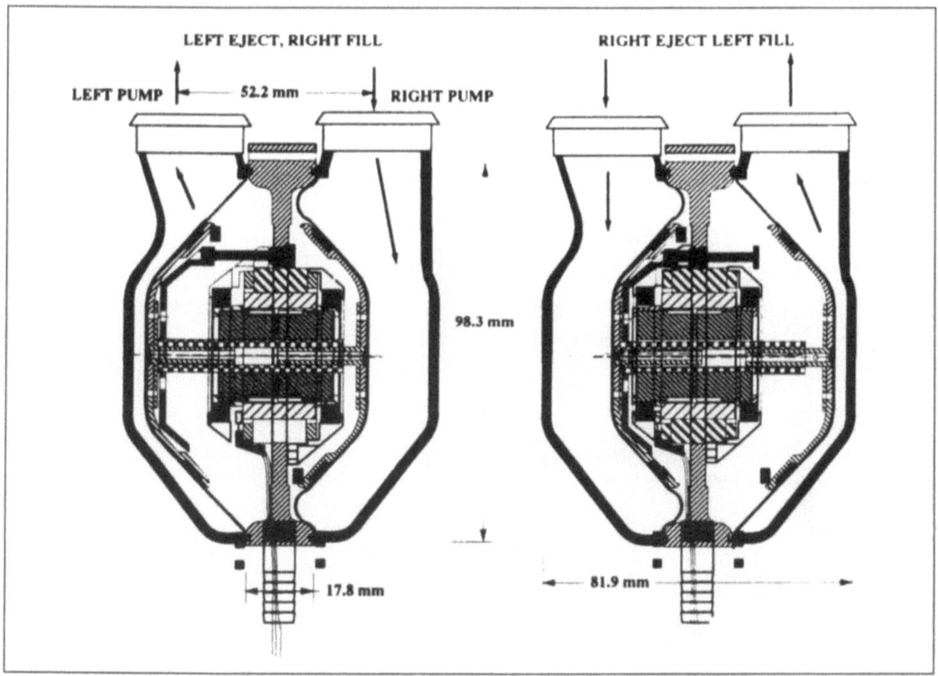

Fig. 4.   Baylor total artificial heart in left ejection and right fill phase (left side) and right ejection and left fill phase (right side) (1).

Mambrito in Rome. An example of this type of implantable orthotopic artificial heart is shown in Fig. 6.

In a Korean artificial heart design the motor moves itself in a pendulous motion by an epicyclical gear train (Fig. 7). In this design a compliance chamber is not necessary, moving the motor instead of pusher plates has the advantage of saving dead space occupied by the motor.

A special feature of the last six systems in Table 2 is the unidirectional rotating motor. Not reversing the rotational direction decreases the energy consumption and results in better long-term durability. The TCI-Heart Mate system uses as a gear a combination of cam and followers; in the total artificial heart under development at the Helmholtz Institute in Aachen a brushless DC motor drives a planetary reduction gear, which generates a hypocycloidic crank motion for both piston rod bearings. The piston rods actuate the pusher plate (Fig. 8).

A unique gear design has been used in a Berlin total artificial heart system developed by Sauer et al. The rotational motion of the motor is transformed by a combination of cogwheel and an inner oval of cogs into a linear motion driving two pusher plates (Fig. 9).

Quite different are the pumping principles of the systems under development by Monties in Marseille and Atsumi in Tokyo.

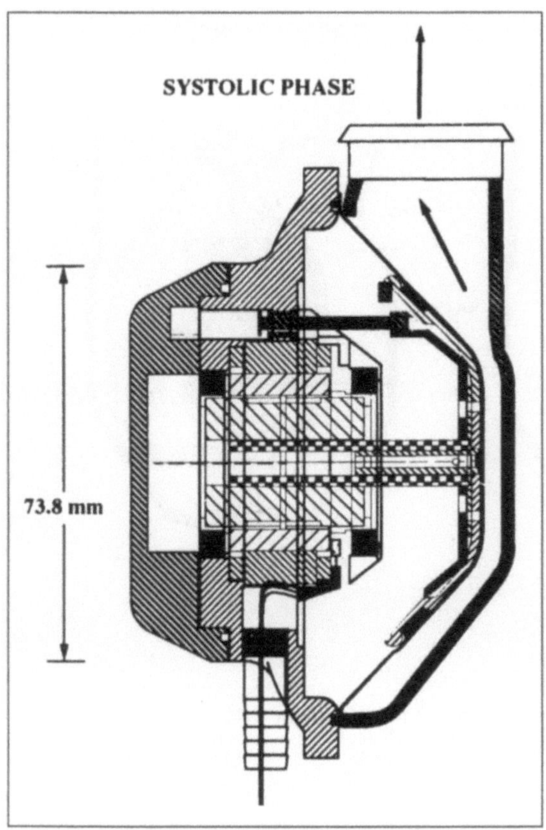

Fig. 5. Baylor left ventricular assist device (1).

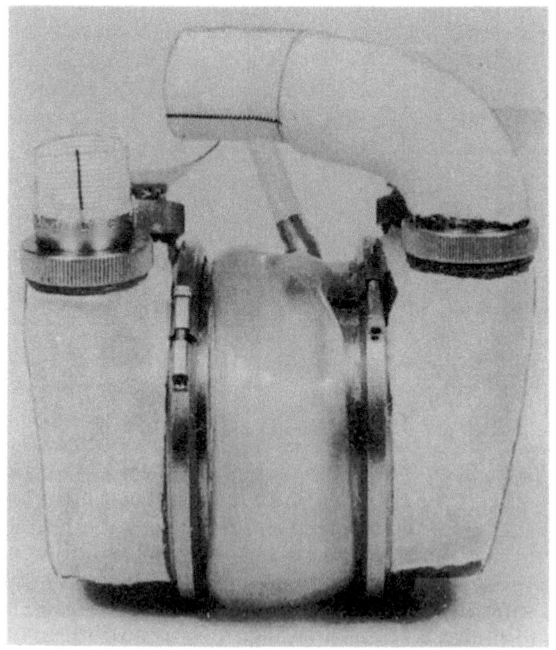

Fig. 6. Implantable orthotopic artificial heart with annular compliance chamber (Hershey) (4).

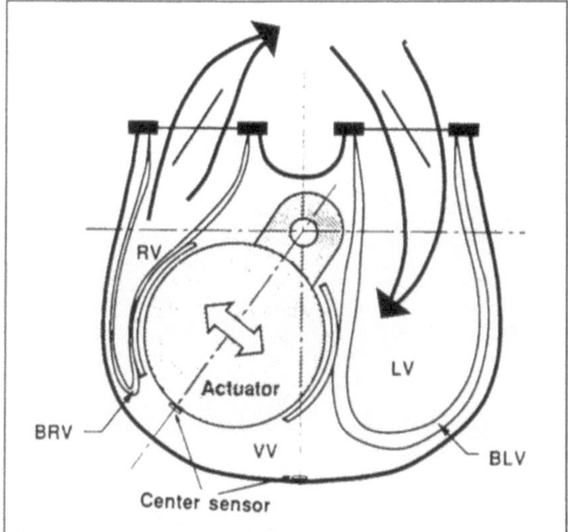

Fig. 7. Korean pendulous artificial heart design (8).

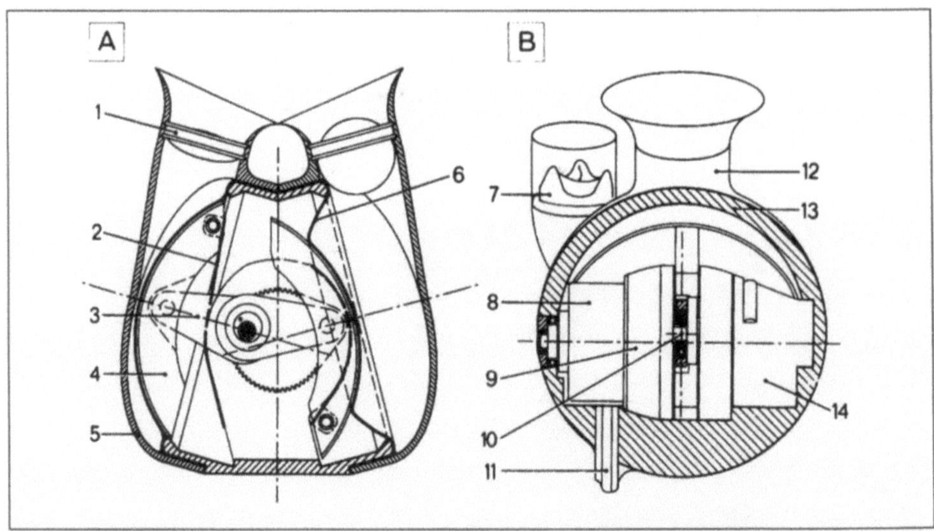

Fig. 8. Aachen total artificial heart (A) cross-sectional view in dispacement axis plane, (B) cross-section perpenticular to (A). 1, inlet disc valve; 2, beam spring; 3, piston rod; 4, pusher plate; 5, pump chamber; 6, diaphragm; 7, outlet leaflet valve; 8, brushless DC-motor; 9, reduction gear; 10, hypocycloidic cranc; 11, vent; 12, outlet with sewing cuff; 13, housing; 14, electronics (10).

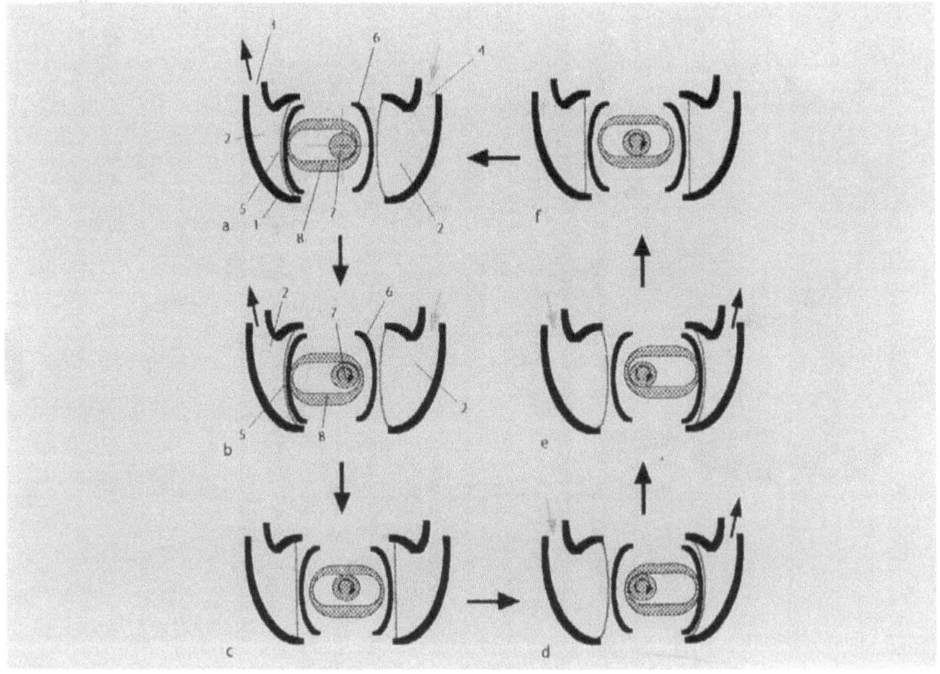

Fig. 9. Artificial heart system with a combination of cogwheel and an inner oval of cogs (11).

The French design uses a low speed, double-lobed hypocycloidal pump without valves. This design is based on the principle of the Maillard-Wankel rotary compressor (Fig. 10).

In the Japanese system a nutating membrane acts as a moving piston. This design requires no heart valves and seals and bearings for the moving axis (Fig. 11).

Electromagnetically activated left vetricular assist devices and total artificial hearts

The direct conversion of electrical energy into the movement of solenoids or magnetical particles in electromagnetic fields can be very efficient and results in extreme system simplicity and thus very high reliability. Systems with electromagnetical energy conversion are listed in Table 3.

The Novacor Baxter implantable left ventricular assist system (Fig. 12) employs a high efficiency balanced solenoid energy converter coupled to a symmetrical dual pusher plate sac-type blood pump. The system has only two moving parts, the symmetrical armature-spring assemblies. The balanced pivoted solenoid armatures perform the actual energy conversion storing mechanical energy in the decoupling springs. The decoupling springs then deliver that energy to the blood pump pusher plates. This system has been under development since the early 1970's and has been used in an ongoing clinical trial as a bridge to cardiac transplantation since 1984. Until April 1995, this left ventricular assist system has been implanted in 312 patients, the duration of support has ranged between 1 and 370 days. Even with more than 10 years clinical application, the system is still under development with the ultimate goal of chronic support. Today the system is not completely implantable. It needs an external vent and percutaneous energy cable, but with a wearable controller, the patients can be discharged from the hospital, allowing them to await a donor heart at home. An example is a patient at the German Heart Institute now supported for more than 600 days after implantation.

Another magnetic actuator has been developed by Kovacs in Tampa. The actuator electromagnet consists of multiple coil windings on a ferromagnetic core geometrically designed to enable both magnetic flux ducting and flux density enhancement in the working air gap of the actuator-pusher plate-diaphragm combination. Dynamic flux enhancement is achieved by the use of critically sized neodymium permanent magnets located in the actuator ferromagnetic structure. This actuator could be used in all kinds of pusher plate blood pumps replacing the mechanical linear motion gearing used for pusher plate displacement. A unique design of a totally implantable ventricular assist system using a vibrating flow pump is under design at the Tohoku University in Japan. An elastic tube with magnets attached on the outside is vibrating in an electromagnetical field with a frequency of 10–50 Hz. Figure 13 shows a schematic illustration of the vibrating flow pump. It consists of inlet and outlet cannulae, a vibrational tube with surrounding electrical coils, and an outflow jellyfish valve. Blood is received from the left side of the pump and ejected into the right side through an inlet portion and the vibrating tube travels 2–5 mm according to drive frequency and output voltage.

A ferrofluidic actuator for an implantable artificial heart has been proposed by Mitamura at the Hokkaido University in Sapporro. This actuator directly drives

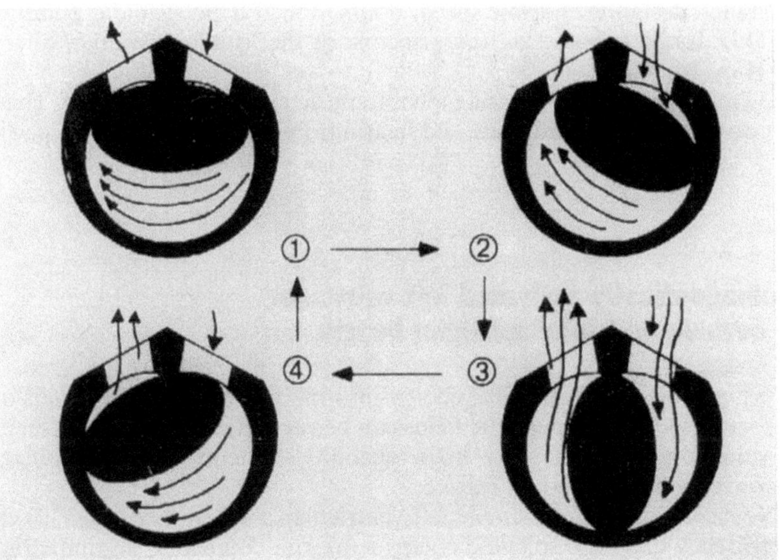

Fig. 10. French design with the principle of the Maillard-Wankel rotary compressor (13).

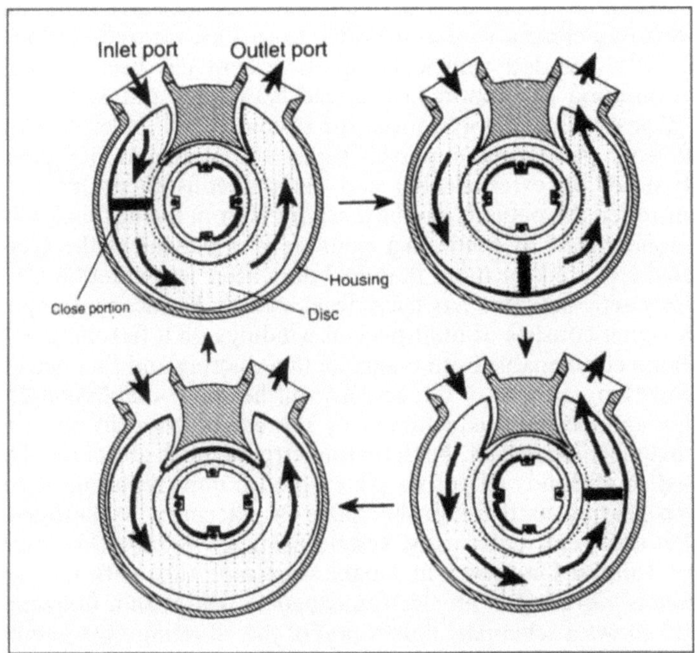

Fig. 11. Japanese system with a nutating membrane (undulation pump) (14).

Table 3. Electromagnetically Activated LVAD and TAH

Developer P.I./Location	System description special features	Status 1995	Ref.
P. M. Portner, Novacor-Baxter Oakland	solenoid-spring pusher plate B.P. wearable controller	long term clinically LVAD	(15, 16) (17, 18)
S. G. Kovacs Univ. of South Florida; Tampa	magnetic actuator direct displacement pusher plate	LVAD in vivo acute	(19)
T. Yambe, H. Hashimoto Sendai Japan	vibrating tube 10–50 Hz oscillation univalved	LVAD in vivo acute	(2B, 21) (22)
Y. Mitamura, T. Wada Sapporo	ferrofluidic activator ferrofl.-piston displacement by controlled magnetic field	feasibility study working labtype	(23)
J. Müller, P. Nüsser H. D. Stahlmann; Berlin	magnetofluidic converter	feasibility study	

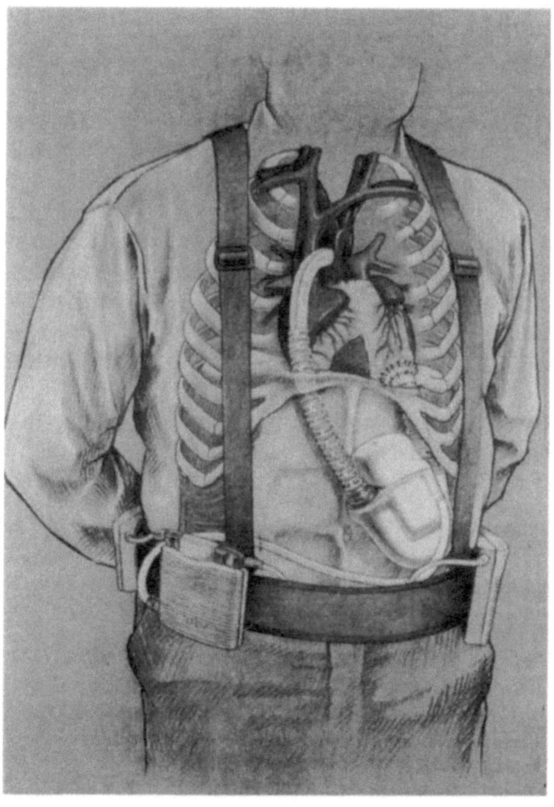

Fig. 12. Novacor Baxter implantable left ventricular assist system (17).

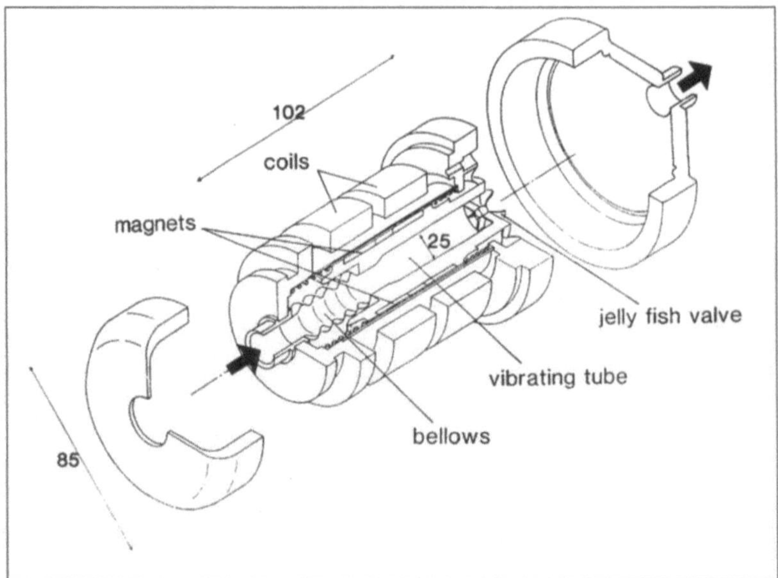

Fig. 13.   Schematic illustration of the vibrating flow pump (22).

magnetic fluids by applying a magnetic field to the ferrofluids. In this feasibility study the magnetic fluid used consists of tiny magnetic particles suspended in kerosene. To apply a magnetic field to the magnetic fluid, a ring solenoid with air gap was made. The magnetic fluid was poured into a U-shaped glass cylinder while a magnetic field was applied, the magnetic fluid was displaced upwards by the magnetic pressure. As a result of this study, the author stated that the ferrofluidic actuator generated a pressure of 9.98 kpa, enough to drive a right blood pump. Although the pressure was not enough to drive the left blood pump, a ferrofluidic actuator for an artificial heart could be made feasible by optimizing the design of the solenoids.

At the German Heart Institute Berlin, another concept of a magneto-fluidic converter is the object of a feasibility study.

Indirect electrohydraulically activated left ventricular assist devices and total artificial hearts

The rotational movement of the electromotor axis can be transformed into the pumping movement of the membranes of displacement pumps with the help of low or high pressure hydraulic coupling. Such systems are listed in Table 4.

The electrohydraulical total artificial heart being developed at the University of Utah consists of a brushless DC motor to drive an axial flow pump that propels

Table 4. Indirect Electrohydraulically Activated LVAD and TAH

Developer P.I./Location	System description special features	Status 1995	Ref.
D. B. Olsen, G. Pantalos University of Utah	reversing DC-Motor axial flow pump diaphragm blood pump	in vivo TAH < 195 d. in vivo LVAD	(24)
O. H. Frazier, R. T. V. Kung THI & ABIOMED Houston	unidirectional DC-Motor centrifugal hydraulic pump fluid switching rotary valve diaphragm blood pump	in vivo TAH < 108 d.	(25)
R. Kiraly, K. Butler CCF & NIMBUS Cleveland	DC-Motor – gear pump high pressure piston magnetic coupling pusher plate blood pump	in vivo TAH < 120 d. in vivo LVAD	(26, 27)
Y. Taenak, NCCRI K. Takahashi Osaka & Tokyo	motor integrated regenerative pump reversible impeller diaphragm blood pump	in vivo acute TAH	(28)
K. Affeld; Berlin	unidir. centrifugal pump periodical axial shift of imp. diaphragm blood pump	LVAD working prototype	(29)
V. I. Shumakov Moskow	reversing DC-Motor axial flow pump diaphragm blood pump		

hydraulic oil to two blood pumps, thus moving their flexible diaphragms and propelling the blood out of the device. The motor rotates in one direction, stops, then rotates in the opposite direction. In contrast, in the ABIOMED total artificial heart a centrifugal pump generating hydraulic pressure operates unidirectionally, whereas hydraulic flow reversal is achieved via a cylindrical rotary valve that alternates the direction of the hydraulic fluid between the left and right pumping chamber (Fig. 14). The energy converter of the Cleveland Clinic-Nimbus total artificial heart consists of a DC motor driving a gear pump that produces high pressure moving a piston in a cylinder that is magnetically coupled with pusher plates of a diaphragm blood pump (Fig. 15). Motor and blood pumps are separated in the concept of a National Cardiovascular Center of Japan electrohydraulic totally implantable artificial heart. The energy converter, a brushless DC motor integrated in a regenerative pump, is implanted in the abdominal region, two blood pumps replaced orthotopically the left and right ventricles. The energy converter pumps silicone oil to alternately push the diaphragms of the blood pumps by bidirectional rotation of the impeller (Fig. 16).

The left ventricular assist device developed by Affeld at the Humboldt University of Berlin uses an electrohydraulic energy converter with only one moving part. This one element consists of an electric motor, an impeller of a centrifugal pump, and a linear electric actuator. The centrifugal pump pumps a transmitter fluid and the linear electric actuator shifts the rotor axially at the end of systole and diastole. The special housing of the centrifugal pump has two flow channels that act as inflow and outflow ducts. Their function is reversed as the result of the axial shift

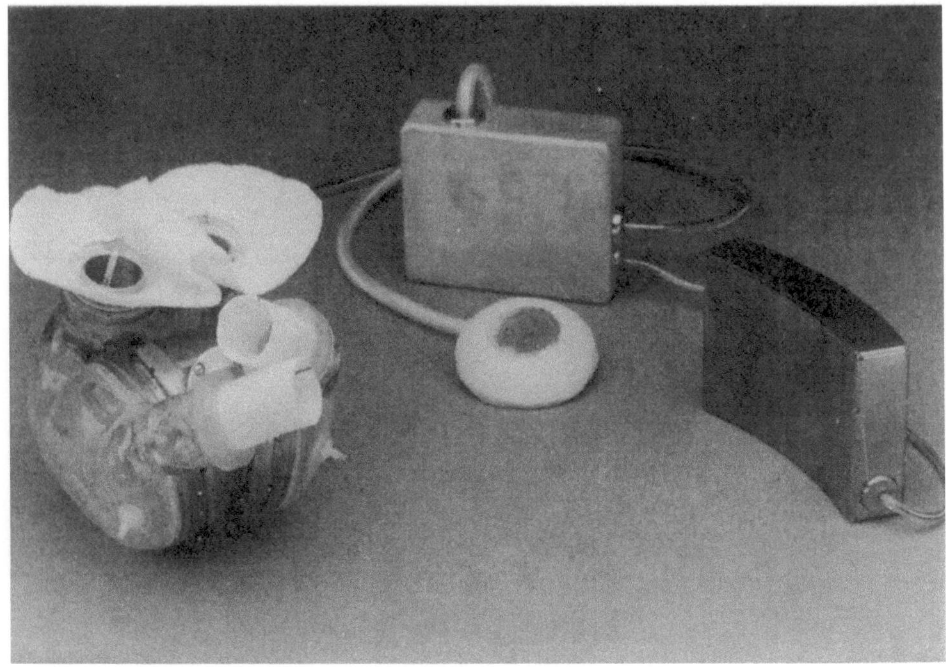

Fig. 14.   ABIOMED total artificial heart system (25).

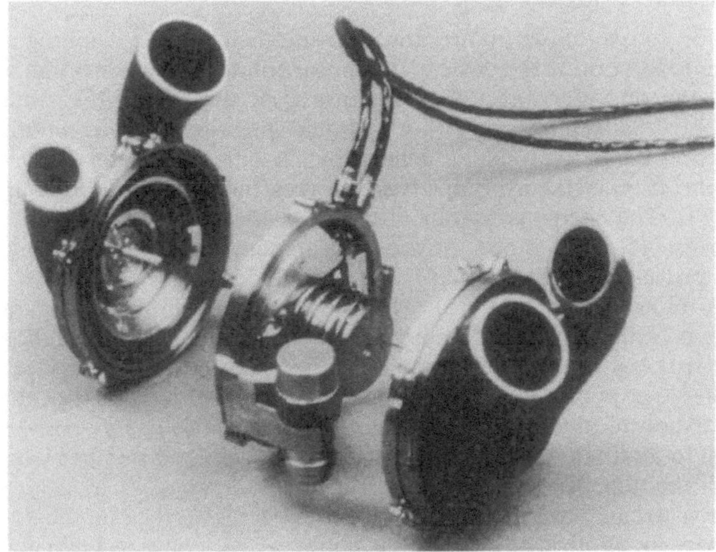

Fig. 15.   Cleveland Clinic-Nimbus total artificial heart (27).

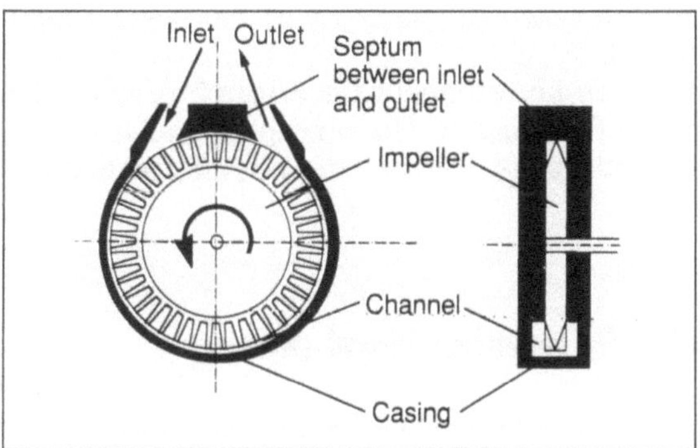

Fig. 16. Regenerative hydraulic pump for the totally implantable artificial heart-National Cardiovascular Center of Japan (28).

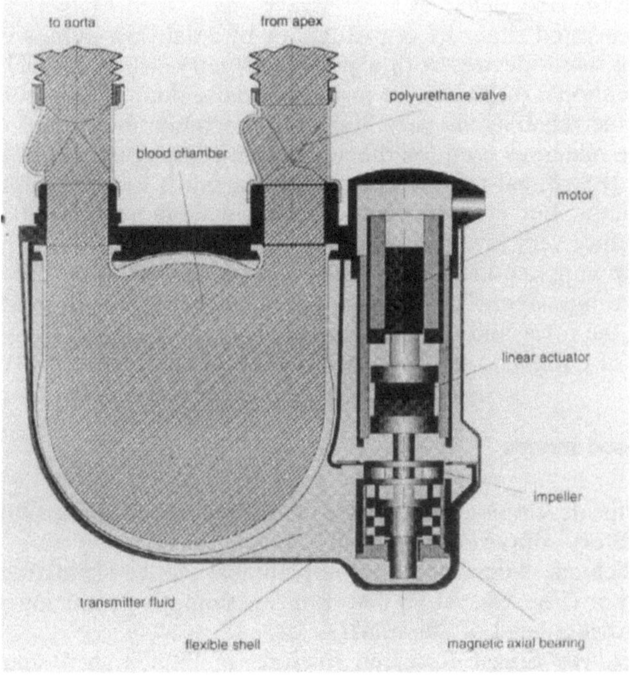

Fig. 17. Left ventricular assist device developed by Affeld at the Humboldt University of Berlin (29).

of the rotor. Systolic flow into the blood pump is achieved by compressing the blood chamber and ejecting the blood. During diastole flow is directed out of the blood pump and into the expansion chamber and the blood chamber is filled. Thus, a pulsatile flow is generated without a change of the rotational direction of the impeller. The rotor combines the function of a centrifugal pump and a valve.

This pump design with only one moving part has a great inherent safety and is very compact (Fig. 17).

There is not too much known about the research progress achieved in Moscow at the research group of Shumakov. His concept is similar to that of the University of Utah, about the status as of 1995 there is not information available.

Directly hydraulically working blood pumps

Rotary blood pumps can be designed as centrifugal pumps (a) with impellers with or without vanes or as axial flow pumps (b) with high speed turbines. The flow produced can be pulsatile or non-pulsatile. At the beginning of the development, the most crucial point was blood trauma and thrombus generation in areas where flow stasis occurred. Because blood is the operating fluid, special attention should be paid to a very careful design avoiding areas of stagnation as well as high shear stresses within the flow field.

The flow generated either by centrifugal or by axial flow pumps is sufficient for left ventricular assist devices with a pump geometry which is much smaller than those of conventional displacement pumps. Because there is only one moving part, the impeller, the reliability is very high, the biocompatibility and especially bio-stability of the materials used for the fabrication of this pump is not poblematic.

In general, centrifugal pumps operate with a much lower spinning speed than axial flow pumps, but even turbines working with more than 30 000 rpm have proven to produce very low hemolysis.

Axial flow pumps require a very close turbine tip clearance and therefore very stiff radial bearings. Centrifugal pumps operate effectively with much larger clearance between the rotor and the housing.

Both types of pumps do not require any kind of heart valve prosthesis.

Centrifugal blood pumps

Research groups developing implantable centrifugal blood pumps for long-term or chronic circulatory support are listed in Table 5.

In Vienna Schima is developing an implantable seal-less centrifugal pump with integrated motor (Fig. 18). At 25 000 rpm this pump is producing a flow of 10 l/min with a pressure head of 100 mmHg.

At the Allegheny Singer Research Institute in Pittsburgh a small implantable centrifugal pump with rotor shaft and seal lubricated at a constant rate with sterile water containing heparin has been developed. The results of animal experiments up to 154 days support the use of a pulse-less centrifugal pump as a ventricular assist device. There were no clinical thromboembolic events, autopsy revealed no infarction or structural change in the brain, kidneys, lungs, liver, intestines nor heart and mean blood values returned to baseline by postoperative day 7 and did not deteriorate thereafter.

At the Baylor College in Houston, a compact seal-less centrifugal pump has been developed which is intended as a long-term ventricular assist device as well as a cardiopulmonary bypass pump (Fig. 19). This pump demonstrated low hemo-lysis and adequate flow performance as a left ventricular assist system. Other cen-

Table 5. Centrifugal Blood Pumps

Developer P.I./Location	System description special features	Status 1995	Ref.
H. Schima, E. Wolner Vienna	Double disc DC-Motor sealless, axleless impeller distance balls	working labtype	(30)
G. J. Magovern Allegheny-Singer Inst. Pittsburgh	LVAD for medium term use 10 ml/h heparinized saline for lubrication	in vivo < 154 d.	(31)
S. Takatani, Y. Nosé G. Noon Baylor College; Houston	Eccentric inlet port (female) pivot bearing secondary vane	in vivo < 28 d.	(32)
T. Yamane, T. Jiyuka Tsukuba – Japan	imp. with mag. suspension and pivot bearings sealless	working labtype	(33)
D. B. Olsen, R. Flach University of Utah University of Virginia	fully magnetically suspended impeller	working labtype	(34)
R. T. V. Kung ABIOMED	fully magnetically suspended impeller	working labtype	
K. X. Quian Taiwan	pulsatile impeller pump	in vivo < 11 d. LVAD & TAH	(35)

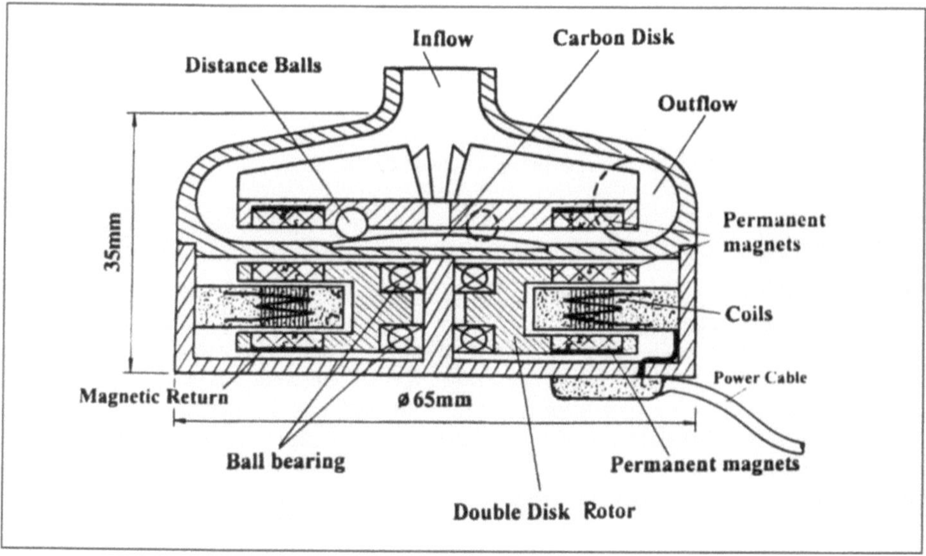

Fig. 18. Implantable seal-less centrifugal pump – Vienna (30).

trifugal blood pumps with magnetically suspended impellers are under development in Japan and the United States aiming at an implantable ventricular assist device.

A pulsatile implantable impeller assist device and a total artificial heart is under development in China at the National Taiwan University. The pulsatility of the blood pressure and flow rate is achieved by introducing a square waveform voltage into the motor coil, thereby changing the rotating speed of the impeller periodically. Two assist pumps with different dimensions have been combined for a biventricular application (Fig. 20).

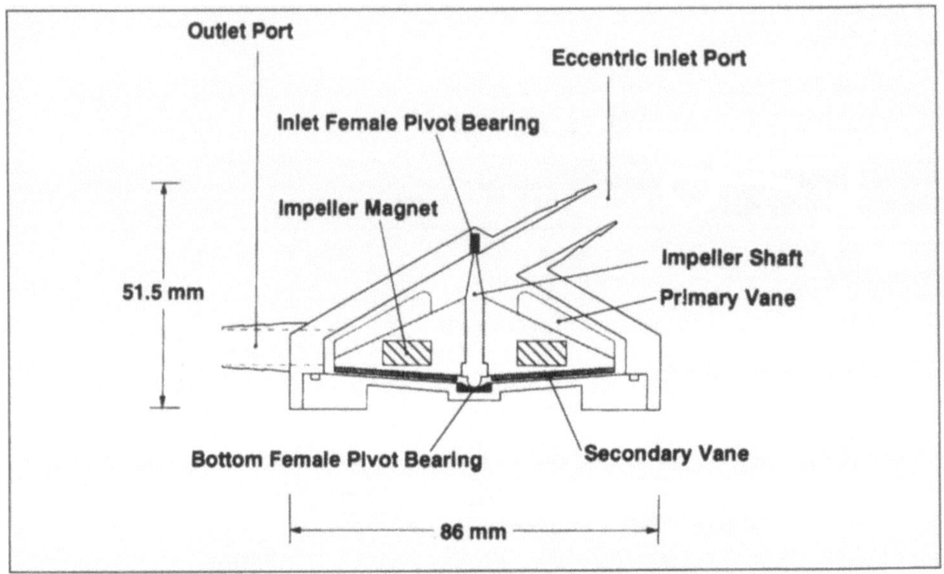

Fig. 19.   Compact seal-less centrifugal pump – Baylor College (32).

Axial flow pumps

Today, axial flow pumps seem to be the smallest devices possible for mechanical circulatory support. With high spinning speed, between 10 000–30 000 rpm, pulseless flow rates of up to 10 l/min at physiological arterial pressures are possible. They are mechanically simple, they do not need flexing polymer membranes or heart valve prostheses, having such a potential for higher reliability and longer durability. A list of ongoing research activities in the field of axial flow pumps is summarized in Table 6.

Jarvik designed a very small axial blood pump with blood immersed bearings (Fig. 21, Jarvic 2000). These pumps, made out of titanium with a diameter of 25 mm, a volume of 25 cc, and a weight of 85 grams, is positioned in the left ventricle across the apex. The patient's remaining left ventricular function is preserved. In first animal experiments the hemolysis rate was unacceptably high, but this problem has been resolved by redesigning the rotor and stator blade configuration. A similar

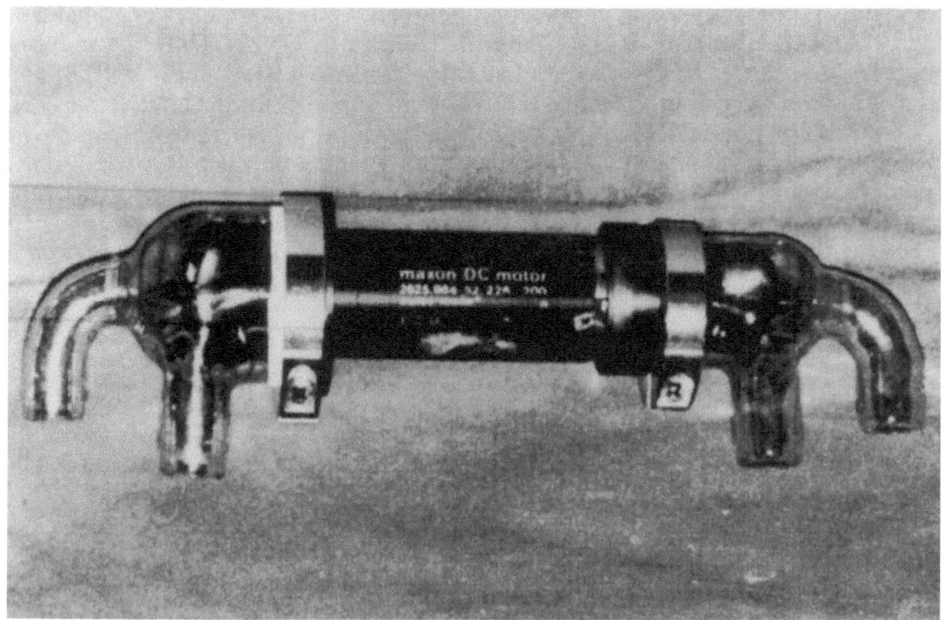

Fig. 20.   Total artificial heart under development in China (35).

Table 6. Axial Flow Blood Pumps

Developer P.I./Location	System description special features	Status 1995	Ref.
R. Jarvik O. H. Frazier (THI) New York	intraventricular pump (IVP) (Jarvik 2000) sealless blood immersed bearings 85 g – 25 ccm; 10 l/min	in vivo < 155 d. in vitro < 3 y.	(36)
Y. Nosé, G. Aber Baylor & NASA Houston	saphire-ruby front-bearings cylindrical circonia rear bear. sealless; 5 l/min. at 100 mmHg	in vivo acute < 9 d.	(37)
K. C. Butler; NIMBUS B. P. Griffith; Pittsb.	ceramic bearings and seals 10 l/min at 120 mmHg	in vivo < 26 d. in vitro long term	(38)
Y. Mitamura, T. Tanaka Sapporo	motor-shaft-impeller ferrofluidic seal, ball-bearings 5 l/min at 100 mmHg	working prototype	(39)
H. Reul, G. Rau HI Aachen	intraart. microaxial blood p. microelectric motor (< 6.5 mm)	working prototype	(40)
R. Kormos, B. P. Griffith M. Umezu Pittsburg & Tokyo	motor-shaft-impeller totally implantable bearing purge system 5 l/min at 100 mmHg	working prototype	(41)

device has been designed in cooperation between the Baylor College of Medicine and the NASA Johnson Space Center in Houston (Fig. 22). Only the inducer/impeller unit moves to generate the bloodflow. The flow straightener in front and the diffuser in the rear of the pump act as bearing supports for the inducer/impeller. The pump has no seals. The flow straightener in front prevents prerotation of the blood caused by the rotational influence of the spinning impeller. It is fixed to the side of the tube and holds a sapphire cup as a front bearing support for the ruby ball spinning with the inducer. The impeller blades contain permanent magnets allowing the impeller to act as a rotor for a brushless DC motor. The motor stator

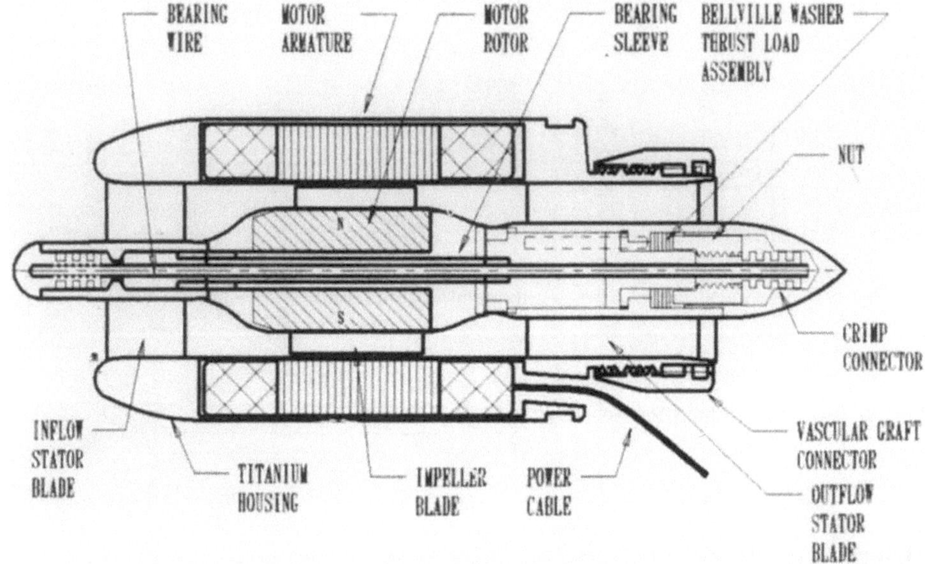

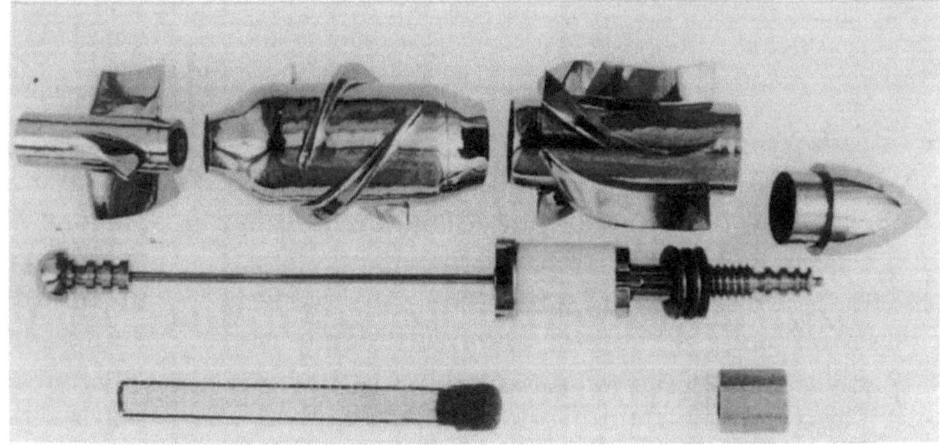

Fig. 21.   Jarvik 2000 (a) schematic illustration, (b) rotor-stator combination (36).

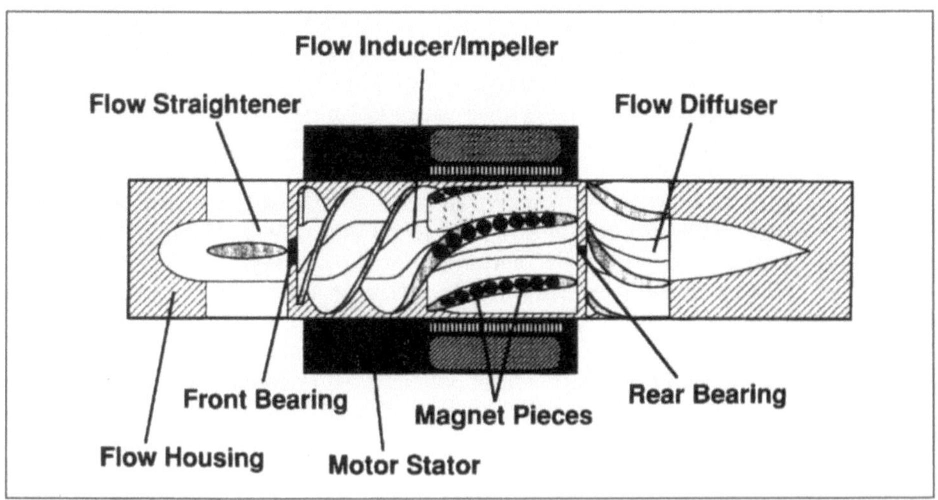

Fig. 22. Axial blood pump – Baylor College of Medicine, NASA Johnson Space Center (37).

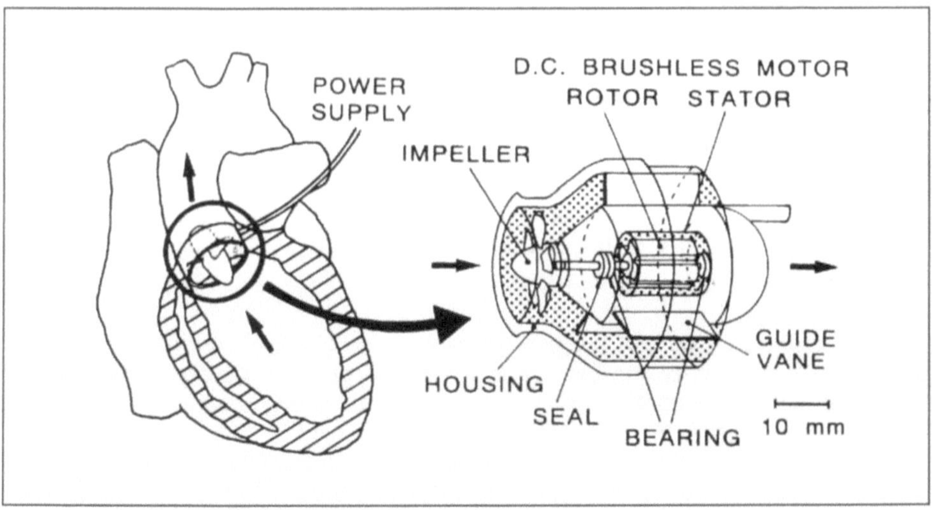

Fig. 23. VALVO pump (39).

is slipped over the flow tube and provides a six-pole rotating magnetic field. Behind the impeller is a diffuser which converts the tangentially directed fluid into an axial flow. The diffuser holds the rear cyclindrical bearing of circonia.

Another axial flow pump is under investigation at the Nimbus Incorporation and the Department of Surgery of the University of Pittsburgh. This design uses titanium for many of the pump components and advanced ceramics for the barings and seals.

A different design is under development in Sapporo at the Hokkaido Tokyo University. This VALVO pump, an axial non-pulsatile blood pump implanted in the aortic heart valve position, consists of an impeller and a motor which are encased in a housing. An impeller with 5 vanes (22 mm in diameter) is used. The impeller is connected to a DC brushless motor, sealing is achieved by means of a ferrofluidic seal (Fig. 23).

At the Helmholtz Institute in Aachen an intra-arterial micro-axial blood pump has been realized. This pump was designed to be introduced through the femoral artery and to be placed within the ascending aorta proximal to the aortic valve. The design speed is 30 000 rpm, resulting in a flow of 4 l/min with a pressure head of 80 mmHg.

The intra-ventricular axial flow pump integrated with a totally implantable bearing purge system is under development in Japanese-American cooperation between the University of Pittsburgh, the Tokyo Women's Medical College, the Waseda University, and the Sun Medical Technology Research Corporation (Fig. 24).

The pump is introduced into the left ventricular cavity via the ventricular apex with the outlet cannula path integrated across the aortic valve. Blood is withdrawn from the left ventricular cavity through several inlet ports at the pump base and is discharged into the ascending aorta. A flange connects the motor to the pump base which is external to the left ventricular apex. In this design a shaft seal is necessary. A purged seal system consisting of a miniature lip seal and ceramic pressure grove journal bearing which also acts as a purge pump, generating more than 3000 mmHg at 10 000 rpm. This purge flow flushes the lip seal and prevents blood backflow into the bearing. The pump produces a flow rate of 5 l/min against 90 mmHg differential pressure at 11 000 rpm.

Thermomechanically activated left ventricular assist devices

The conversion of heat into mechanical forces has been studied with the intention of using nuclear power sources for artificial hearts. Two systems have been designed, a thermopneumatic actuator driven by a Stirling engine, and a Stirling engine coupled with a high pressure hydraulic converter.

As energy storage electrically heated salt highly isolated and encapsulated in a small separated container has been used. After more than 25 years of funding, the National Institute of Health in the United States stopped the program in 1993. With the technology available today, problems with the durability of the systems and the overall efficiency could not be resolved.

Another argument was that the use of implanted capsules with plutonium-238 as an energy source for artificial hearts will not be accepted today by the public.

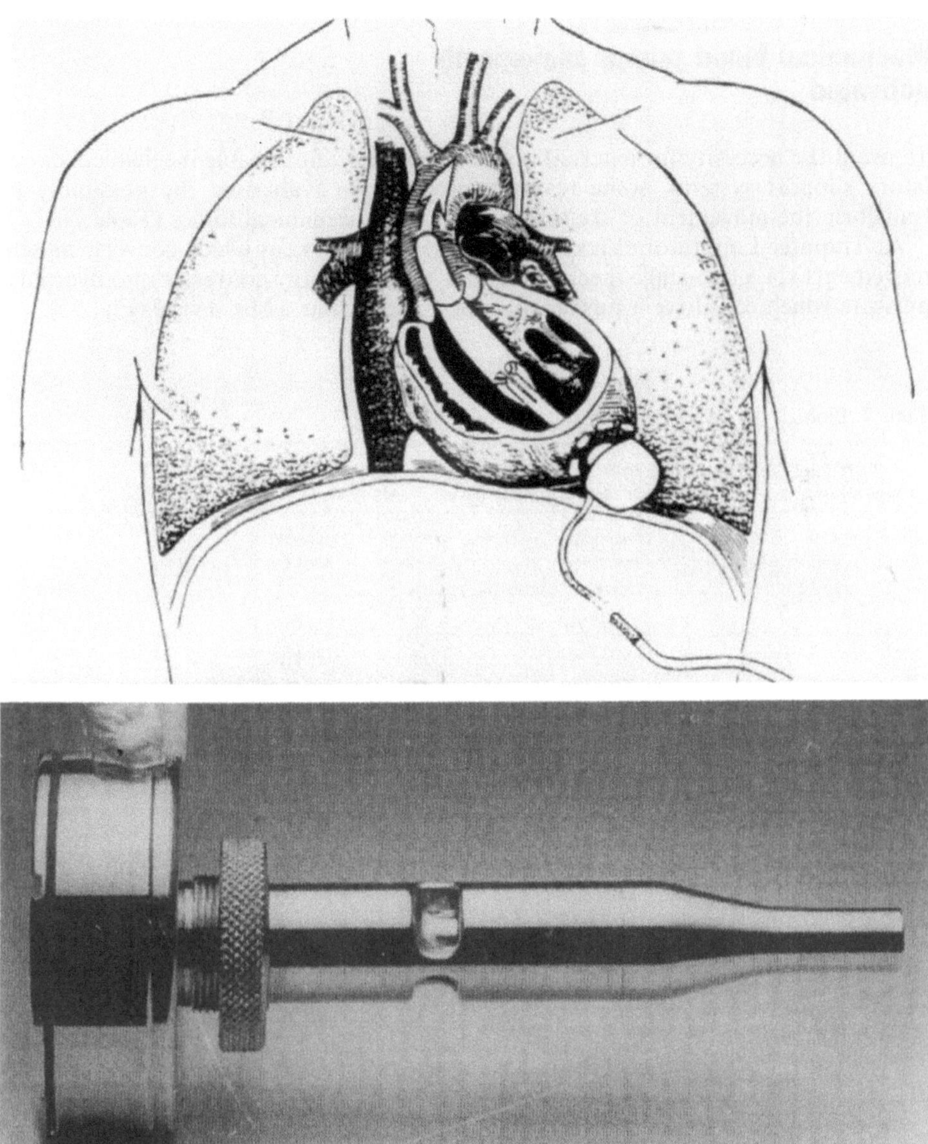

Fig. 24. Intra-ventricular axial flow pump (a) schematic illustration, (b) motor-pump combination (41).

Mechanical blood pumps biologically activated

To avoid the necessity for external power supply for implantable mechanical circulatory support systems, some research projects are evaluating the possibility to transform the movement of skeletal muscles into mechanical forces (Table 7).

At Thoratec Laboratories a system is under development which converts muscle movements via a two-stage mechanical to hydraulic energy converter into hydraulic pressure which can drive a pusher plate of a ventricular assist device (Fig. 25).

Table 7. Biologically activator mechanical blood pumps

Developer P.I./Location	System description special features	Status 1995	Ref.
D. J. Farrar, J. D. Hill Calif. Pacific Center & Thoratec Lab.	two-stage hydraulic energy converter, driven by skeletal muscle pusher plate blood pump	ex vivo working prototoype	(42)
G. Takatani, Y. Nosé Houston	roller screw linear actuator driven by latissimus dorsi pusher plate blood pump	in vitro working prototype	(43)
H. Mizuhara, T. Ban Kyoto	by muscle contraction compressed pneum. chamber diaphragm blood pump		(44)

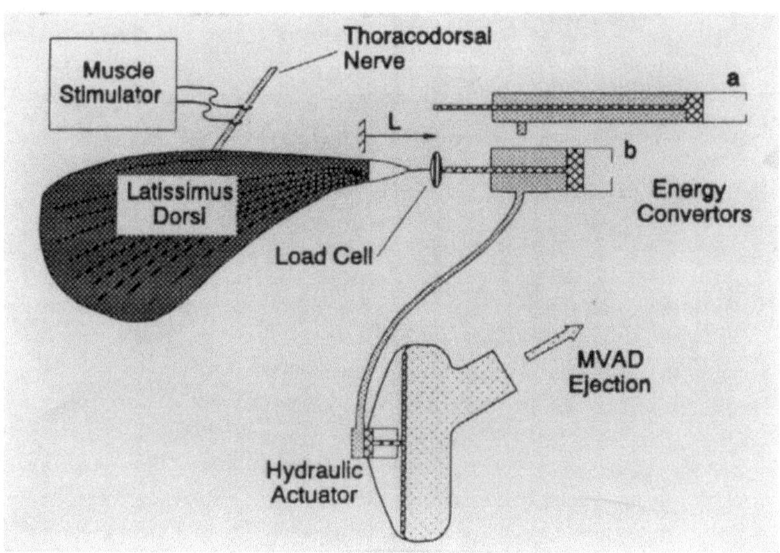

Fig. 25.   Mechanical to hydraulic energy converter – Thoratec Laboratories (42).

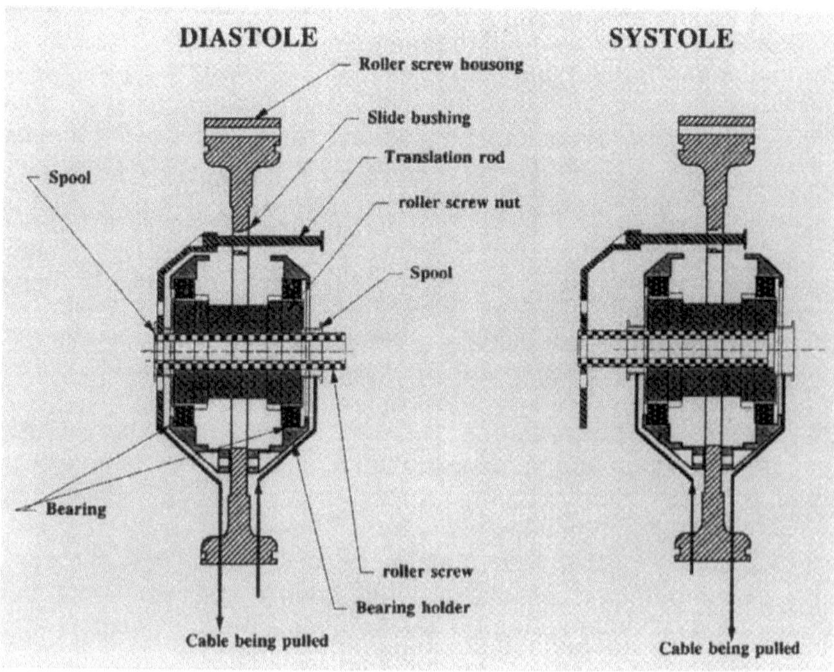

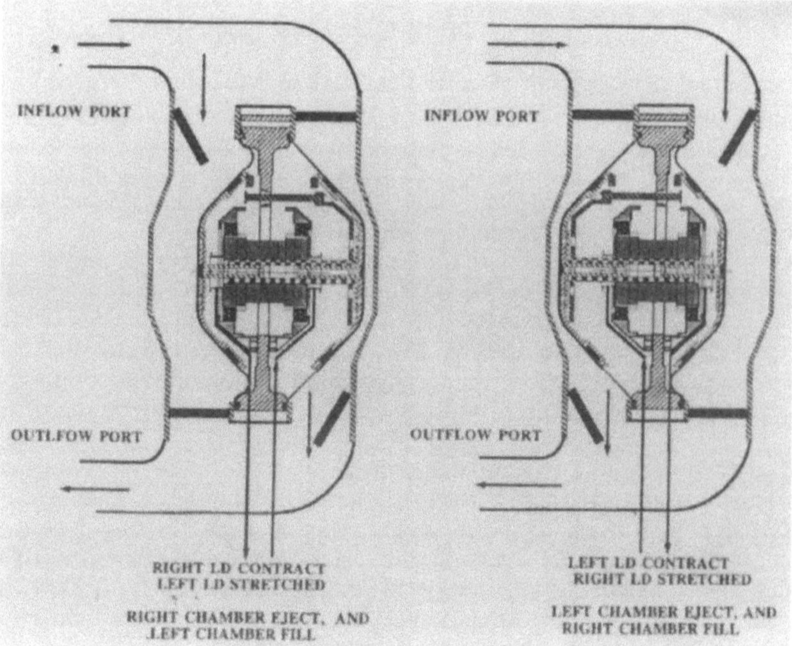

Fig. 26. Roller screw linear muscle actuator (a) energy converter, (b) double chamber assist pump (43).

A double chamber ventricular assist device with a roller screw linear muscle actuator driven by the left and right latissimus dorsal muscles has been developed in Houston at the Baylor College of Medicine (Fig. 26). The prototype of this ventricular assist device can provide flows of 2–4 l/min against an afterload of 100 mmHg, a compliance chamber is not required because of the double chamber design of the pump. With this performance, the muscle power requirements are not exceeding 3–4 watts over the systolic cycle.

A Japanese research group in Kyoto is developing a pneumatic chamber which is inserted beneath the muscle and compressed by contractions of the muscle so that muscle contractor power is converted into pneumatic pressure. Of importance is the optimal insertion position of the chamber and the influence of chamber size on generated pneumatic pressure. The pneumatic chamber was able to generate power sufficient to drive a right ventricular diaphragm assist device.

Summary

A completely implantable mechanical circulatory support system or total artificial heart consists of a blood pump (two blood pumps) with an energy converter, compliance chamber (volume compensator), internal batteries, internal controller, transcutaneous energy and data transfer system, and external supply and monitoring systems.

Two implantable LVADs with electrically-driven displacement pumps entered worldwide clinical trials. These systems, the Novacor Baxter and HeartMate TCI, have been under development since the early 1970's, the ultimate goal of a fully implantable assist system, has not been reached yet. Today's configuration needs power supply by a percutaneous cable; instead of a compliance chamber the systems are vented to the open air by percutaneous tubing. Transcutaneous energy transmission systems and especially the volume compensator needed with these type of pumps are still not available for clinical use.

Implantable artificial hearts with a pair of displacement pumps and electrically-driven energy converters are at the beginning of the in vivo testing period. After satisfying results, including animal survival for up to 6 months, the device readiness testing period is planned to start in 1997. If the long-term durability tests and animal experiments have proven the mechanical reliability and biocompatibility of the systems, first clinical applications can be expected at the beginning of the new century.

Even after 25 years of development, there are quite a lot of problems to be solved. The most important are listed in Table 8. Mechanical and chemical durability of the materials used, their biocompatibility in terms of blood contact and tissue contact as well as the electromechanical components are still not fulfilling the high standards necessary in long-term clinical application for a life-sustaining device. Size and weight of the implantable components have to be further reduced, in most cases fail-safe features are not yet incorporated.

So this first generation of mechanical circulatory support systems will hopefully complete their development within the next 5–10 years.

Nevertheless, today's clinical results with the left ventricular assist devices in bridge-to-transplant patients have proven the feasibility of using these devices as alternative to cardiac transplantation, important information has been gathered

Table 8. MCSS: Technical problems 1995

Durability	
– membrane	flexlife, degradation
– gearing	wear, corrosion, ...
– bearing	wear, seizure
– sealing	wear, seizure
– encapsulation	fluid permeation
biocompatibility	
– blood contact	thrombus formation, cellular trauma
– tissue contact	cell ingrowth, infection
– body fluids	chemical degradation
power supply	
– batteries/TETS	heat dissipation, efficiency cycle life
control	
– electronics	reliability, ...
– sensors	long term stability, ...
size & weight	
– compactness of design	device volume / pump output
– anatomical fit	location of components
fail-safe features	

in this first clinical period which started in 1984 (Novacor). Questions about the acceptance of the device by the patient, the biocompatibility for timespans up to 650 days, and the rehabilitation process under the device could be answered.

During recent years, a second generation of circulatory support systems, direct hydrodynamic pumps, are under development.

Both principles to convert electrical energy in flow and pressure, centrifugal and axial flow pumps, have been applied in the new concepts.

Compared with the system for implantable displacement pumps, the list of components, and therefore possible problems, is much smaller. For hydrodynamic pumps, the size and weight as well as the ratio (device volume/flow produced) is much smaller.

Presently discussed obstacles are the thrombus formation around seals and bearings, the mechanical wear and seizure of the bearings, and the blood trauma produced by high speed spinning turbines with still imperfect fluid dynamics.

Rotational pumps are producing pulseless flow, but long-term animal experiments have proven the physiological compatibility of this kind of flow. Under discussion are possibilities to convert the pulseless flow in a physiological pulsed pattern.

Durability problems are minimized with these systems because they only have one or two moving parts. Biocompatibility and biostability of the materials used is also less problematic because an elastic polymer material is not required.

The conversion of muscle power into mechanical force to drive blood pumps is still at the beginning. Some ideas have been formulated as concepts, some laboratory type models have been built to evaluate whether the power delivered by the muscle will fulfill the requirements of the blood pumps in terms of energy delivered and long-term function.

The efforts required to develop implantable artificial hearts and heart assist devices exceeded by far all expectations which were formulated at the beginning of artificial heart research in the United States in the 1960's. The delay in time and the enormous increase in expenses should be kept in mind when trying to foresee future developments.

But it seems to be certain that an implantable artificial heart which will replace the necessity of heart transplantation will be realized sooner or later, evolving new technologies will help to achieve the ultimate goal of a so-called "forgettable" device for patients with endstage heart failure.

References

1. Takatani S, Orime Y, Tasai K, Ohara Y, Naito K, Mizuguchi K, Makinouchi K, Damm G, Glueck J, Ling J, Noon G, Nosé Y (1994) Totally implantable total artificial heart and ventricular assist device with multipurpose miniature electromechanical energy system. Artificial Organs 18 (1): 80–92
2. Takatani S, Shiono M, Sasaki T, Glueck J, Noon GP, Nosé Y, DeBakey ME (1992) Development of a totally implantable electromechanical total artificial heart: Baylor TAH. Artificial Organs 16 (4): 398–406
3. Orime Y, Takatani S, Tasai K, Ohara Y, Naito K, Miziguchi K, Meier D, Wernicke JT, Damm G, Glueck J, Noon GP, Nosé Y (1994) The Baylor total artificial heart; Flow visualization studies. ASAIO J 40: M499–M505
4. Snyder A, Rosenberg G, Weiss W, Pierce W, Pae W Jr., Marlotte J, Nazarian R, Ford S (1991) A completely implantable total artificial heart system. ASAIOI Transactions 37: M237–M238
5. Snyder AJ, Rosenberg G, Weiss WJ, Ford SK, Nazarian RA, Hicks DL, Marlotte JA et al (1993) In vivo testing of a completely implanted total artificial heart system. ASAIO J 39: M177–M184
6. Okamoto E, Tomoda K, Yamamoto K, Mitamura Y, Mikami T (1994) Development of a compact, highly efficient, totally implantable motor-driven assist pump system. Artificial Organs 18 (12): 911–917
7. Mambrito B, Arabia M, Chieco S, Ferrazzi P, Ferri E, Fierli M, Glauber M, Meli M, Zagara M (1994) The Italien Artificial heart Program. Artificial Organs 18 (7): 533–537
8. Hee Chan Kim, Byoung Goo Min (1992) Cardiac output regulation in the moving actuator total artificial heart without a compliance chamber. ASAIO J 38: 846–850
9. Myers TJ, Dasse KA, Macris MP, Poirier VL, Cloy MJ, Frazier OH (1994) Use of a left ventricular assist device in an outpatient setting. ASAIO J 40: M471–M475
10. Kaufmann R, Reul H, Rau G (1994) The Helmholtz Total Artificial Heart Labtype. Artificial Organs 18(7): 537–542
11. Sauer IM, Frank J, Spiegelberg A, Bücherl ES (1995) A new energy converter for a total artificial heart. Int. J. Artif. Org. 18 (8)
12. Goa H, Smith LM, Krymkowski MG, Kohl RJ, Schmidt DH, Christensen CW (1992) In vitro assessment of the Milwaukee Heart and right to left balance. ASAIO J 38: M722–M725
13. Montiès JR, Havlik P, Mesana T, Tourres JL, Demunck JL: Development of the Marseille pulsatile rotary blood pump for permanent implantable left ventricular assistance. Artificial Organs 18(7): 506–511
14. Abe Y, Chinzei T, Isoyama T, Ono T, Mabuchi K, Imanishi K, Kouno A, Atsumi K, Fujimasa I, Imachi K (1995) Basic study to develop the undulation pump for practical use: Antithrombogenicity, Hemolysis, and flow patterns inside the pump. Artificial Organs 19(7): 691–693
15. Miller PJ, Green GF, Chen H, Ramasamy N, LaForge DH, Jassawalla JS, Ream AK, Oyer PE, Portner PM (1983) In vivo evaluation of a compact, implantable left ventricular assist system (LVAS). ASAIO Transactions 29: 551
16. Daniel MA, Lee J, LaForge DH, Chen H, Billich J, Miller PJ, Ramasamy N, Strauss LR, Jassawalla JS, Portner PM (1991) Clinic evaluation of the Novacor totally implantable ventricular assist system. ASAIO Transactions 37: M423–M525
17. Miller PJ, Billich TJ, LaForge DH, Lee J, Naegli A, Ramasamy N, Jassawalla JS, Portner PM (1994) Initial clinical experience with a wearable controller for the Novacor left ventricular assist system. ASAIO J 40: M465–M470

18. Pristas JM, Wonowich S, Nastala CJ, Gifford J, Conner EA, Borovetz HS, Griffith BP, Portner PM, Kormos RL (1995) Protocol for releasing Novacor left ventricular assist system patients out-of-hospital. ASAIO J 41: M539–M543

19. Kovacs SG, Reynolds DG, McKeown PP; Augereau PG, Wasselle JA, Ondrovic LE, Aiba M (1992) A magnetically actuated left ventricular assist device. ASAIO J 38: 38–46

20. Nitta S, Yambe T, Sonobe T, Naganuma S, Kakinuma Y, Kobayashi S, Tanaka M, Matsuki H, Abe K, Yoshizawa M, Kasai T, Hashimoto H (1995) Totally implantable ventricular assist system using a vibrating flow pump. Artificial Organs 19(7): 676–679

21. Yambe T, Tanaka A, Maekawa T, Hashimoto H et al. (1995) Fractal dimension analysis of the oscillated blood flow with a vibrating flow pump Artifical Organs 19(7): 729–733

22. Naganuma S, Nitta S, Yambe T, Kobayashi S, Tanaka M, Hashimoto H (1995) Gas exchange efficiency of a membrane oxygenator with use of a vibrating flow pump. Artificial Organs 19(7): 747–749

23. Mitamura Y, Wada T, Sakai K (1992) A ferrofluidic actuator for an implantable artificial heart. Artificial Organs 16(5): 490–495

24. Tatsumi E, Diegel PD, Holfert JW, Dew PA, Crump KR, Hansen AC, Khanwilkar PS, Rowles JR, Olsen DB (1992) A blood pump with an interatrial shunt for use as an electrohydraulic total artificial heart. ASAIO J 38: M425–M430

25. Kung RTV, Yu LS, Ochs BD, Parnis SM, Macris MP, Frazier OH (1995) Progress in the development of the ABIOMED total artificial heart. ASAIO J 41: M245–M248

26. Harasaki H, Fukamachi K, Massiello A, Chen J-F, Himley SC, Fukumura F et al. (1994) Progress in Cleveland Clinic – Nimbus total artificial heart development. ASAIO J 40: M494–M498

27. Rintoul TC, Butler KC, Thomas DC, Carriker JW, Maher TR, Kiraly RJ, Massiello A et al. (1993) Continuing development of the Cleveland Clinic – Nimbus total artificial heart ASAIO J 39: M168–M171

28. Masuzawa T, Taenaka Y, Tatsumi E, Choi WW, Toda K et al. (1995) Development of an electrohydraulic total artificial heart at the National Cardiovascular Center, Osaka, Japan ASAIO J 41: M249–M253

29. Affeld K, Bailleu A, Buß A, Diluweit J, Friedrichsen U, Gadischke J, Hanitsch R, Hetzer R, Huber A et al. (1994) A new electrohydraulic energy converter for a left ventricular assist device. Artificial Organs 18(7): 479–483

30. Schima H, Schmallegger H, Huber, L, Birgmann I, Reindl Ch, Schmidt Ch et al. (1995) An implantable Seal-less centrifugal pump with integrated double-disk motor. Artificial Organs 19 (7): 639–643

31. Reddy RC, Goldstein AH, Pacella JJ, Cattivera GR, Clark RE, Magovern GJ Sr (1995) End organ function with prolonged nonpulsatile circulary support. ASAIO J 41: M547–M551

32. Ohara Y, Makinouchi K, Orime Y, Tasai K, Naito K, Mizuguchi K, Shimono T et al. (1994) An ultimate, compact, seal-less centrifugal ventricular assist device: Baylor C-Gyro pump Artificial Organs 18(1): 17–24

33. Yamane T, Ikeda T, Orita T, Tsutsui T, Jikuya T (1995) Design of a centrifugal blood pump with magnetic suspension. Artificial Organs 19(7): 625–630

34. Kim HC, Bearson GB, Khanwilkar PS, Olsen DB, Maslen EH, Allaire PE (1995) In vitro characterization of a magnetically suspended continous flow ventricular assist device. ASAIO J 41: M359–M364

35. Qian KX, Wang SS, Chu SH (1995) In vivo studies of pulsatile implantable impeller assist and total hearts. Artificial Organs 19(4): 328–333

36. Jarvik RK (1995) System considerations favoring rotary artificial hearts with blood-immersed bearings. Artificial Organs 19(7): 565–570

37. Wernicke J-T, Meier D, Mizuguchi K, Damm G, Aber G, Benkowski R, Nosé Y, Noon GP, DeBakey ME (1995) A fluid dynamic analysis using flow visualization of the Baylor/NASA implantable axial flow blood pump for design improvement. Artificial Organs 19(2): 161–177

38. Kameneva MV, Antaki JF, Butler KC, Watach MJ, Kormos RL, Griffith BP, Borovetz HS (1994) A Sheep model for the study of hemorheology with assisted circulation. Effect of an axial flow blood pump. ASAIO J 40: 959–963

39. Yamazaki K, Okamoto E, Yamamoto K, Mitamura Y, Tanaka T, Yozu R (1992) The valvo-pump, an axial blood pump implanted at the heart valve position: Concept and initial results. Artificial Organs 16(3): 297–301

40. Sieß T, Reul H, Rau G. (1995) Concept, realization, and first in vitro testing of an intraarterial microaxial blood pump. Artificial Organs 19(7): 644–652
41. Yamazaki K, Kormos R, Mori T, Umezu M, Kameneva M, Antaki J, Outa E, Litwak P et al. (1995) An intraventricular axial flow blood pump integrated with a bearing purge system. ASAIO J 41: M327–M332
42. Farrar DJ, Reichenbach StH, Hill JD (1995) Mechanical advantage of sekletal muscle as a cardiac assist power source. ASAIO J 41: M481–M484
43. Takatani S, Takami Y, Nakazawa T, Jacobs G, Nosé Y (1995) Double chamber ventricular assist device with a roller screw linear actuator driven by left an right latissimus dorsi muscles. ASAIO J 41: M475–M480
44. Mizuhara H, Koshiji T, Nishimura K, Nomoto S, Matsuda K, Tsutsui N, Kanda K, Ban T (1995) Applicability of the latissimus dorsi muscle in situ as a biomechanical energy source. ASAIO J 41: M495–M499

Author's address:

Dr. E. Hennig
Deutsches Herzzentrum Berlin
Augustenburger Platz 1
D-13353 Berlin, Germany

Prospects for permanent mechanical circulatory support

J. T. Watson

National Heart, Lung, and Blood Institute, National Institutes of Health, USA

In the United States heart failure remains a common cause of death and disability and is the single largest hospital discharge diagnosis. Some 3 to 4 million U.S. citizens suffer this condition and the age-adjusted death rate for both men and women has doubled over the last two decades. The risk of premature death for all heart failure patients is 60–70% at 5 years. For patients with advanced heart failure the 1-year survival is 40–50%. Cardiac transplant is a desirable treatment for many of these patients but is application is limited (1).

Treatment options

Medical treatment using angiotensin converting enzyme inhibitors, prolongs life about 6 months for patients with selected indications but does not normalize survival (2). Cardiac transplantation has not been the subject of randomized trial but is considered the "desirable standard" of treatment. The current cardiac transplant 1-year survival rate is just over 80%, whereas 5-year survival data is tabulated at 50–60%.

In the United States (US) and worldwide the number of donor hearts per year has remained stable at 3500 and seems it may decline even with liberalized procurement policies. The US waiting list is over 3300 candidates. Overall the average candidate for transplantation has a less than 1-in-15 chance of receiving a donor heart, a 40% risk of death while waiting during the first year, and a 15% risk of death during the first year after operation. The limited success with medical therapy and the continuing lack of donors for cardiac transplantation are the compelling reasons to continue research on alternative treatments, such as mechanical circulatory support or donor hearts from genetically altered animals (3), for patients with end-stage heart failure.

Permanent circulatory support

Permanent circulatory support is a viable alternative treatment for heart failure if the patients are informed of expected device lifetime and possible adverse events. They must be assured it is safe, provides clinical benefit with a useful quality of life, in a reliable and cost-effective manner. Because of the recognized need for and demonstrated progress on mechanical circulatory support systems, the NHLBI is supporting research and development of implantable total artificial hearts (TAH), innovative ventricular assist systems (IVAS) and genetically enhanced cardiovascular implants. The latter program is focused on improving the biocompatibility and clinical utility of all permanent cardiovascular implants.

Research programs

Implantable TAH systems

Research on the first generation of implantable total artificial heart systems began in the U.S. in 1988 and has now progressed to a final design stage preparatory to reliability testing. The evolution of these design concepts is based on the resourceful work from many worldwide artificial organs programs over the last several decades.

These implantable artificial heart systems are all electrically powered, designed for a 5-year lifetime, with a cardiac output range of 3–8 liters per minute, that provides physiological systemic pressures with normal cardiac filling pressures. There are five active U.S. programs: two are supported by nonfederal funds at Baylor Medical College and in Milwaukee, and three are funded by the government.

Current research activities are divided into two phases. Phase I, 1993–1996, of the current program is to complete the system design using a comprehensive quality control program for laboratory, clinical and device manufacture (4). By 1996, a limited number of hermetically sealed TAH systems will be tested by each research team in animals for periods of 2 months and bench tested submerged under saline for at least 3 months. The three prototype systems under development are outlined below: Hershey Medical Center working with the 3M Corporation have designed a system ultilizing a brushless DC motor to drive a mechanical roller screw actuation mechanism. This approach supplies alternating left and right actuation of the respective blood pump diaphragms.

Nimbus Corporation collaborating with the Cleveland Clinic Foundation also use a DC motor to drive the gear pump of an electro-hydraulic system, which is magnetically coupled to a follower piston that alternately actuates the left or right pusher plate supporting the blood pump diaphragms.

Both of these systems require a volume compensation mechanism attached to the energy converter to balance differences of 10–15% between the left and right-sided outputs of the artificial blood pumps.

A centrifugal pump used in the Abiomed and Texas Heart Institute (THI) system generates a unidirectional flow which is shuttled back and forth by a linear hydraulic valve, to actuate the left and right blood pump. This design is unique because volume compensation is accomplished on the blood side using a diaphragm control mechanism in the inflow to the right ventricle.

In the fall of 1996 the TAH systems showing the most promise by peer-review of actual laboratory and animal results will enter "readiness" testing during Phase II of this Program. The second phase (1997–2000) is for formal, rigorous tests of the 2-year reliability of the systems and their biocompatibility in animals as a prerequisite to initiating clinical trials.

The first TAH clinical experience with a permanent heart replacement is expected after the year 2000, although some implantable TAH experience may be gained as bridge-to-cardiac-transplant during the 1990s.

Innovative ventricular assist systems

Research on completely implantable ventricular assist systems (VAS) was formulated in 1977. The implanted components included a blood pump and energy converter in an un-vented configuration, an energy transmission mechanism and an automatic controller with rechargeable batteries. Primary power was derived from an externally worn battery pack. Ten separate NHLBI VAS programs were planned and implemented 1977–1980. These activities were targeted creating new knowledge and technologies which would eventually integrate into complete implantable systems. By 1984, five different system concepts emerged from this vanguard project demonstrating potential as an implantable VAS.

Four systems entered "device readiness testing" to formally quantify 2-year reliability in laboratory tests and biocompatibility performance in animals. Each system was remotely monitored by the NIH for physiological cardiac output and blood pressure. Devices were submerged in body-temperature saline and tested for 2 years of continuous operation without maintenance.

All four teams from the device readiness testing program have entered FDA-regulated clinical trials with an advanced paracorporeal or "vented" ventricular assist system. Two of these systems have pre-market approvals from the FDA Cardiovascular Panel of experts. One system is the Abiomed BVS 5000 for hospital-based patients, while the second, the Thermocardiosystem, Inc. Heartmate is battery powered and provides complete ambulatory freedom for heart-failure patients awaiting a donor for cardiac transplantation. Under a FDA investigational device exemption, Novacor is conducting a worldwide trial of its N100, a smaller vented version of the N120 supported by the NHLBI. And the Hemopump, the first clinically safe continuous flow pump, developed by Nimbus, Inc., continues to be clinically evaluated. Collectively, these four developers represent the state-of-the-art in ventricular assist device design and clinical application in the U.S.

The clinical results are quite interesting. A tabulation of bridge-to-cardiac-transplant patients at a few centers disclosed that of 298 circulatory support patients, 180 (60%) received transplants, and 161 of the total (54%) were discharged from the hospital. That is, 89% of the transplanted patients were discharged with fewer hospital days than conventional transplant patients and survival at 1 year was 90%.

"Bridge" patients on experimental, battery powered, vented systems have complete ambulatory freedom but the patient must maintain continuous battery power through a percutaneous lead. Of these patients, some are leaving the hospital and functioning well at home. They participate in moderate exercise activities, fly in airplanes and hold their regular jobs such as a German patient who works in the family bakery.

The fact that VAS systems designed in 1977 are today safe and provide clinically effective circulatory support with a good quality of life has led to the start of a new program titled "Innovative Ventricular Assist System" (5). Last year the NHLBI released a program announcement to stimulate innovation in ventricular assist systems having a 5-year lifetime and designed for adult men and women with heart failure. These systems will incorporate recent advances in the understanding of circulatory support requirements, mechanisms, physiology, materials science, bioengineering, quality control, and manufacturing.

The program was open to all concepts, including pulsatile and continuous flow systems powered by electric, thermal, or biological sources. The aim of this new program is to develop a new generation of devices that will be permanent assist systems so that patients will not need to receive transplanted hearts for which the demand for donor hearts far exceeds the supply. It is estimated that long-term assist devices of this type will be life saving for 25 000–35 000 individuals annually in the U.S.

Research contracts were awarded to six investigative teams that propose to achieve this aim employing a variety of innovative techniques, each of which will require extensive basic bioengineering efforts and animal testing to demonstrate their capabilities. Nimbus, Inc. in Sacramento together with the University of Pittsburgh plans to develop a pump with ceramic bearings that are lubricated by the plasma. It will be able to deliver either pulsatile or non-pulsatile blood flow. The Cleveland Clinic Foundation collaborating with Ohio State University and other investigative teams will focus on the development of a centrifugal pump with blood lubricated bearings to deliver non-pulsatile blood flow. It will be driven by a specially designed motor that is highly efficient and small in size. Transicoil, Inc. in Pennsylvania in collaboration with the Texas Heart Institute will be focusing on a rotary blood pump that is immersed within the ventricle of the natural heart with bearings lubricated by the blood to provide either pulsatile or non-pulsatile blood flow. Abiomed, Inc. in Massachusetts is collaborating with the Columbia Presbyterian Medical Center in New York to develop a system that is a hybrid of biologic augmentation and mechanical assistance in such a way as to eliminate blood contact with artificial surfaces, thus avoiding any thromboembolic effects. Whalen Biomedical, Inc. in Cambridge, Massachusetts togehter with the University of Utah will perform research and development on a muscle-powered heart assist system that will not require an external power source. The Pennsylvania State University in Hershey will develop an improved electro-mechanical ventricular assist system with long-life bearings and an adaptive control technique to deliver pulsatile blood flow.

Each program is in the early stages of research and experimentation. No human subject studies are involved. Obstacles such as thrombogenicity, reliability, size, and efficiency are challenging, and the research and development supported by this program will require intensive efforts and collaboration by all the investigative teams. The total cost of this program over the 5 years will be approximately $ 27 million.

Genetically enhanced cardiovascular implants

Risks of complication such as thrombosis, infection, bleeding, and intimal hyperplasia increase with the duration of the implant. To control and prevent these complications, new activities are in place to stimulate interdisciplinary research that improves healing and defense mechanisms to CV trauma and lessen injury for implants (6). The general concept is to use tissue engineering approaches employing genetically altered cells that perform biocompatibility functions such as preventing thrombosis or other complications.

The research teams include expertise in bioengineering and biomedical science. Projects include improving biocompatibility by attaching cells to the implant that are capable of locally controlling the implant microenvironment and research on hybrid organs, sometimes called "organoids", for systemically treating cardiovascular disorders by delivery of antiproliferative or other agents. The results of this research will broadly apply to circulatory support systems.

One project will improve the biological and biocompatibility properties of vascular stents using microporous biodegradable biomaterials. These stents are capable of delivering recombinant adenoviral vectors directly to the underlying tissue. These vectors will genetically modify endothelial cells in situ and enhance their ability to re-endothelialize, to retard neointimal hyperplasia and to augment their antithrombotic capabilities, by overexpression of prostaglandin H synthase or similar mechanism.

Another project proposes to develop a polymer-biomaterial coated metallic retrievable coronary stent that serves as a drug delivery platform for releasing specific agents to vascular endothelial and smooth muscle cells. The drug agents would regulate the genetic expression of these cells to produce substances that inhibit thrombosis and neointimal hyperplasia using factors such as antisense oligonucleotides.

A third project is developing a method to coat the inside of ventricular assist devices with genetically engineered vascular endothelial and smooth muscle cells. These cells will secrete antithrombotic agents like prostacyclin and endothelial-derived relaxing factor, also known as nitric oxide (NO), to decrease the incidence of thromboembolic complications that occur in some patients with ventricular assist devices. Adenovirus-based vector transformation of cells will enhance prostaglandin H synthase, NO production by expression of the NO synthase gene and of the gene which encodes for a co-factor needed during NO synthase production.

References

1. Braunwald E, Katz AM, Abboud FM, Cohn JN (1994) Proceedings of the National Heart, Lung, and Blood Institute Task Force on Heart Failure. Bethesda, MD
2. The SOLVD Investigators (1991) Effect of enalapril on survival in patients with reduced left ventricular ejection fractions and congestive heart failure. N Engl J Med 325:293–302
3. Nowak R (1994) Xenotransplants Set to Resume. Science 266:1148–1151
4. Request for Proposals (RFP) NHLBI-HV-92-28 (1992) Phased Readiness Testing of Implantable Total Artificial Hearts, Issued by the National Heart, Lung, and Blood Institute, Bethesda, MD.
5. Request for Proposals (RFP) NHLBI-HV-94-25 (1994) Innovative Ventricular Assist System (IVAS), Issued by the National Heart, Lung, and Blood Institute, Bethesda, MD.
6. Request for Applications (RFA) NHLBI-HL-93-019 (1993) Genetically Enhanced Cardiovascular Implants, Issued by the National Heart, Lung, and Blood Institute, Bethesda, MD.
7. Carrel A, Lindbergh CA (1935) The culture of whole organs. Science 81:621–623
8. Koh GY, Soonpaa MH, Klug MG, Pride HP, Cooper BJ, Zipes DP, Field LJ (1995) Stable fetal cardiomyocyte grafts in the hearts of dystrophic mice and dogs. J Clin Invest 96:2034–2042

Author's address:
Watson, John T., PhD
National Heart, Lung & Blood Institute
2 Rockledge Center Ste 9044
6701 Rockledge Drive MSC 7940
Bethesda, MD 20892-7940
USA

Quality of life with ventricular assist devices

W. Albert, S. Kiekbusch, K. Köller, R. Hetzer,

German Heart Insitute Berlin, Berlin, Germany

In 1958, concepts and guidelines for the development of artificial hearts were presented by Akutsu et al. (1) and first attempts with temporary mechanical circulatory support to heart transplantation were made by Cooley and Liotta in 1969 (2). The first bridging to heart transplantation with left ventricular support systems took place in 1978 by Norman et al. (3). In the same year, Reemtsma et al. (4) conducted a study on bridged patients proving that the survival rate was good. Pneumatic paracorporeal ventricular assist devices were successfully used by Hill (5) and an implantable left ventricular assist device by Starnes (6) in 1984.

Since that time, surgical techniques, indication criteria, and management of complications have been modified in accordance with growing experience. The increasing discrepancy between the number of patients needing heart transplantation and the shortage of available donor organs affects the use of assist devices. Whereas the primary intention was a short-term bridging of patients to heart transplantation, the large number of patients now requires more long-term assist devices. There is at present in Berlin a patient who has lived with an assist device already for 635 days.

A very important issue with new technologies in health care is their evaluation with respect to the achieved quality of life and, with shortness of resources, their cost-effectiveness in comparison to alternative procedures (for example assist devices vs. heart transplantation). Clinicians agree that the outcome of clinical trials can only insufficiently be defined by traditional criteria, such as mortality and the degree of morbidity. Of equal importance is the patients' ability to remain contributing, functioning members of society and experience physical, emotional and social well-being. The patient himself has a right to form an opinion of the effectiveness and outcome of a proposed treatment.

Quality of life has been defined as a multidimensional concept that embraces a wide range of physical and psychological characteristics and limitations which describe an individual's ability to function and derive satisfaction (7). It comprises various dimensions:

1) Cognitive functioning, dependent on neuropsychological status, low cardiac output, surgery, thromboembolism, hemorrhages and medications with cerebrotoxic effects, it influences complex cerebral functions, such as memory, concentration, fluency of thinking processes, information-processing etc. This impairment is a specific source of affective reactions and communication disturbances and, furthermore, it influences the quality of responses to questionnaires and interviews (Bornstein et al) (8).
2) Emotional functioning with emphasis on distress, such as depression, anxiety, anger/hostility and somatiform expressions of affective dysregulation as well as positive feelings like vigor, hoe etc.
3) Social functioning, i.e., integration into the social environment.
4) Quality of partnership refers to aspects of communication, emotional support, intimacy and sexual functioning

5) Physical functioning, i.e., ability to carry out daily activities, self-care, specific limitations, etc.

6) Work status and, in a wide spread sense, personal productivity

The quality of life dimensions on the one hand encompass objectively measurable skills and actions, as well as psychic reactions that can only validly be assessed by experienced professionals; on the other hand, the subjective assessment by the patient himself, measured by self-rating questionnaires, as individualized quality of life, is equally important. In individual appraisal processes patients are comparing therie current level of functioning with former or expected levels, in this way they evaluate to what extent they are content with specific treatment procedures.

In the last decade, quality of life assessment approaches gained a high degree of differentiation in respect to specific illnesses, treatment procedures, and measuring instruments. Measuring instruments of general use with single indexes are being replaced by profiles including several independent dimensions or the development of test-batteries involving multiple validated and reliable instruments for measuring very specific domains of quality of life. The aim is to gain increased effectiveness of measurement concerning hypothesis-defined domains, adequate depth and broadness in order to target trial-related issues, adaptation to the time-related courses of treatment and aspects of patients' motivations and constraints.

Operalisation of health-related quality of life in patients with mechanical circulatory assist systems is impressingly affected with these challenges. There is a need for a specific investigation rationale.

We started in 1991 a project at the German Heart Institute Berlin to observe, analyze and understand the psychological processes during mechanical circulatory support and to evaluate outcome and quality of life after subsequent heart transplantation. Up to June 1996, Hetzer and coworkers performed 157 biventricular assist implantations for bridging to heart transplantation with the Berlin Heart System, and 54 patients received a left ventricular assist device (19 Heart Mate, 35 Novacor). Heart tranplantation was performed with 60% of Berlin Heart patients (73% discharged), also 60% in the Novacor group (91% discharged), and 67% in TCI (84% discharged).

Patients and methods

By random selection, 47 patients on BVAD and 24 patients on LVAD were included in the study and complete data collected during the assist period. Eleven patients in the BVAD-group died from infections, bleeding, cerebral complications, etc. compared to four in the LVAD-group. Five LVAD patients were weaned successfully. The demographic data and clinical characteristics are presented in Table 1. BVAD patients were younger with significantly more women than in the LVAD group. The mean bridging time in LVAD is twice as high than with BVAD.

The frame for this work was an explicit psychotherapeutic setting embedded in a treatment concept with regular team conferences (comprising nurses, surgeons, and psychiatrists). Aim of our work was to offer patients a "holding function" by supporting them with basic information about the impact of the treatment, focus on specific conflicts and stress reactions, offer relaxation techniques and support for family members. According to various psychologic disorders psychopharmacologic agents were administered. Data collection and testing was involved in this

Table 1

	Patients	
	BVAD	LVAD
	Biventricular Assist Device n = 36	Univentricular Assist Device n = 20 (14 Novacor, 6 TCI)
Women	12	2
Men	24	18
Mean age	35.3 years	44.65 years
Diagnosis:		
Dilative Cardiomyopathy	26	17
Ischemic Cardiomyopathy	10	3
Bridging time	mean: 73 days range 23 – 130 days	mean: 162 days range 15 – 388 days

therapeutic setting thus avoiding "artificial examinations", patients, were informed about their test performance, the relevance of deficits and their remission course. This was important for their motivation to participate, and patients could achieve more feelings for internal focus of control, i.e. to be able to influence their status and not to remain in a fatalistic position.

The psychiatric evaluation was performed with the AMDP-inventory (9), an excellent validated psychiatric rating scale, by well-trained examiners and corresponding diagnoses were defined according to DSM III-R.

Assessment of neuropsychological dysfunctions is a complex field of inquiry in respect to adequate techniques, standardized procedures and proper interpretation (see summaries in (10, 11).

There are few formalized batteries for general clinical use for brain damage, like the Halstead-Reitan battery or the Luria-Nebraska neuropsychological battery, providing precise information about quality and quantity of cerebral organic disabilities.

The complexity of these batteries did not allow their use in MSC patients. We focused on three tests with a high degree of sensitivity to cognitive impairment: The Benton Test (12, 13): it is a sensitive test of visual inattention and deficits of the immediate span of recall and spatial organisation problems. The Bender Gestalt (14) test involves capacities of visuomotor response and verbal concept realization and discriminates quite well between cerebral brain damage and psychiatric disorders. Bender scores are also sensitive in documenting changes over time associated with cerebral oxygenation status (Krop et al., 15). To test working memory and attention, the Digit Span – a subtext from the Wechsler Intelligence Scales – was selected yielding a high degree of sensitivity for diffuse brain damage (Wechsler, 1981, 16).

Assessing emotional functioning during MCS, we used the Profile of Mood States (POMS) (17), a self-rating scale with the dimensions depression, irritability, psychic fatigue, and vigor.

The "Giessen Beschwerde-Bogen" (GBB) (18), is an extensive validated and reliable self-rating instrument to score differentially and economically bodily complaints, grouped in the dimensions cardiac, rheumatic and epigastric complaints, exhaustion/fatigue, and psychic impairment induced by overall complaints.

POMS and GBB-scores important domains of quality of life during mechanical circulatory support from the subjective point of view of the patients, whereby psychiatric expert ratings and neuropsychological testing provide objective domains of quality of life.

Considering the importance of coping, we included a coping questionnaire. Coping is a decisive factor for successful adaptation to illness and related treatment procedure with an important impact on quality of life. According to their transactional stress-solving concept, Lazerus and Folkman (19) define coping as "... constantly changing cognitive and behavioral efforts to manage specific external and/or internal demands that are appraised as taxing or exceeding the resources of a person".

The Freiburg questionnaire of coping (FKV) (20) is a self- and expert-rating questionnaire emphasizing specific illness and treatment stress factors; it is being scientifically tested in cardiac and transplanted patients. Five independent dimensions measured are computed: religiosity or spiritual engagement, distraction and self-encouragement, achieving adjustment to problems, denial and wishful thinking and depressive withdrawal.

During treatment with MCS, patients were examined three times a week, and data were analyzed according to two predefined time periods: the initial period after MCS-implantation (day 0–14) and the stabilization period – lasting from the 30th day after implantation to transplantation.

The rationale for choosing two research periods is based on preliminary experience in therapeutic work in patients with biventricular support (see Fig. 1).

In an initial or short-term period after implantation, we observed an overwhelming dominance of disorders with organic etiology resulting from complex interaction of extracorporeal circulation, metabolic, neuropsychologic dysfunctions and cerebrotoxic medication effects and cerebromicrobolic events. Beside this, acute psychic shock reactions contribute to behavioral disorders with psychomotoric excitation or a withdrawal from the environment comparable to a "possum reflex".

The following so-called adaptation period is characterized by rapid remission of organ-induced symptomatology and an increase of intensive psychic stress reactions. Patients show a high degree of psycho-vegetative tension, anxiety and panic reactions, dissociative episodes and diffuse bodily sensations. Step-by-step, patients tend to restore their cognitive and emotional inner world to gain self-control. These processes are largely fluctuating day-by-day according to quality and intensity, and then follows a period of stabilization. Now reactive psychic syndromes are predominant caused by realization of the traumatic stress of MCS, the violation of body integrity, future social and economic consequences, and in some cases, the fear of family conflicts. Patients are forced to adapt to the clinical setting and develop adequate coping strategies.

Due to these processes data analysis was performed separately for two distinct periods: the initial period (IP) and the stabilization period (SP). During IP there were extensive shifts in organic mental syndromes, for example, one patient, for some days, suffered from delirium followed by an organic hallucinosis and later on

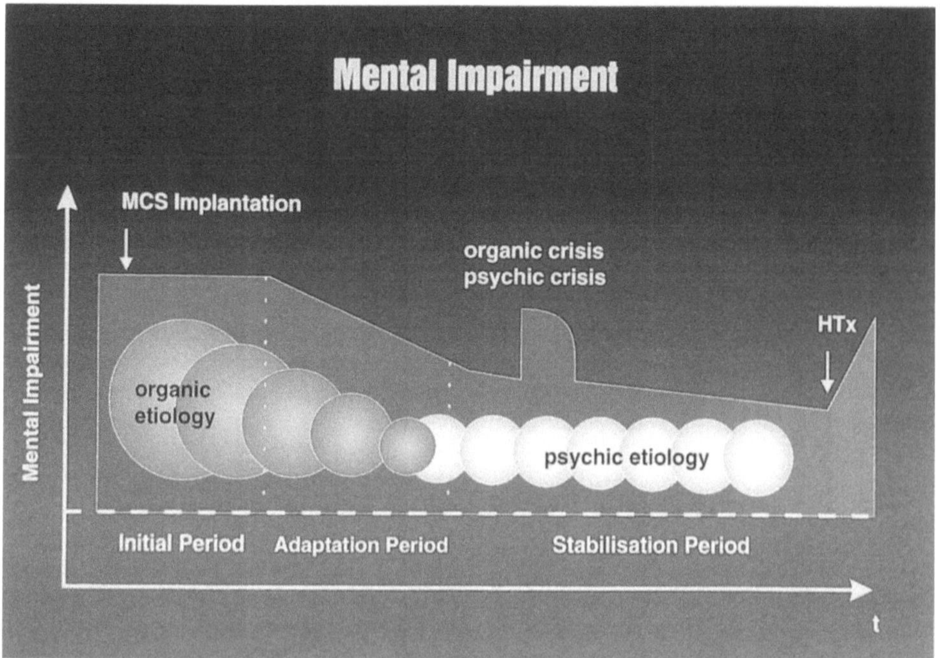

Fig. 1

from an organic anxiety syndrome. According to this, one patient would receive different diagnoses, which were cumulated in both assist groups and then statistically analysed.

The same analyzing procedures were performed for psychiatric neuropsychological disturbances during the stabilization period. Quality of life assessment is based on self-ratings with POMS, GBB, and FKV was possible in only 30 out of 56 patients. The 26 "drop outs" were mostly impaired by severe organic complications. Due to the reduced number of patients, the assist group as a whole was compared with cardiac rehabilitation patients and healthy persons.

The follow-up study of Qolife after heart transplantation was a retrospective examination of a group of patients formerly bridged with the Berlin Heart biventricular assist device and assessment was performed 2 to 4 years after heart transplantation (mean 2.9 years). There were no relevant differences in demographic data compared to the BVAD group in the prospective study.

We used the SF-36 health survey from the medical outcomes study (MOS) (21) providing a profile of eight scales comprising health concepts for physical functioning, role functioning – limited by physical impairment, bodily pain, general health, vitality, social functioning, role-functioning – limited by emotional impairment, mental health. Finally, patients estimated their overall health and the resulting life satisfaction in added questions.

Decriptive statistics were used to obtain frequencies as well as distribution characteristics on questionnaire subscales. Differences between group were analysed by means of t-tests.

Results

Initial period on MCS

Organic mental syndromes during the initial period on MCS were found in 69.4% of BVAD patients and 60% of LVAD patients. The difference is not significant. The distribution of diagnoses were similar in both groups: 14% developed a delirium with an early or delayed onset, 11% an organic delusional syndrome or an organic hallucinosis, and 62% an organic mood syndrome. Through adequate medical management and psychopharmacologic treatment the disorders gradually remitted. Apart from the etiologic shift from predominant organic factors to more genuine psychological causes, about 50% of the initially depressive or anxious patients remained in a state of mood disorder during the stabilization period.

Stabilisation period on MCS

Organic mental syndromes were now observable in close connection with somatic complications like bleeding, severe infections, device malfunction etc.: Seven patients on BVAS and two patients on LVAD showed transient episodes.

Neuropsychological impairment was computed by a simple summary variable – an impairment index – where patients score if their performance was below a test-specific normal range.

On this basis 58% of the BVAD patients showed impaired performance compared to 30% of the LVAD patients (p < 0.0001). Similar differences in favour of

Table 2

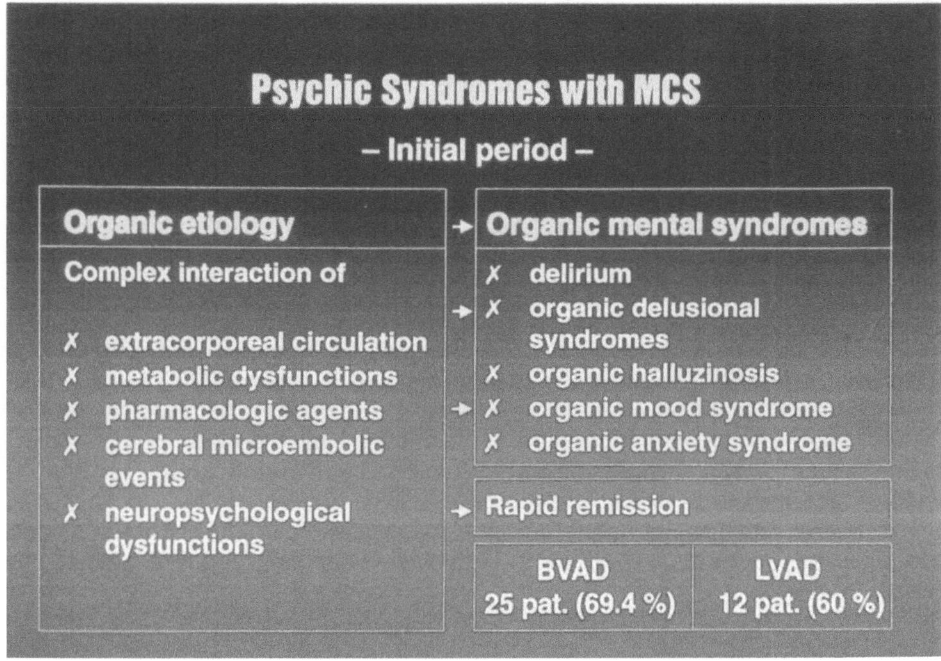

Table 3

Neuropsychological impairment and neurologic defects
-stabilization period-

	BVAD	LVAD
neuropsychological impairment (Benton-Test, Bender-Gestalt-Test, Serial Digit Span)	21 pts	6 pts
neurologic defects	6 pts	1 pt

Table 4

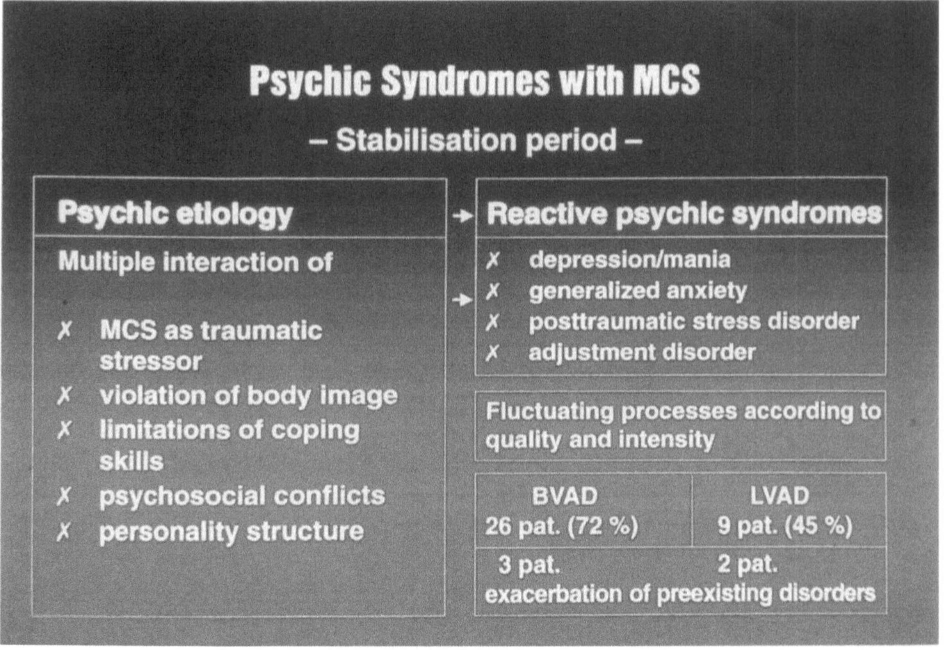

LVAS treatment were found in respect to severe neurologic deficits due to cerebral bleeding or embolic stroke (device-related or septic thrombembolisms): Six BVAD patients vs. one LVD patient.

Assessing psychogenic reactions revealed a great deal of diagnostic uncertainties due to rapid fluctuating processes. A precise allocation to the clearly defined diagnostic categories of DSM III-R was difficult. The specific clinical features and the diagnostic guidelines of DSM III-R provided four illness categories as useful: major depressive episode and manic episode, generalized anxiety disorder, post-traumatic stress disorder and adjustment disorder with all subtypes.

In general, there were significantly more patients suffering from psychic syndromes in the BVAD group (26 patients – 72%) than in the LVAD group (nine patients – 45%). A major depressive episode was diagnosed in 11 BVAD patients vs. Three LVAD patients, whereby BVAD patients were characterized by elevated symptom severity and occasional psychotic features. Adjustment disorders with a combination of depression and anxiety, physical complaints and often withdrawal was diagnosed in 10 BVAD vs. two LVAD patients. Generalized anxiety was found more often in the LVAD group (three vs. one). Posttraumatic stress disorder with distressing recollection of the event and anxious dreams was diagnosed in four BVAD vs. one LVAD patient.

In the quality of life domain: emotional distress, assessed by the Profile of Mood States, the MCS patients achieved impressive positive results (see Fig. 2). In the subscale depression, they showed a lower score (i.e., better mood) than a cardiac rehabilitation control group (patients after bypass surgery or infarction). Irritability levels were significantly lower (p < 0.01) in MCS patients, no relevant differences were found in the subscale psychic fatigue. The vigor level (high scores indicate

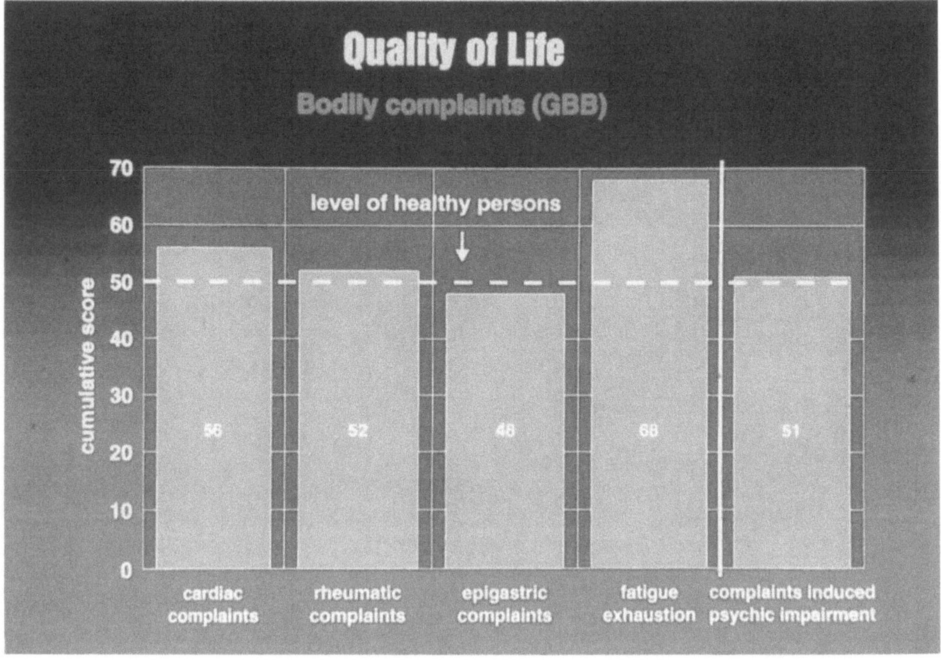

Fig. 2

elevated vigor) in MSC patients is nearly two times higher than in the control group (p < 0.01).

Results with the Giessen complaints questionnaire (see Fig. 3) indicated equal levels in the subscales cardiac, rheumatic, and epigastric complaints in MCS patients compared to healthy controls. Clear negative scores were derived in the dimension fatigue/exhaustion. In the scale overall psychical impairment induced by all complaints, surprisingly, there were no differences between MCS patients and controls.

Analysing coping patterns from the Freiburg questionnaire of coping, a polar distribution could be delineated: the prominent coping feature is depressive withdrawal and the scale comprising religious and spiritual coping skills exhibited the lowest levels (see Fig. 4). Denial and wishful thinking is slightly more often used than active problem solving or self-encouragement to deal with the stressful situation.

Follow-up study

The scores of the group of biventricular assisted patients with subsequent heart transplantation in the dimensions of the SF-36 health survey were compared to a group of serious chronically ill patients (CIP) (168 patients) and a healthy control group (HC) (638 patients) (see Fig. 5). In the scale physical functioning our study group showed reduced activity levels, close to chronically ill patients, and reported severe role impairment due to physical limitations. Bodily pain scores exceeded the levels of both groups used for comparison, indicating massive impairment in daily life and work due to pain.

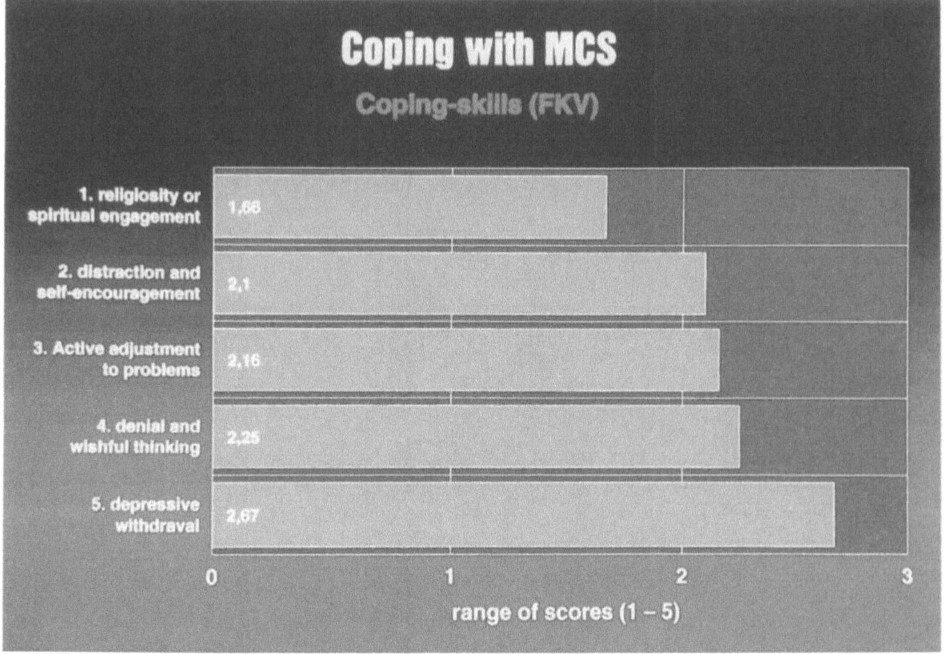

Fig. 3

Quality of Life-Follow-up
SF-36 Health Survey
BVAD + HTx-patients (45 pat.)
serious chronic ill pat. (168 pat.)
normal persons (638 pat.)
* : p < 0.01
SF-36 Scale Score
100
90
80
70
60
50
40
30
20
10
0
65
57,7
79,8
58,21
64,87
75,85
48,95
44,39
69,38
Physical Functioning
Bodily Pain
Role Functioning
Physical Limitations

Fig. 4

Quality of Life-Follow-up
SF-36 Health Survey
BVAD + HTx-patients (45 pat.)
serious chronic ill pat. (168 pat.)
normal persons (638 pat.)
psychiatric ill patients (163)
* : p < 0.01
SF-36 Scale Score
100
90
80
70
60
50
40
30
20
10
0
76,3
77,25
82,7
51,92
59,6
75,96
84,01
40,22
Mental Health
Role Functioning
Emotional Limitations

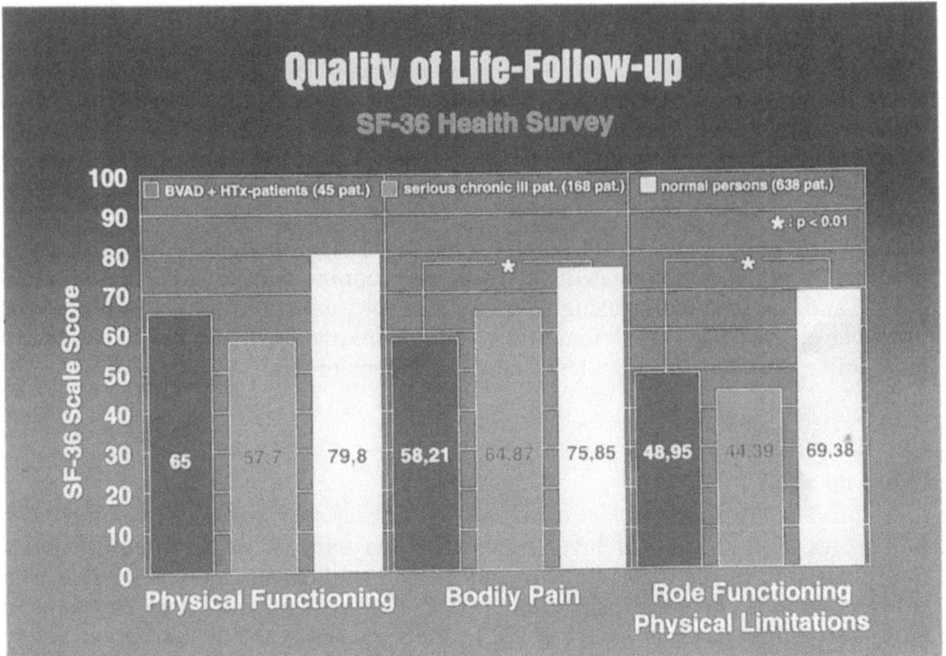

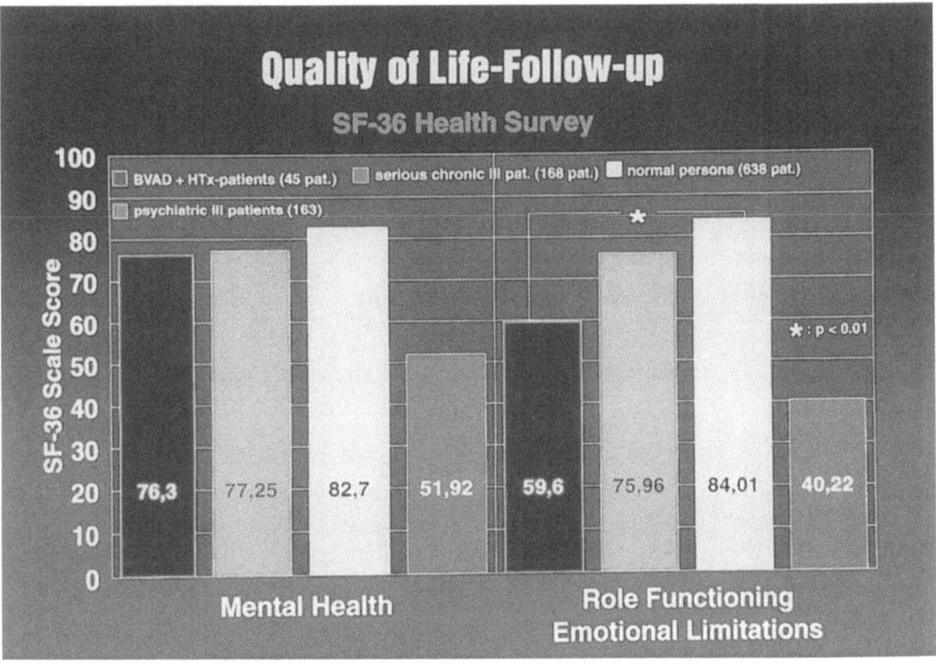

Fig. 5

Quality of Life-Follow-up
SF-36 Health Survey
100
90
80
70
60
50
40
30
20
10
0
SF-36 Scale Score
BVAD + HTx-patients (45 pat.)
serious chronic ill pat. (168 pat.)
normal persons (638 pat.)
* : p < 0.01
*
73,9
79,65
91,31
57,87
50,1
67,19
Social Functioning
General Health Perceptions

Fig. 6

Quality of Life-Follow-up
SF-36 Health Survey
100
90
80
70
60
50
40
30
20
10
0
SF-36 Scale Score
BVAD + HTx-patients (45 pat.)
serious chronic ill pat. (168 pat.)
normal persons (638 pat.)
* : p < 0.01
*
73,9
79,65
91,31
57,87
50,1
67,19
Social Functioning
General Health Perceptions

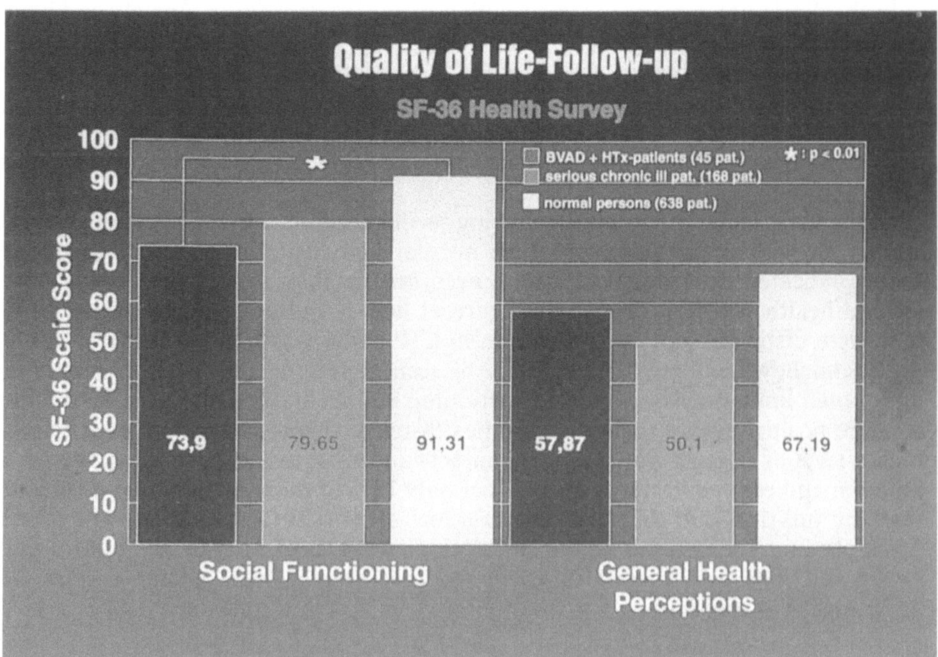

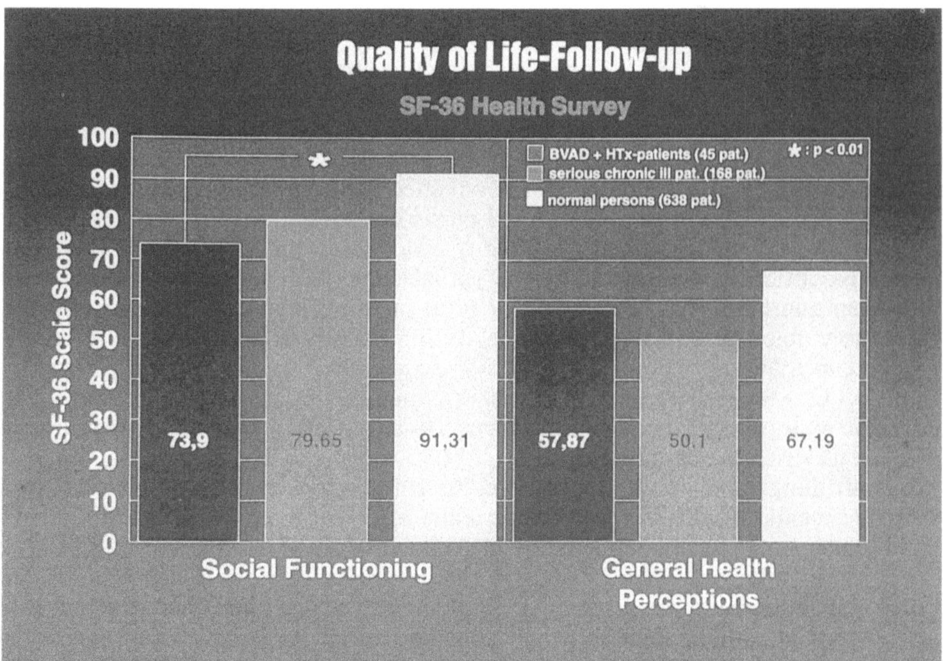

Fig. 7

In the dimension general mental health – including depression, anxiety and being positively affected – the values of the study group (76.3) indicate some emotional distress of moderate quality (see Fig. 6). The differences between the study group and healthy controls are small and far from the levels of psychiatric patients (p < 0.001). In contrast to this, the patients reported severe restrictions in work or daily activities attributed to emotional limitations (59.6 vs. 75.9 in CIP and 84 in HP).

In the scale social functioning referring to the negative impact of physical health and/or emotional problems on their normal activities and work performance, scores indicated extensive restrictions, even severer than in CIP (see Fig. 7). But general health perceptions including current health, outlook and resistance to illness were distinctly more positive than in CIP (57.8 vs. 50.1). An explanation for these somehow incoherent results may be seen in specific appraisal processes: the undoubted limitations in physical functioning and mental health are in dissonance to more positive future social life and health-related expectations: patients desire a higher level of engagement in social contacts and wish to return to adequate occupational and economic status. But in fact only 18% of the transplanted patients are working full-time due to the social insurance system in Germany and the refusal of employers. The positive health perceptions were confirmed by the final overall health and life-satisfaction index, where the assist/transplanted patients scored with 2.1 (range: 1 = excellent to 5 = bad)!

Discussion

First results to psychologic effects of mechanical circulatory support were presented by Ruzevich et al. (22) in a retrospective study after heart transplantation. Refering to the assist period only, 16% of the patients remembered to be burdened by emotional affects, fears about survival were rare, and patients emphasized their confidence in the staff. In contradiction, Abou-Avdi et al. (23) from the Texas Heart Institute group evaluated emotional effects to be worse than physical effects in 92% of their patient population and persisting posttraumatic stress reactions in 50%. However, retrospectively designed questionnaires reflect primarily situational cognitive attitudes, influenced by the actual state, with low correlations to real experience in the past due to denial or positive reinterpretation. Shapiro (24) prospectively observed 17 LVAD recipients during the bridge period: Seven developed organic mental syndromes and six a major depression, two serious family problems. Kendall (25) found high level of psychiatric impairment at initial assessment, with organic improvement quality of life increased but in many patients depression and behaviour disturbances persisted.

Confirming these results in the present study about two-thirds suffered from organic mental syndromes for a short time after assist implantation. Frequency and diagnostic patterns were equally distributed in BVAD and LVAD patients.

However, after remission of organic complications with cerebral-psychiatric impact and fading away of prolonged traumatic shock reactions, 3 to 4 weeks after assist implant, major depressive episodes and mixed affective disturbances with features of posttraumatic stress symptoms significantly more often occurred in BVAD patients (26). Besides these quantitative differences in psychopathology, BVAD pat. showed in psychotherapeutic work a higher degree of psychic desorganization with reduced verbal-communicative capacities. They expressed threatening fears of fractionation and suffered from ubiquitous bodily sensations: psychosomatic patterns which characterizes early human development periods. The violation of body image and the manipulations in blood pressure, human development periods, pulse regulation, specific noise and vibrations induced by "cold rings and pumps" were responsible for these processes. Accordingly, it is encouragement and reassurance of orientation to reality that correct distored cognitions.

LAVD patients clearly exhibited a lower incidence of these profound reactions and, furthermore, showed significantly fewer neuropsychological impairment. Psychopharmacologic treatment with anxiolytics, antidepressants and neuroleptics was necessary in both groups to form a basis for interpersonal therapy.

The differences between the two MCS groups may be due to the greater immobilization of BVAD pat. who achieved a lower physical exercise level than LVAD patients, i.e., limited walking, self-care restrictions and, in consequence, more negative self-control perceptions. Analyzing the decreased chance of survival in BVAD vs. LVAD, Portner et al. 1989 (23), Frazier et al. 1992 (26) emphasized the severity of heart failure and the complexity of two implanted devices as causative factors. These factors are also responsible for the discrepancies in psychic reactions.

More than 50% of patients recovered on MCS (LVAD > BVAD) to such an extent that they were able to self-evaluate their psycho-somatic status. Their quality of life ratings were impressively positive: they expressed low levels of emotional distress and bodily complaints. Surmounting their life-threatening experience, they obviously mobilized intensive "elan vital" with a hopeful outlook, providing active coping processes. These results are consistent with recent research of the Pittsburgh group (27).

Dew et al. (30) emphasized the impact of out-patient care of assist patients in improving life quality to a level equal to other patients on the waiting list for HTX.

Quality of life some years after assist implant and subsequent heart implantation is mainly characterized by limitations in social functioning which the patients attribute to physical and emotional impairment despite good health perceptions and a hopeful outlook. The achieved quality of life is not different from that of patients treated by heart transplantation alone; a preceding assist period does not influence the longterm outcome in any specific way. This is confirmed by Reedy (31) and Birovljev (32), who stated equal successful long-term results in transplant patients despite pre TX duration of assist devices or use of uni- or biventricular mechanical support. Finally, it must be emphazised that patients were globally very satisfied with their life some years after assist and subsequent heart transplantation, their values were even slightly more positive than those in a normal population.

References

1. Akutso T, Kolff WJ (1958) Permanent substitutes for valves and hearts. Trans Am Soc Artif Intern Organs 4: 230–235
2. Cooley DA, Liotta D, Hallman GL, Bloodwell RD, Leschman RD, Milliam JD (1969) Orthotopic cardiac prothesis for two staged cardiac replacement. Am J Cardio (24): 723–730
3. Norman JC, Cooley DA, Kahan BD, et al (1978) Total support of the circulation of a patient with postcardiotomy stone-heart syndrome by a partial artificial heart (ALVAD) for 5 days followed by heart and kidney transplantation. Lancet 1: 1125–1127
4. Reemtsma K, Drusin R, Edie R, et al (1978). Cardiac transplantation for patients requiring mechanical circulatory support. N Engl J Med 298: 670–671

5. Hill JD, Farrar DJ, Hershon SS, et al (1986) Use of prosthetic ventricle as a bridge to cardiac transplantation for postinfarction cardiogenic shock N Engl J Med 314: 626–628

6. Starnes VA, Oyer PE, Portner PM, et al (1988) Isolated left ventricular assist as a bridge to cardiac transplantation. J Thorac Cardiovasc Surg 96: 62–71

7. Shron VA, Shumaker SA (1992) The integration of health quality of life in clinical research: Experiences from cardiovascular clinical trials. Progress ion Cardiovascular Nursing 7: 21–28

8. Bornstein RA, Hammer D, Sterling R, Steng J, Lewis R, Magorien R (1990) Neuropsychological impairment in candidates for cardiac transplantation. In: Willner AE, Rodewald G (eds). Impact of cardiac surgery on the quality of life. Plenum Press, New York: 231–235

9. Arbeitsgemeinschaft für Methodik und Dokumentation in der Psychiatrie: Das AMDP-System. Manual zur Dokumentation psychiatrischer Befunde (1971), Springer Verlag Berlin

10. Lezak MD (1983) Neuropsychological assessment. Oxford University Press

11. Margolin DJ (1992) Cognitive neuropsychology in clinical practice. Oxford University Press, New York

12. Benton AL (1990) Der Benton Test, Hans Huber Verlag, Bern

13. Benton AL, Spreen O (1964) Visual memory test performance in mentally deficient and brain damaged patients. Amer I Ment Defic 68: 633–633

14. Bender L (1938) A visual motor gestalt test and its clinical use. New York

15. Krop H, Cohen E, Block AJ (1972) Continous oxygen therapy in chronic obstructive pulmonary disease: neuropsychological effects. Proc Ann Conv APA, 7: 663–664

16 Wechsler D (1981) WAIS-R manual. Psychological Corporation, New York

17. McNair D, Lors M, Droppleman LF (1971) Eits manual for the Profile of Mood Sates. Educational and Industrial Testing Service, San Diego

18. Brähler E, Scheer J (1983) Der Giessener Beschwerdebogen – Handbuch. Hans Huber Verlag, Bern

19. Lazarus RS, Folkman S (1984) Stress, Appraisal and Coping. Springer, New York

20 Muthny FA (1988) Freiburger Fragebogen zur Krankheitsverarbeitung. Handbuch. Beltz-Verlag, Weinheim

21. Ware JE, Sherbourne CD (1992). The MOS 36-item short form health survey I. Conceptual framework and item selection. Med Care, 30: 473–483

22. Ruzevich SA, Swarz MT, Reedy JE, et al (1990) Retrospective analysis of the psychologic effects of mechanical circulatory support. I Heart Lung Transplant 9: 209–212

23. Abou-Awdi NL, Frazier OH (1992) Quality of life of patients on LVAD support. In: Walter PL (ed) Quality of life after open heart surgery. Kluwer Academic Publishers, Dordrecht, pp 397–401

24. Shapiro PA, Lewin H, Oz M (1994) Left ventricular assist devices: Psychosocial burden and implication for heart transplant programs. Presented at the Third Biennial Conference on Psychiatrie, Psychosocial and Ethical Issues in Organ Transplantation, Richmond, VA, October

25. Kendall K, McCarthy PM, Sharp JW, Vargo RL (1994) Quality of life for hospitalized implantable left ventricular assist device patients. Cleveland Clinic Foundation, Cleveland OH, unpublished manuscript

26. Albert W, Bittner A, Hetzer R (1994) Psychosomatic reactions during mechanical circulation with Berlin Heart Assist Device in bridging to heart transplantation. Presented at the Third International Conference on Circulatory Support Devices for Severe Cardiac Failure, Pittsburgh, PA, October

27. Portner PM, Oyer PE, Pennington DG et al (1989). Implantable electrical left ventricular assist system: bridge to transplantation and the future. Ann Thorac Surg 47: 142–150

28. Frazier OH, Rose EA, Macmanus Q et al (1992). Multicenter clinical evaluation of the Heartmate 1000 IP left ventricular assist device. Am Thorac Surg 53: 1080–1090

29. Kormos RL, Murali S, Dew MA, Armitage JM, Hardesty RL, Borovetz HS, Griffith BP (1994). Chronic mechanical circulatory support: Rehabilitation, low morbidity, and superior survival. Ann Thorac Surg 57: 51–58

30 Dew MA, Kormos RL, Roth LR, Armitage JM, Pristas JM, Harris RC, Capretta C, Griffith BP (1993) Life quality in the era of bridging to cardiac transplantation: Bridge patients in an outpatient setting. ASAIO J 39: 145–152

31 Reedy JE, Pennington DG, Miller LW et al (1992). Status I heart transplant patients: conventional vs ventricular assist device support. J Heart Lung Transplant 11: 246–252

32 Birovljev S, Radovancevic B, Burnett CM et al (1992). Heart Transplantation after mechanical
    circulatory support: four years' experience. J Heart Lung Transplant 11: 240–245
33 Schepank H (1987) Psychogene Erkrankungen der Stadtbevölkerung. Springer, Berlin New
    York

Author's address:
W. Albert
Psychosomatic Dept.
German Heart Institute Berlin
Augustenburger Platz 1
13353 Berlin, Germany

Lessons from the heart: Ethical reflections on the clinical trials of the Jarvik-7

R. C. Fox

Sociology Department, University of Pennsylvania, Philadelphia, USA

At the center of my sociological reflections on ethical aspects of permanent mechanical circulatory support is the extensive, first-hand study that medical historian Judith P. Swazey and I conducted from 1983 through 1988 on the Jarvik-7 artificial heart experiment, which we reported in our co-authored book, "Spare Parts" (3). Our study of what we came to think of as the "rise and fall" of the Jarvik-7 in the United States, included participant observation and in situ interviewing at the University of Utah Medical Center in Salt Lake City, and at the Humana Corporation's Audubon Hospital in Louisville, Kentucky, as well as a running content analysis of the way the attempts to implant the Jarvik-7 device in a series of patients were presented in professional medical and scientific journals, and in the media.

A Short Story of the Jarvik-7 artificial heart experiment

This chapter in the continuing quest to replace a failing human heart with a manmade substitute was a short-lived one. It was confined to the 1980's when, for the first time, surgeons removed the hearts of five patients with end-stage cardiac disease and replaced them with a device intended to permanently assume the functions of the human heart. Spawned by these experiments, artificial hearts were also implanted, as they had been several times before, in over 400 people awaiting a human heart transplant, as a temporary "bridge" that might keep them alive until a donor heart could be procured. The Jarvik heart was used for 150 of these bridge implants; other devices were employed for the 250 additional ones.

This artificial heart experiment began clinically on December 2, 1982, when Dr. William C. DeVries and his team at the University of Utah Medical Center in Salt Lake City removed the heart of Dr. Barney Clark, a 61-year-old dentist from Seattle, Washington, and implanted in him the pneumatically powered, "tethered" device called the Jarvik-7 heart. The telemetry equipment that monitored and recorded Dr. Clark's slowly deteriorating biological life with an artificial heart showed that the Jarvik-7 beat steadily 12.912.499 times for 112 days. Then, on March 21, he was pronounced dead from circulatory collapse caused by multiorgan system failure, and the drive unit powering the artificial heart was turned off.

Dr. DeVries, who moved a few months later to the Heart Institute at the Humana Corporation's Audubon Hospital in Louisville, Kentucky, implanted the Jarvik-7 heart in three more patients during 1984 and 1985. His fourth and final patient-subject, Jack Burcham, died 10 days postoperatively from a massive hemorrhage caused by a cardiac tamponade. Patients two and three, William Schroeder and Murray Haydon, lived respectively for 620 and 488 days with their artificial hearts, and during those months underwent a variety of finally fatal complications such as infections, hemolytic anemia, renal and respiratory insufficiency, bleeding, and blood clotting. A fifth Jarvik-7 implant was performed in April 1985 by Dr. Bjarne Semb at the Karolinska Hospital in Stockholm, Sweden; his patient, 52-year-old Leif Stenberg, had been in a stroke-induced coma for 2 months when he died of respiratory and vascular failure 299 days after his implant.

The implantation of a permanent total artificial heart ended quietly and unofficially in the United States after DeVries performed the fourth and what proved to be the final implant in the series of seven that had been authorized on a case-by-case approval basis by the Food and Drug Administration (FDA). When William Schroeder, the second and longest survivor of the recipients, died in August 1986, most of those involved in the experiment acknowledged privately that it was, and should be finished. Although no explicit formal decisions or declarations to that effect were made, a de facto moratorium on the use of the Jarvik-7 as an artificial device existed from then on.

In January 1990, the FDA issued a recall notice to Symbion, Inc., the manufacturer of the Jarvik-7 heart, withdrawing the agency's approval of the investigative use of the device, of the small Jarvik-7-70 model, and of the company's ventricular assist device as well. The FDA cited various respects in which the company had violated the requirements for the production of an experimental device and its use by investigators – including deficiencies in manufacturing quality control, monitoring of research sites, training of personnel and reporting of adverse reactions. On balance, the FDA concluded, "the risks to patients were outweighing the benefits".

In using a synoptic account of the Jarvik-7 experiment as a reference point for my remarks at this symposium, it is not my intention to imply that no progress in the development of a permanent mechanical support for persons with terminal heart failure has been made since the demise of the Jarvik-7, or that all the circumstances that surrounded the clinical trials of this device are inevitable concomitants of any such undertaking. But this case throws into high relief ethical issues concerning the conduct and regulation of scientifically, medically, and morally competent patient-oriented clinical research, and the drive to sustain life and "rebuild people" through organ replacement that are not confined to the Jarvik-7, and that are important to re-examine.

Getting Into Clinical Trials

To begin with, the Jarvik-7 study dramatically poses a question associated with clinical research that is as perennial as it is basic: namely, had the experimental work done with the device in the laboratory and in the barn on animals advanced sufficiently – conceptually, technically, and empirically – to warrant initiating clinical trials of the device with patients as subjects? The answer to the crucial question of when the time has come to move from the laboratory to the clinic is never scientifically or ethically simple. The intellectual excitement of investigators about the therapeutic promise of the experiments in which they are engaged, their sense of clinical urgency about finding means to save the lives of desperately ill patients and of effectively treating their conditions, the emotional and material vested interests that they, the institutions with which they are affiliated, and the organizations funding their work may have in their gaining recognition as pioneers of a therapy, along with attention from the media, may inflate the hopefulness of researchers, lead them to over-estimate the therapeutic status of a new procedure, drug, or device, and propel them too quickly into clinical trials.

Currently, for example, the field of gene therapy seems to have reached such a juncture. More than a hundred gene therapy trials are now en route, galvanized by the effervescence of molecular biology and genetics; the desire to find remedies for conditions that range from cystic fibrosis and severe combined immunodeficiency disease, to cancer and AIDS; the involvement of many academic centers and the U.S. National Institutes of Health in this area; the hundreds of millions of dollars that pharmaceutical and biotechnology companies have invested in it; and by media "hype". Lately, some biomedical leaders in the field have been expressing concern over the rush to clinical trials that is occurring, and the possibility that these trials are taking place at the expense of more basic, long-term, high quality laboratory research on vectors and in cell biology which need to be better understood if genetic treatments are to produce safe, effective, and enduring therapeutic benefits (4).

By any criteria, the 1982 launching of clinical trials with the Jarvik-7 model of a total artificial heart was premature, and unwarranted by the results of its performance in the calves and sheep on which it had been previously tried. With the exception of one animal who lived for 268 days after being implanted, none of the animals survived more than 5 months, and most of them died much earlier. The chief causes of the morbidity and death of the animals derived from persistent problems with biomaterials, the durability of some components of the device, and the pneumatic power supply from blood clotting, and from lethal infections due to penetration of the animals' skin by the device's air hoses. Pneumothorax, respiratory failure, and brain death resulting from hypotension and acidosis also figured among the reported causes of death in a series of 35 animals implanted with the Jarvik-7 by the Utah artificial heart team between 1980 and 1982.

The Utah group's justification for their decision to move the Jarvik heart into clinical trials was based on their positive interpretation of their results compared to the maximum 1-week survival of animals with a total artificial heart that had prevailed in the 1970's; on their argument that because they had learned all that they could from healthy animals unsusceptible to end-stage cardiac disease, man had become the "animal of necessity" (8); and on their scientifically unfounded expectation that the human body might prove to be more "tolerant" of the device than the bodies of calves and sheep, and that complications would therefore be less severe and more clinically controllable.

A cluster of converging factors helped to catapult the Jarvik heart from the laboratory and animal barn to the operating room and surgical intensive care unit of the Utah Medical Center and subsequently, of the Humana Hospital Audubon in Louisville, Kentucky. Foremost among them was a strong, competitive desire to "win the race" with other artificial heart teams, and gain the individual, institutional, and national priority and prestige that would come with pioneering the first implants of a permanent replacement for the human heart. Along with surgeon William DeVries's personal and professional ambition, and his desire to rescue persons with end-stage cardiac disease from death, the American Mormon precepts, world-view, and sense of mission in which he was raised played a significant, largely implicit role in his drive to clinically trail-blaze the implantation of the Jarvik-7 heart. In ways that go beyond the scope of this presentation, the Mormon ethos of the University of Utah and of the Salt Lake City community in which it is embedded was also an underlying force in that institution's commitment to Jarvik-7 clinical trials. Of special relevance were the importance that Mormonism attaches to health; its view of the human body as a tabernacle; its concept of science and scientific research as an organized way of seeking and expressing "intelligence", which it considers the "glory of God"; and its belief in a cosmic principle of eternal progression that spans this life and the life that comes after it (1, 3, 7). However, in other respects, the University of Utah's motives for clinically launching Jarvik-7 total artificial heart implants were very similar to what impelled the Humana Corporation, one of the United States's largest investor-owned, for-profit, health care companies, its affiliated Humana Hospital Audubon, and Humana Heart Institute International (a private group practice) to recruit William DeVries, and offer to underwrite the costs of an artificial heart program of up to 100 implants. Utah and Humana were both interested in promoting themselves as well as medical research, technology, and care – in enhancing their corporate image, professional reputation, and financial status through their involvement with the Jarvik-7. In the end, the clinical trials of this total artificial heart resulted in the deaths of all its human recipients, not only from their grave cardiac disease, but from the device-borne complications that had led to the deaths of the calves and sheep who were its prior animal-subjects. Would the same outcome be likely to occur with the post-Jarvik-7 permanent mechanical support devices now under investigation? If so, would it be biomedically sound and humanely defensible at this stage in their development to move them from the laboratory to the clinic? In my opinion, the ethical answer to the second question is, "No".

Misconducted Clinical Trials

In what surgeon Francis D. Moore has termed the "black years" phase of early clinical trials with mortally ill patient-subjects (5), when the experimental new therapies being tried are fraught with uncertainty and risk, and the failure and death rates accompanying them are exceedingly high, the justification for what is ventured lies above all in the clinically relevant knowledge, understanding, and technique that may be forthcoming. Although it is hoped that the experimentation will directly and immediately benefit the patients who participate in such trials, often this does not come to pass, as the Jarvik-7 case tragically illustrates. What is more troubling however, is the fact that from their inception and throughout the duration of the Jarvik-7 trials, the chief surgeon-implanter-investigator and his entourage did not exhibit the competence necessary to generate, analyze, and publish scientifically reliable and valid findings based on their endeavor.

DeVries himself had little prior experience or trained expertise in designing or conducting patient-oriented clinical research. The protocol for the first implant of the artificial heart that he submitted to the Institutional Review Board (IRB) at the University of Utah Medical Center was inadequate in many scientifically crucial ways, as were the several revised versions of it that he wrote in response to the IRB's criticisms. The Board became so concerned about the deficiencies of the protocol and DeVries's seeming inability to satisfactorily remedy them that they overstepped their role and took collective responsibility for turning the research proposal into a more acceptable scientific plan. In Louisville, DeVries became associated with a community hospital (Humana Audubon) that was not accustomed to doing clinical research. In considering the protocols for the implants of the Jarvik-7 heart that he performed there, the hospital's relatively new and inexperienced IRB relied heavily on the Utah IRB, uncritically accepting its prior review and approval of the protocols for DeVries's first implant in Salt Lake City, and his application to do a second one.

The research that accompanied the conduct of four implantations of the Jarvik-7 heart (one at the University of Utah Medical Center, and three at Humana Audubon Hospital) had serious limitations and flaws. It was highly empirical, unfocussed, trial and error research that entailed the omnivorous collection of reams of data. The gathering and monitoring of the data were computerized, but the information collected was not framed and ordered by a well thought out, well designed research plan. Nor were the data systematically and continually analyzed along the way. Only a few, relatively unilluminating articles were ever published from all the material that was amassed.

"Ignorance" about how to design and execute competent and meaningful clinical trials "is the biggest form of misconduct," Richard Peto, Oxford University's renowned expert on the subject, has declared (6). In his view, and in mine as well, this form of ignorance – which probably occurs more frequently than falsifying, fabricating, or plagiarizing scientific data – is not only intellectually regrettable, it is also morally blameworthy. As I have written elsewhere, "the Jarvik-7 story has come to exemplify for me the wrongdoing and damage that incompetent clinical research entails" (2).

Shortcomings in Overseeing the Clinical Trials

These questionable features of the Jarvik-7 clinical trials took place under the supposedly watchful eyes of an unusually large number of observers and of gatekeepers, who had the direct or indirect capacity to influence the course of this clinical experiment – its initiation, continuation, and conclusion.

The trials were accompanied by massive, thickly descriptive, and theatrically prominent print and electronic media coverage throughout their three-year trajectory. The media treated their unfolding as a "big story" about the advance of medical technology and heroic medicine, infused with moral messages concerning the human heart, its meaning, what it was like to excise it and to live without it, and such cardinal American values as courage, optimism, innovation, and the determination to overcome adversity and limitations. The media attention was augmented by the news dispatches and conferences, and the public relations activities orchestrated by the University of Utah Medicine Center and by the Humana Corporation's Audubon Hospital.

The evolving details of the artificial heart implants were also closely followed by senior administrative officials and physicians at the institutions where they took place; the members of their Institutional Review Boards; a wider community of cardiovascular and cardiac surgeons (especially those involved in cardiac replacement); a variety of non-physician experts in areas such as medical ethics and health law; the Food and Drug Administration's Division of Cardiovascular Devices, and its advisory panel; and by senior officials of the National Institutes of Health and the artificial heart program of its National Heart, Lung, and Blood Institute.

Although in each of these settings there were persons who had strong doubts about the medical scientific and clinical justification for launching the trials of the

Jarvik-7 heart, the merits of the protocol on which it was based, and the qualifications of the principal investigator to conduct and direct the research, only a few individuals were willing to express their reservations and concerns publicly, or to overtly recommend deterring action. The social controls that could have been exercised over these clinical trials were weakened and delayed by the zeal with which the vision of creating a viable total artificial heart was pursued, by the power of its symbolic significance, and by the various forms of personal, professional, and institutional self-promotion and self-protection that it brought into play.

The Lessons

These trials with the Jarvik-7 heart should not have occurred at the time, in the way, and under the auspices that they did. They have ended, but the efforts that have been made since the early 1920's to permanently replace the human heart with an artificial one go on. Perhaps this goal is as hubris-ridden and unattainable as Icarus's legendary attempt to fly as high as the sun on the wings of feathers and wax invented and fashioned by his father, Daedalus. Whatever their outcome, however, if clinical trials with other models of a total artificial heart ensue, those who conduct them should be mindful of the ethical faults and moral wrongs that accompanied the ascent and the descent of the Jarvik-7 heart, and they should not repeat them.

References

1. Fox RC (1984) It's the same, but different. A sociological perspective on the case of the Utah artificial heart. In: Shaw MW (ed) After Barney Clark. Reflections on the Utah artificial heart program. University of Texas Press, Austin, pp. 68-90
2. Fox RC (1995) Experiment perilous. 45 years as a participant observer of patient-oriented clinical research. Perspectives in Biology and Medicine: in press
3. Fox RC, Swazey JP (1992) Spare parts. Organ replacement in American society. Oxford University Press, New York and Oxford
4. Marshall E (1995) Gene therapy's growing pains. Science 269: 1050-1055
5. Moore FD (1968) Medical responsibility for the prolongation of life. JAMA 206: 304-306
6. Nowak R (1994) Problems in clinical trials go beyond misconduct. Science 264: 1538
7. O'Dea TF (1957) The Mormons. University of Chicago Press, Chicago
8. Swazey JP (1978) Protecting the animal of necessity: Limits to inquiry in clinical investigation. Daedalus 107: 129-145

Author's address:
Renée C. Fox, Ph.D.
Sociology Department
University of Pennsylvania
3718 Locust Walk
Philadelphia, PA 19104-6299
USA

Discussion Session, Afternoon of October 22, 1995

Robicsek: This was certainly an appropriately enlivening and controversial finishing of a very interesting program today. While the title of the afternoon session was permanent mechanical support, I believe only part of the program was really aimed at permanent support. We spent a good portion of the time on "bridging". The entire subject reminds me of a famous quotation of Galenus, who said "This medicine will cure all those who are ill, with the exception of those who are incurable. You can recognize those who are incurable because they all die." So I think we found the panacea today. I learned a lot. I learned that the best way to improve your life, so you can go fishing, gardening, be happy, is to have a permanent artificial heart implanted. All of the patients looked very happy with the exception of Bud Frazier's cow. We also learned that some of the patients, while happy, have been quite ungrateful, because they can cohort and queue them, but if they get a visit from Tante Jutta from Katzenellenbogen, that they don't come to Prof. Hetzer to show themselves. We also learned from Prof. Loisance that in France being a bachelor is an indication for a heart transplant, because that is cheaper than a wife. I didn't understand some portions of his lecture, he said that the cost is 970 francs a day. Then I wonder, why did I have to pay for a dinner on the Champs Elysées double of the demand. We learned from Bud Frazier, I would love to ask him the name and address of the stock broker who makes $ 50.000 with a permanent implantable heart, but I don't think he's going to tell us. Anyway, I'd like to ask our last speaker, Dr. Fox, a question. It was a very provocative lecture, but you took somehow the easy way out by bashing the Jarvick heart and then stopped a little bit short of commenting on the present situation. Will you just go a step further? You warned us to avoid the mistakes. What do you like and what do you not like about what you've heard during this very informative session today?

Fox: Well, I was going to add a line to my paper saying that I am reassured that the Icarus complex is not as characteristic of this group as I had depicted in the group that I spoke of. I think this is a very flamboyant, and in some ways, perhaps, even an unfair case to present, but because it is a case which magnifies certain issues. I still think it could be more important to think not about what kinds of phenomenon are inherent to the process of clinical investigation and particularly that phase of it where one moves in the early stages from the laboratory to the clinic. I have been privileged to watch all of my life as a sociologist of medicine the way in which men and women who have chosen the life of clinical investigating wrestle with these kinds of issues. The issue about it being always premature at a certain level to move from the laboratory to the clinic, because of the high level of uncertainty that is involved and because the patients who become your first subjects are so mortally ill that not only the morbidity, but the mortality rate is going to be excruciatingly high, is something that every person who does this kind of clinical research has to grapple with. Also the issue about clinical research companies being a moral matter and not just an intellectual matter, I think is something again that is worthy of our attention. That is not just some kind of malady that afflicted the Jarvick-7 experimental process, nor the problem of oversight, which is not simple. As a matter of fact, Dr. Watson can speak more about that than I can. Just having a certain number of regulatory bodies in place, or having good informed voluntary consent forms, does not necessarily take care of the intricacies of the regulation of the kind of research we're talking about-from inside the consciences of the investigators and from inside their institutions. I'll go out on a limb. I'm a sociologist trying to understand what I have listened to for the last two days and I have a layperson's biomedical knowledge, but I'm impressed both by the progress that has been made and with the prudence with which the people I've heard present at this meeting spoke of what they are doing, what their hopes are, and what they are intending to do as their next step. So I heard nothing that set off moral alarm bells in me. In fact, quite to the contrary, in Dr. Watson's presentation what they have funded is certainly not to leap out of the laboratory onto the level of human trials. Even though the great excitement at this meeting is the possibility that the left ventricular devices may help a patient's heart to, if not heal totally, the muscle strength to return and so forth. They may turn out to be therapeutic devices in and of themselves. Everybody framed that hope with great caution and with scrupulous plans about studying the process coming to understand it better from a basic science point of view as well as from a clinical level. So, I'm not your moral judge. I'm not even an ethicist, even though Dr. Hetzer would like to think so. But, for whatever my opinion is worth, if I had come as a sociologist to study you, I would not have found the same patterns as the ones that I reported in this short paper.

Robicsek: Any questions from the audience on this subject? Dr. Watson, do you accept this new idea which Professor Hetzer's group is advocating, the device as a bridge, a bridge not to transplantation, but a bridge towards well-being. How does the FDA look at this, to us in the States, a novel indication?

Watson: Well, I can't speak for the FDA, but I can speak for NIH. I think they find it very exciting. My final comment in discussing the future focus on two ideas: 1) that we can actually use these systems to study the natural history of heart failure, that's what Dr. Hetzer's group is doing by identifying this group of patients that we discussed this morning, and 2) the advent of a lot of the advances in molecular and cellular biology will have some synergism with these systems and that in the operating room we may have the molecular biologist there with the surgeons doing some vector implanting, or whatever it might be, to help restore and regenerate the myocardium. We saw this patient today. I've waited 20 years to see a patient like that. That was terrific. I think there is a lot of excitement about the prospects for the future.

Robicsek: Do you think that the bridge to health concept will be accepted as an indication in the States?

Watson: Yes, I do. I think Alexis Carrel was right when he first proposed it back in the 1920's and 30's.

Fox: Could I ask a question about molecular biology therapy. There is a great deal of exuberance not only in this field, but in others, about the relationship between molecular biology and prospects in medicine. It would greatly improve clinical care. As I understand it, there is still an enormous hiatus between what we have learned on the level of molecular biology and the conceptual and empirical possibility of translating that onto the clinical level. It's a dream, but you present that as if we're closer to it than I would suppose that we are. The notion, and even the point of now talking about the molecular biologist in the OR pushes me even further. It's a hope and a dream, but I watch medical students, for example, being trained to be physicians at this point and one of the big problems is this enormous gap between what they're learning in molecular biology and between what they have to know in order to take care of patients where much of molecular biology has no relevance whatsoever to the everyday practice of medicine.

Watson: Well, my response, if I may, is that [the wait for] gene therapy is probably a period of about 12 years from the beginning of that. Actually I think this next week in Science the first results on the ADA deficiency studies of Dr. Anderson will come out and in the following few the one from Jim Wilson on cystic fibrosis will come out. So the process is beginning and we're at the very pioneer stage of gene therapy.

Fox: Dr. Wilson is one of the people who has recently said that we should go back to the laboratory and work more on cell biology and vectors because, although he goes forward with that work, he's one of the people who feels that gene therapy in trials are somewhat premature even though he's got a vested interest in saying otherwise.

Robicsek: I'd like to ask Drs. Körfer and Loebe a question. Both of you presented quite a wide array of different devices in your respective patient groups. Why do you change from one device to the other? Do you use the device according to the patient characteristics, according to the clinical situation, or just because you believed at one point of your studies that one device was better than the other.

Hetzer: Maybe I can answer this question. Professor Körfer has left already, but I know the development of his program and ours here in Berlin. You have to look at it in its historical context. We started in 1987 when we twice used the total artificial heart developed by Professor Bücherl. At that time I thought its handling and implantation was just too complicated for mere bridge to transplantation. At the same time the same group had developed external pneumatically driven pulsatile pumps, which for the purpose of bridge to transplant served as well, if not better, because you had control of the pump bladders. If thrombosis developed, you could change the chamber, and so on. We used this pump for a long time. I think the development in Professor Körfer's program was very similar. He started off with centrifugal pumps, then acquired the Abiomed. He was not happy with the Abiomed in every instance, so he acquired the Thoratec, which is very similar to the Berlin Heart, and finally went to the implantable Novacor and TCI pumps, as we did, for the, let's say, greater comfort which these patients experienced and the somewhat longer support periods one could thus provide them. Although we also had patients with the Berlin Heart system who were on this pump for more than 240 days, but they were more restricted in their mobility, it is more uncomfortable, and also, as our psychologists have shown, the psychological impact of a pump which is outside the body is obviously much more detrimental to the patient than a pump were the larger parts are implanted. I think you have to look at this in a historical way, which was first of all determined by the availability of pumps, secondly by improved patient quality of life, and the progressive need for longer use because of the increasing discrepancy between donor availability and the number of patients waiting. I think these are very important criteria.

Robicsek: Do you now use one device or do you alternate between two devices?

Hetzer: No. Those left ventricular assist pumps, like the TCI or the Novacor, can be used very well in acutely ill patients, provided that the cardiac shock condition is not too profound. Once the patient is acidotic or is in pulmonary edema, the mere unloading of the left ventricle will probably not be sufficient in the acute phase due to transiently elevated pulmonary vascular resistance. We have observed that in such instances you may be confronted with right ventricular failure or at least right ventricular insufficiency. Now when we have a patient who presents, let's say, unconscious, in pulmonary edema, and anuric, we give him an external biventricular system because it can handle this very profound situation better than mere left ventricular assistance with an implantable device. So we presently use three different systems.

Robicsek: Looking at your patient material, while it was not spelled out, I somehow distinguish two completely different groups with a lot of overlapping. One where you use the device as a lifesaving device on that particular day to pull the patient through, as a later bridge, or out of the operating room or out of the hospital, or whatever. And then you very consciously injected the concept, you didn't say so, but I had the feeling that you say that under some circumstances the device could be used in patients whose lives may not be immediately threatened, but as a treatment device for managing heart failure. Did I overread you or you said that?

Hetzer: We have not used a device in this second condition. We are considering it. Those four patients who Dr. Loebe presented, those older patients in whom we implanted this pump with the prospect of permanent use, were all patients who fulfilled the criteria of having the acute need for mechanical support, i.e. all of them were on catecholamines and all were in failure. These patients were beyond our transplant inclusion criteria, that means that otherwise the decision would have meant letting them die. We gave them the alternative of a permanent system, but as you have seen, those patients obviously were not only acutely ill, they were also too sick in many systems. The initial experience in four patients has shown very well the limitations for applying this concept. I think it is very important, as I mentioned in my short preamble today, that we come to a conclusion about which patients probably do not qualify for such a chronic device even at an older age and what degree of polymorbidity a patient may have and still go through such a procedure. But those four patients were still clear candidates for an assist device.

Robicsek: Dr. Frazier, considering the atmosphere in Europe in this field and the research possibilities in the United States, do you believe in that particular matter, are you lucky or are you unlucky that you work in Houston rather than working in Berlin, concerning this subject.

Frazier: Well, both. I do to some degree envy the situation here in that there is a certain amount of clinical freedom, although I think the restrictions that we have are for the most part viable ones and have become a bit more tolerable. There are still certain limitations that I'm concerned about, specifically the hemopump, which I think is a type of technology that could help patients in a wide variety of cardiovascular collapse, that we don't have access to in spite of the fact that we've done all the initial research work on it. But I think it's important to design trials that do show some effect, not only in the social climate that was alluded to by Dr. Fox, but also by the milieu of economic concerns. I think one of the good things about the FDA study is, that we compared really comparable patients, i.e., in comparable states of heart failure and we showed not only an improvement in the clinical outcome, but if it were thoroughly analyzed, an improvement in the economic outcome. So, I'd like to be here, particularly if I were 30 years old, it'd be a good place to be, but at my stage, I think I'll stay in Texas.

Portner: I'd just like to make a comment because I'm amazed at the restraint of my friend, Bud Frazier. The reality, as you know, is that all new things are evaluated first in Europe. That's great for the European investigators. I think that it's unfortunate for us in the U.S.

Robicsek: It is fortunate, or unfortunate, or both.

Portner: I think it's unfortunate. It depends on your point of view, obviously, whether it's fortunate or unfortunate.

Frazier: Well, I certainly agree to that. I'm so used to this problem in America. I hope the Europeans have the foresight to not come under the total clinical control of forces that are really deleterious to medicine, because it does result in much of our clinical studies being done in Europe. It's hard to do a good study in America. The one thing that we've had in America that's really been sort of on the forefront will all end up in Europe.

Fox: If I may comment on this. The mood in our country at the present moment, particularly in the present political climate, is contrary to a long-standing American tendency to think that the best way to handle things, not just in the medical sphere, but in many others, is to allow a completely unbridled kind of individualism and the play of the free market to proceed and that out of this will come the best kind of behavior, intellectually, morally, economically, and politically. There's always this tremendous issue about overregulating and what role the Federal Government should play versus local authorities versus the consciences of individual investigators, and so forth. Without indicting medical professionals, I think a society should not assume that these ethical issues that we are referring to are so simple that you can depend purely on individual consciences. The person who is involved in this investigation has to try to design some responsible ways of overseeing the work and making sure that the research is properly conducted.

Robicsek: I have to take an issue with myself, because from the sociologists's viewpoint, everything should be nice, neat, and regulated, but this regulation is tied to devices. The feeling of the clinician is that we are facing similar problems by the hundreds, day by day, which are not regulated. What do you think of this new movement, which is still going on, if I'm not mistaken, that new operations and new clinical intervention procedures should be regulated as well as devices?

Fox: That's not new.

Robicsek: So far it didn't occur.

Fox: I think Dr. Watson, who was discussing that, maybe has something to say about this feeling that devices are seen differently as other forms of therapeutic intervention, and so forth, but I don't think devices have been singled out.

Robicsek: Yes, I mean, artificial heart, yes, heart transplantation, no, at the same institution. We have total freedom of indication and whatever on heart transplants, but our hands are, if not tied together, but tied separately on devices.

Fox: You have a good point there. I'm very concerned as a matter of fact about the slippery slope that I see in organ transplantations going down at this point in the frantic attempt to do something about getting organs in order to deal with the organ shortage. That is not scrutinized or commented on.

Robicsek: The pigs are coming. Professor Loisance.

Loisance: I just would like to give a word of caution. You give the feeling that everything is fine in Europe. We don't have any laws about sexual harassment, as you have in the U.S., but we nevertheless have control of what we are doing in Europe. If you believe that we are totally free, in that case, you are wrong. We also deal with an administration. I think that the difference is that there is probably more interconnection between the administration and the clinicians. Clinicians still have control on administrative decisions. For example, each new material needs an EC mark and to get an EC mark, you have to fill out tons of paperwork, too. Less probably than in the U.S., but nevertheless, you have to complete the whole procedure. We are not totally free. The control you have in the U.S. did not prevent the Jarvick story which means that there is some dysfunction in the American system.

Robicsek: We all know that the tragedy in Sweden quoted by Dr. Fox really originated because they couldn't do heart transplantations in Sweden. So that was the indication for the Jarvick heart.

Watson: I would agree on the comment about the United States' FDA being somewhat dysfunctional. My plea is for scientific-based regulation rather than bureaucratic-based regulation. One comment I'll make about the Jarvick situation which Dr. Fox mentioned in her presentation, the National Heart, Lung, and Blood Institute did write to the FDA recommending against the Jarvick trial. Also, a representative of the Heart, Lung, and Blood Institute went to Utah and talked with all the principles, recommending against the trial. It was privately funded. We have two research systems: one with private funding and one with public funding. This was supported with private funds that were actually obtained from a small foundation located in Washington, DC, ironically. Actually, in Bethesda, Maryland, right near the NIH.

Robicsek: Dr. Hennig, we always used to say that medicine is behind industry and technology. We doctors use glass tubes and rubber tubing and carry the patients 4 to 5 floors up for an X-ray. I think we are right now speaking about the highest level of technology, if not in medicine, then in cardiovascular medicine. Do you think we are up to a level of the industry or behind 5, 10, or 15 years.

Hennig: Well, I believe the problems in the development of artificial hearts have always been underestimated. We have never had the high technology support by the industry that is needed for this development. You know, I guess that development is always driven by the anticipation of economic gains. To date, and also in the future, the development of artificial hearts will always be in small laboratories in combination with small companies. Many years ago we tried to begin a German research program together with AEG Telefunken, Siemens, Messerschmidt-Bölkow-Blohm and on the polymeric side with Hoechst, but it didn't work. After two or three years of enthusiastic research supported with millions of DMs from the German government, all of the companies stopped their work because they did not expect financial success, they didn't see a market. It's the same today.

Robicsek: What is the driving force in development today, the economy, or science...

Hennig: For technical development, it's the economy. If you see the development during the last years, advances in electronics are driven by computers, advances in batteries are driven by computers, advances in biomaterials, well, there aren't many because it's not so important for the industry.

Robicsek: Professor Hetzer, do we try to solve the problem with one million here or one million there which could involve billions of dollars in health expenditures. What is the answer?

Hetzer: Well, I would like to say something to what Hennig was saying. I think it's very true that in the past it was not easy to convince companies to participate. The first time that Dr. Watson came to my facility was when we made an attempt to convince a strong German company, Daimler Benz, to join a program with us. Some specialists in this big company finally decided that this would have no future. Of course, it has a future once a big, strong company stands behind it and offers all its technical possibilities and potential. Also, that's what I tried to bring into the discussion today, I think we are really now at a point where we have to think about implants, pumps that last for maybe five years or so, which are easy to implant, which are small, and which are much less costly than the ones available today. Each time when I am asked after presentations that I give elsewhere, I say that I assume that in a few years we will have implants about the size of an implantable defibrillator and also at approximately the same cost of such a device. I think it will be mandatory to have something like this, since this was also the content of the presentation of Prof. Dietz. I think if you want to go on in the heart disease population, we have to focus more on chronic failure. This will be the issue of the future. The answer at present, in my estimation, is not transplantation and not xenotransplantation, which I think, although it is optimistically considered presently, is years away from realization. I think if something shall be done, mechanical pumps of a reasonable size and cost have to be developed. I think this should actually be an interesting concept for a big company, because I assume there will be a market and a large one at that, even if the pumps become rather inexpensive in the future.

Portner: I'd like to comment on both of those points. I think it's more complex than whether a market is there or not. I think the real issue that either a large company looks at or an investor who might be interested in investing in these technologies is profit. The people who invest in small companies are interested in not just if there is a market, but also in the return on their investment. The problem, and I've thought this for a long time, is that until there is actually a reasonably large scale clinical experience, it's very hard for those kind of financial investors to see a return that's near enough in their spectrum to justify putting a large amount of money in. I'm not as familiar with the situation in Europe, but I'd be very surprised if it's very different. Typically the investor in the United States expects a return within three years. In this field that's not a very realistic expectation. I'd point out that there is one big company who has made an investment, namely Baxter and there's one company which has been very successful in raising a large amount of money on the public market, which is TCI. Once there is a reasonable level of success and these devices become more commonly used, it'll be much easier for future researchers to find that kind of support in either the investment community or in large companies. So, it's one of those chicken and egg problems where you have to have the success in order to have the support. The other point that I'd make is that it takes a very large amount of money to get to the point where you're successful. I mean, I think you can do development on a low scale in a university setting or in a small company setting, but once it comes to requiring the kind of infrastructure that will allow real commercial success of one of these technologies, it takes a very large amount of money, ten times as much as developing it.

Robicsek: Are there any questions from the audience. Professor Hetzer, any closing remarks?

Hetzer: I would like to ask once again what kind of patients we would consider for such a chronic implant. Professor Loisance?

Loisance: I pointed out a few options on my last slide. We have to speak with the cardiologists and try to arrive at a consensus. We can either choose a cardiac transplantation candidate or a non-cardiac transplantation candidate. For this type of study I would prefer to deal with transplantation candidates. Starting a study with the worst category of patients, the sickest patients, might lead to underevaluating the impact of this technology.

So I would prefer to start with transplantation candidates. We definitely need to get the cardiologists involved, because they control the patients and take good care of them. There is a population of good transplantation candidates who will never be transplanted because of the organ shortage situation. It's not unethical to propose a protocol in which patients eligible for transplantation, normally listed for transplantation, but who are very unlikely to undergo transplantation, should be defined as group one in a randomized protocol and remain on the transplantation list. If a critical situation should then develop, a mechanical system would be implanted.

Hetzer: Yes, that's what we do anyway.

Loisance: And the second arm of the study would involve elective implantation whereby the patient would be allowed to undergo transplantation for any reason. But the end point of the study would be very simple data, duration of life, quality of life, and obviously the cost issue. What was unacceptable in Sweden was that the patients could not undergo transplantation there. If you perform elective implantation to keep the patient indefinitely on the system, for ethical reasons the option of transplantation should be possible.

Robicsek: What you are proposing is the American system. That is what we're doing.

Hetzer: That's what we're doing also.

Loisance: We have never started a prospective randomized study on stable patients eligible for transplantation.

Hetzer: You see, it is not so easy to put a stable patient on such a support system. We handle our own list of patients with about 300 patients. But presently those patients are not in the condition that they will readily accept a mechanical system without urgent need. I would not either, if I were a patient. So, how can you conduct a randomized prospective study with such patients? A pump is implanted on an emergency basis only if the patient is in danger of dying.

Frazier: Well, I think most of us are not as fortunate as the French in having these patients not die. We see a lot of sick people in Houston also. Maybe they just need to drink more wine or something. Anyway, we have sick people. I have about 60 people on our waiting list and we've got about 4000, I think, waiting in America now. So, for some reason, what you say is true. I can't explain it and I don't intend to. However, in spite of your experience, there are a lot of other people who are dying. So we'd like to know how we can wish that away, maybe it's Lourdes or something else. But, I think as far as selecting patients, you can select transplant patients because there are sub-groups of transplant patients that have high mortality. For example, in one large group in America, survival was measured in black females who were CMV negative at the time of transplantation. They had, I believe, 2 year survival, I may be misquoting this paper, but it was 1- or 2-year survival, 20% percent. A very low prognosis. They were of all blood types, they weigh over 200 pounds. In America 50% of those patients listed for transplantation in 1992 died before they were transplanted. I think these are patient sub-groups that we could randomize in an ethical way and in a constructive way. Now the time of randomization to transplant must be at the time of implantation, that is to say, the patient shouldn't be compared to when they're transplanted, but at the time that they are randomized. The other large group that we are looking at right now is the non-transplant group. There are a lot of patients, and I think I saw one of them in your slide of survivors, he was an older man, but he was healthy looking. You could look at him and tell he still had good muscle tone, he was still pretty sturdy. I think there are patients in that sub-group who don't readily qualify for heart transplantation, but they are still very strong. Dr. Cooley is 75 and he operates every day and Dr. De Bakey is 87 and he's still operating. So, there are a lot of strong older patients who wouldn't qualify for heart transplantation who could be randomized in a study. In addition to these two sub-groups, and considering the impact of the work this morning, I do think we have to particularly look at bridge to recovery. I think that's the most exciting thing; looking at bridge-to-recovery patients in a prospective way. So, there are four studies right there that we could conduct in a prospective randomized manner.

Watson: In terms of the clinical trial which seems to be coming in Europe, I agree with the careful consideration of all factors and the possibility of having a disinterested data review group, with Dr. Fox or similar people on it, for example, that would oversee the trial and give feedback to the steering committee.

Portner: We have talked to heart failure cardiologists who don't see an ethical problem with doing a randomized trial such as Professor Loisance talked about. I mean, you have to pick a subset of patients in heart failure who have very high mortality. Such a group could be patients with V02 max below 12 and low serum sodium where you have already identified two-year survival of 10 to 15%. So, I think there are cardiologists who feel that that's not an unethical thing to do. Only if you do not do it as a permanent implant, but you do it with the possibility of a crossover at some period of time to transplantation. I think the other thing that needs to be emphasized is that sometimes we talk about these alternatives as though these mechanical devices are immediate alternatives to transplantation. In fact, if you believe the epidemiological studies which were discussed by Dr. Dietz and have been by many others, for every patient who gets a transplant today, there are at least 10 or maybe 20 who could benefit. So, what you're doing is, because of the inherent or implicit comparison with transplantation, you're denying a large number of patients the opportunity to perhaps have a therapy which could be beneficial.

Closing remarks

Hetzer: I did not want to interrupt the discussion and take over this place from my friend and mentor, Francis Robicsek. I think we have to come to an end. I have the feeling that this was a very long day and that you are looking forward to having a little rest and see something other than the audience. I think it was a very interesting meeting for us yesterday with the pediatric program, where much more experience needs to be acquired and many more improvements and things have to be done before we can safely use such pumps in every single case. I think this morning it was very good to talk about this concept of weaning which was, and still is, a surprising experience for us. I think luck was with us and we are happy to see that this opens a very new field of research in looking at things with good patient outcome. As you probably saw, the situation of being confronted with patients, who do not qualify for transplantation, and whom we have to condemn to die, because we cannot do anything bothers me very much. Therefore we were thinking about using alreadily available pumps now for permanent support. I believe we have to find a solution in one way or the other without overstretching this concept and also overextending the economical means on the one side and the social mores and public acceptability and acceptance of such a concept on the other. I strongly believe that we will have to deal with this issue very much in the near future.

I thank you very much for coming. The audience was very patient until the very last moment. In particular I thank all the speakers and panelists and the gentlemen who accepted the chairmanship and guided the panel discussion. I would like to especially thank Drs. Fox and Watson for making such a long trip to share their very important opinions with us. I would like to thank my co-workers, my secretaries, who always do a good job, and Mr. Jessen from the organizing company. He gets better each time when I work with him and everything is perfect, at least I haven't heard any complaints from our guests. I would also like to thank the medical industry for supporting our meeting. I wish you a safe trip home, and for those of you staying, a nice evening in Berlin. Thank you very much.

Author Index

W. Albert, MD
German Heart Institute Berlin
Augustenburger Platz 1
13353 Berlin
Germany

V. Alexi-Meskishvili, MD
German Heart Institute Berlin
Augustenburger Platz 1
13353 Berlin
Germany

S. Däbritz, MD
Department of Thoracic
and Cardiovascular Surgery
Klinikum RWTH
Pauwelsstraße
52057 Aachen
Germany

R. Dietz, MD
Franz-Vollhard-Klinik
Max-Delbrück-Centrum
Wiltbergstraße 50
13125 Berlin-Buch
Germany

A. El-Banayosy, MD
Department of Thoracic
and Cardiovascular Surgery,
Heart Center
North Rhine-Westphalia,
Georgstr. 11
32545 Bad Oeynhausen
Germany

O. H. Frazier, MD
Texas Heart Institute
M.C. 3-147
P.O. Box 20345
Houston, TX 77225-0345
USA

R. C. Fox, PhD
Sociology Department
University of Pennsylvania
3718 Locust Walk
Philadelphia, PA 19104-6299
USA

M. Glauber, MD
Department of Cardiac Surgery
Azienda Ospedaliera
I-24100 Bergamo
Italy

E. Hennig, PhD
German Heart Institute Berlin
Augustenburger Platz 1
13353 Berlin
Germany

R. Hetzer, MD, PhD
German Heart Institute Berlin
Augustenburger Platz 1
13353 Berlin
Germany

T. R. Karl, MD
Victorian Paediatric Cardiac
Surgical Unit
Royal Children's Hospital
Flemington Road
Parkville, 3052, Melbourne
Australia

U. Kühl, PhD
Med. Clinic of Internal Medicine
Benjamin Franklin Hospital
Department of Cardiology
Freie Universität Berlin
Hindenburgdamm 30
12200 Berlin Steglitz
Germany

M. Loebe, MD
German Heart Institute Berlin
Augustenburger Platz 1
13353 Berlin
Germany

D. Loisance, MD, PhD
Centre de Recherches
Chirurgicales Henri Mondor
Faculté de Médecine
8, rue du Général Sarrail
F-94000 Créteil
France

G. Minzioni, MD
Department of Cardiac Surgery
IRCCS Policlinico S. Matteo
27100-Pavia
Italy

J. Müller, MD
German Heart Institute Berlin
Augustenburger Platz 1
13353 Berlin
Germany

P. J. del Nido, MD
Department of Cardiac Surgery
Children's Hospital
300 Longwood Ave.
Boston, MA 02115
USA

G. Wallukat, MD
Max Delbrück Centre
for Molecular Medicine
Cardiology
Robert-Rössle-Str. 10
13125 Berlin
Germany

J. T. Watson, PhD
National Heart, Lung and
Blood Institute
2 Rocklege Center Ste 9044
6701 Rockledge Drive MSC 7940
Bethesda, MD 20892–7940
USA